Ambulatory Practice

Guest Editors

DAVID W. RAMEY, DVM
MARK R. BAUS, DVM

VETERINARY CLINICS
OF NORTH AMERICA:
EQUINE PRACTICE

www.vetequine.theclinics.com

Consulting Editor
ANTHONY SIMON TURNER, BVSc, MS

April 2012 • Volume 28 • Number 1

SAUNDERS an imprint of ELSEVIER, Inc.

W.B. SAUNDERS COMPANY
A Division of Elsevier Inc.

1600 John F. Kennedy Boulevard • Suite 1800 • Philadelphia, Pennsylvania 19103

http://www.vetequine.theclinics.com

VETERINARY CLINICS OF NORTH AMERICA: EQUINE PRACTICE Volume 28, Number 1
April 2012 ISSN 0749-0739, ISBN-13: 978-1-4557-4507-4

Editor: John Vassallo; j.vassallo@elsevier.com

Veterinary Clinics of North America: Equine Practice (ISSN 0749-0739) is published in April, August, and December by Elsevier Inc., 360 Park Avenue South, New York, NY 10010-1710. Business and Editorial Offices: 1600 John F. Kennedy Blvd., Suite 1800, Philadelphia, PA 19103-2899. Subscription prices are $257.00 per year (domestic individuals), $397.00 per year (domestic institutions), $126.00 per year (domestic students/residents), $299.00 per year (Canadian individuals), $496.00 per year (Canadian institutions), $346.00 per year (international individuals), $496.00 per year (international institutions), and $172.00 per year (international and Canadian students/residents). To receive student/resident rate, orders must be accompanied by name of affiliated institution, date of term, and the signature of program/residency coordinator on institution letterhead. Orders will be billed at individual rate until proof of status is received. Foreign air speed delivery is included in all *Clinics* subscription prices. All prices are subject to change without notice. **POSTMASTER:** Send address changes to *Veterinary Clinics of North America: Equine Practice,* 3251 Riverport Lane, Maryland Heights, MO 63043. Customer Service (orders, claims, online, change of address): Elsevier Health Sciences Division, Subscription Customer Service, 3251 Riverport Lane, Maryland Heights, MO 63043. Tel: 1-800-654-2452 (U.S. and Canada); 314-447-8871 (outside U.S. and Canada). Fax: 314-447-8029. E-mail: journalscustomerservice-usa@elsevier.com (for print support); E-mail: journalsonlinesupport-usa@elsevier (for online support).

Reprints. For copies of 100 or more of articles in this publication, please contact the Commercial Reprints Department, Elsevier Inc., 360 Park Avenue South, New York, NY 10010-1710. Tel.: 212-633-3812; Fax: 212-462-1935; E-mail: reprints@elsevier.com.

Veterinary Clinics of North America: Equine Practice is covered in *MEDLINE/PubMed (Index Medicus), Excerpta Medica, Current Contents/Agriculture, Biology and Environmental Sciences, and ISI*

Printed and bound by CPI Group (UK) Ltd, Croydon, CR0 4YY
Transferred to Digital Print 2012

Contributors

CONSULTING EDITOR

ANTHONY SIMON TURNER, BVSc, MS
Diplomate, American College of Veterinary Surgeons; Professor, Department of Clinical Sciences, College of Veterinary Medicine and Biomedical Sciences, Colorado State University, Fort Collins, Colorado

GUEST EDITOR

DAVID W. RAMEY, DVM
Chatsworth, California

MARK R. BAUS, DVM
Grand Prix Equine, Bridgewater, Connecticut

AUTHORS

MARK R. BAUS, DVM
Grand Prix Equine, Bridgewater, Connecticut

STEPHANIE S. CASTON, DVM
Diplomate, American College of Veterinary Surgeons - Large Animal; Assistant Professor, Department of Veterinary Clinical Sciences, College of Veterinary Medicine, Iowa State University, Ames, Iowa

ANN E. DWYER, DVM
Partner, Genesee Valley Equine Clinic, PLLC, Scottsville, New York; Clinical Associate, Flaum Eye Institute, University of Rochester Medical Center, Rochester, New York

A.T. FISCHER JR, DVM
Diplomate American College of Veterinary Surgeons; Chino Valley Equine Hospital, Chino Hills, California

RON FRIEDMAN, MS, DVM
Diplomate, American College of Theriogenologists; The Oregon Equine Reproduction Center/ Friedman Veterinary Service, Lake Oswego, Oregon

SUSAN S. GILLEN, DVM
Gillen Equine Veterinary Clinic, Pleasant Grove, California

MIKE GRAPER, DVM
Private Practice, Cornerstone Equine Services, Rhinelander, Wisconsin

DEREK C. KNOTTENBELT, OBE, BVM&S, DVM&S, MRCVS
Diplomate, European College of Equine Internal Medicine; Professor of Equine Internal Medicine, Philip Leverhulme Hospital, University of Liverpool, Neston, United Kingdom

ROBERT P. MAGNUS, DVM, MBA
President, Wisconsin Equine Clinic and Hospital, Oconomowoc, Wisconsin

JOHN S. MITCHELL, DVM
Equine Associates, Boca Raton, Florida

PHILIPPE MOREAU, DVM, MS
Diplomate, European College of Veterinary Internal Medicine - Companion Animals;
Diplomate, European College of Veterinary Neurology; Medi-Productions, SAS,
Limoge, France

WILLIAM MOYER, DVM
Diplomate, American College of Veterinary Sports Medicine and Rehabilitation; Large
Animal Clinical Sciences, College of Veterinary Medicine and Biomedical Sciences,
Texas A&M University, College Station, Texas

STEPHEN E. O'GRADY, DVM, MRCVS, APF
Northern Virginia Equine, Marshall, Virginia

DAVID W. RAMEY, DVM
Chatsworth, California

CLAUDIA SANDOVAL, DVM
Fairfield Equine Associates, LLC, Newtown, Connecticut

CLAUDIA TRUE, DVM
Woodside Equine, LLC, Ashland, Virginia

HARRY W. WERNER, VMD
Equine Practitioner; Practice Owner, Werner Equine, LLC, North Granby, Connecticut

Contents

> Current economic conditions make the practice of equine medicine challenging. The downward trend in the US economy has had a huge impact on horse owners and equine veterinarians alike. Horses are expensive to keep; as such, economics are the driving factor in the problem of the unwanted horse. Under these conditions, efficient equine ambulatory practices are well-suited to weather the economic storm. As contributors to this issue note, one can practice high-quality medicine and surgery without the overhead and expense of a large clinic. Ambulatory practitioners face formidable challenges but they also have opportunities to establish and secure a good future.

> The horse owner not only expects outstanding care for his horse; he also recognizes and appreciates a well-run equine practice. A well managed ambulatory equine practice supports the ideals of both high standards of care and mobility. A poorly managed practice will ultimately impact the care that an equine veterinarian attempts to provide the horses in his or her care. Without careful attention to profitability and efficiency, the practice's ability to grow and develop with emerging therapies and technologies is impossible. A poorly managed practice will significantly contribute to the frustration that an equine veterinarian feels after working long hours and receiving only nominal pay.

> The mobile equine practitioner must provide high levels of care while serving the needs of the horse owner, managing the intricate needs of a business and maintaining a balanced home life. Technological advances in the past several decades have provided many useful tools to help the mobile equine veterinarian provide uncompromising levels of care, maintain an open line of communication with his or her clients and colleagues, produce sophisticated images of any part of the horse's body, and create detailed medical records, while generating an invoice that captures all fees incurred at the time of service.

A healthy group of loyal clients is of the utmost importance for a healthy practice. Knowing the clients' expectations and making every effort to exceed them when clients meet with the veterinarian or visit the clinic will result in continued client satisfaction. Clients will show loyalty to a veterinarian when they perceive that the care provided suits them and their animal and exceeds their expectations.

The scope of medical problems encountered by the equine ambulatory practitioner is immense, but it is certainly possible to practice high-quality equine medicine in a field setting. However, hospital referral should be offered to clients for conditions not conducive to successful treatment in the field. When surgical or hospital referral is not an option, it is imperative that the ambulatory practitioner not only offer humane alternatives but also inform and educate horse owners on equine suffering and welfare issues so that clients do not have unreasonable expectations of a positive outcome.

A successful ambulatory equine practice strives for efficiency in all areas, from vehicle fuel economy to inventory overhead. While elective procedures can usually be scheduled with maximum efficiency in mind, horses and their penchant for trouble mean that surgery can add an inherently inefficient component to the practitioner's schedule. Still, surgeries can add a level of challenge and interest to ambulatory practice, and good surgical skills can serve as something that can distinguish the practitioner and increase his or her reputation in the local and regional equine community.

Wounds are common in horses and wound care is an important aspect of ambulatory equine veterinary practice. An approach to wound care is described with emphasis on evaluation and prioritization of damaged structures at initial exam and the principles of wound healing. The relative value of some wound treatments and practices are discussed. A logical and useful method of caring for wounds can be used based on the normal wound-healing process while factoring potential complicating issues into the equation.

Lameness and performance evaluation can be one of the most reward-ing aspects of equine veterinary practice. There is a misconception that it depends on new sophisticated and expensive diagnostic modalities, but knowing where and when to use these modalities form the real art of equine lameness practice. The art is vested in knowledge of horsemanship, an understanding of anatomy and function, and inquir-ing senses to sort out what the horse and his handlers are telling you. The ability to determine a horse's lameness problem will be one of the most endearing experiences the equine ambulatory clinician can pro-vide for his or her clientele.

Hoof care and therapeutic farriery are valuable and important aspects of equine ambulatory practice. Developing, establishing and sustaining solid relationships with the horseshoeing community are essential for the overall health of the horse. Good relationships with the horseshoe-ing community can help the ambulatory veterinarian develop his or her practice, and serve as a consistent source of continued learning.

Equine dermatology is a highly visual specialty and a high number of conditions can be diagnosed with a detailed history and physical examination alone provided that these are performed carefully. Addi-tional tests can be used to confirm or rule-out possible differentials in almost all cases. The correct diagnosis enables focused treatment to be undertaken and gives the owner a realistic prognosis. Short cuts are usually counterproductive!

The equine eye can be examined with simple portable equipment and many pathologic conditions can be diagnosed with stall-side tests. Inexpensive digital cameras are effective for imaging the periorbit and anterior segment. Ambulatory practitioners can institute many effective treatments, including installation of subpalpebral lavage tubes for delivery of topical treatments for corneal disease, and standing ocular surgery using regional anesthesia and sedation. Prompt diagnosis and appropriate treatment of ocular problems can be sight saving and is an invaluable service to patients and clients.

VETERINARY CLINICS: EQUINE PRACTICE

THE CLINICS ARE NOW AVAILABLE ONLINE!

Access your subscription at:
www.theclinics.com

Preface
Ambulatory Practice

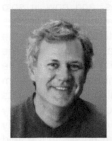 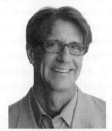

David W. Ramey, DVM   Mark R. Baus, DVM
Guest Editors

The horse, arguably the most important animal in human history, was cared for long before there were veterinarians. Before there were veterinarians, there were farriers (not the same as today's horseshoer, but from L. *ferrarius* "of iron"), and individuals with a keen interest in horses. The world's first veterinary school was founded in Lyon, France, in 1761, specifically to advance the care available for horses. In the subsequent centuries, equine medicine progressed rapidly, allowing for precise diagnoses and effective treatments that were unimaginable in previous decades.

For most of history, treatment of horses has been directed by individual practitioners, who, armed only with their personal knowledge, observations, and experience, willingly attended to the health needs of horses. But as veterinary knowledge and expertise increased, so did the ability of veterinarians to deliver care, as well as the number of individuals trained to deliver such care. Thus, the 20th century saw an explosion in facilities providing care for horses, from an increasing number of veterinary schools to large private hospitals staffed with dozens of veterinarians, many with board certifications in various specialties.

While horses have inarguably benefited from the explosion of knowledge and information, and developments in equipment and technology, the practice of equine medicine is still firmly carried on the backs of individual ambulatory practitioners. According to their 2011 member survey, the American Association of Equine Practitioners estimates that roughly 40% of its members practice by themselves, and another 24% practice with just one or two other veterinarians. Such practitioners are generally the first veterinarians that horse owners entrust with their horse's health (akin to a family practice physician), and there is no need for many of the cases that they see to move beyond the primary care offered in the field.

Equine ambulatory practice presents unique challenges to its practitioners that go far beyond medicine, surgery, and preventive care. Practitioners have to balance life away from practice with the demands of clients. Money spent on equipment

Vet Clin Equine 28 (2012) xi–xii
doi:10.1016/j.cveq.2012.03.004
0749-0739/12/$ – see front matter © 2012 Elsevier Inc. All rights reserved.

purchases are balanced against money available for much needed vacations; the time devoted to a colicky horse may be time taken away from a school play, or a baseball game; each has its benefits, as well as costs, both financial and emotional.

After a one-year internship at Iowa State University, Dr David Ramey has practiced exclusively in an ambulatory setting, at times with employees, and now in solo practice. Dr Mark Baus was a co-owner of a large referral hospital and now practices by himself. We feel that there has been a need for information directed at the practitioners who make up the backbone of equine medical practice, and, with the assistance of other practitioners, have tried to fill that need. We have tried to provide insight and perspective on a variety of aspects of equine ambulatory care, from medicine and surgery, to considerations when purchasing equipment, to thoughts about the client communications that are so critical for a successful ambulatory practice. Information on the diagnosis and treatment of specific conditions is readily available; the thoughts and suggestions of practitioners who treat horses in the field are not. Thus, there is little information on specific techniques, but much in the way of accumulated years of experience. We are grateful for the assistance and contributions of all of our authors to this issue of *Veterinary Clinics of North America: Equine Practice*, including several ambulatory practitioners, several whom have never been previously published. We hope that their perspectives and insights can help equine ambulatory veterinary develop both their approaches and their skills in this unique and challenging area of veterinary practice.

David W. Ramey, DVM
9615 Andora Avenue
Chatsworth, CA 91311, USA

Mark R. Baus, DVM
Grand Prix Equine
434 Main Street South
Bridgewater, CT 06752, USA

E-mail address:
ponydoc@pacbell.net (D.W. Ramey)
mbaus@grandprixequine.com (M.R. Baus)

Equine Ambulatory Practice: Challenges and Opportunities

David W. Ramey, DVM

KEYWORDS

- Equine • Equine ambulatory practice • Advantages
- Doctor-client relationship • Equine veterinarians • Horses

According to the 2011 American Association of Equine Practitioners' membership survey, approximately 40% of equine veterinarians practice alone and another 24% practice with one or two other veterinarians. As such, the primary care of the horse is almost literally carried on the backs of practitioners who work by, and for, themselves.

In the early 21st century, the practice of equine veterinary medicine appears to have become somewhat dichotomous. While a significant majority of those veterinarians still practice in small general practices, there are also large, multiperson practices that offer horse owners advanced imaging, surgery, and round-the-clock care that cannot be practically provided in the field. Given that larger, more well-equipped equipped practices can provide services that are unavailable to solo practitioners, it may seem to some that the days of the solo practitioner are limited. However, while medicine rapidly changes and current economic conditions present formidable challenges, equine ambulatory practice offers unique advantages and its practitioners are uniquely positioned to thrive.

ADVANTAGES OF AMBULATORY PRACTICE

Everything in life seems to be some sort of a balancing act. For practitioners of equine medicine, balance includes the decision about what type of practice will make for a satisfying veterinary career. As such, an equine practitioner may find that ambulatory practice provides significant advantages over larger group practices.

Ambulatory practice affords veterinarians the autonomy to practice medicine as they see fit. Being one's own boss is usually thought of as one of the biggest advantages to practicing alone; even practicing with another person allows the individual great autonomy. The ambulatory practitioner can usually set his or her own rules and provide services independent of supervision. There are no partners to convince, no managing veterinarian/owner to persuade, and no convincing superiors

The author has nothing to disclose.
9615 Andora Avenue, Chatsworth, CA 91311, USA
E-mail address: ponydoc@pacbell.net

Vet Clin Equine 28 (2012) 1–9
doi:10.1016/j.cveq.2012.01.005
0749-0739/12/$ – see front matter © 2012 Elsevier Inc. All rights reserved.

to buy into new choices or directions. In a small ambulatory practice, there is a sense of ownership that may be impossible to develop in a group practice.

Staffing an equine ambulatory practice is entirely at the discretion of the ambulatory practitioner. One can choose to have part-time or full-time employees or no employees at all! Further, in an intimate small-practice setting, employees may take a more personal interest in the business, since a good deal of the responsibility for the success of the business falls on them. Conversely, practitioners may elect to eschew potential employees altogether, or even work with a spouse as per many other family businesses.

The lack of a set schedule is a very appealing aspect of ambulatory practice. Having the flexibility to see horses at one's own convenience (emergencies notwithstanding) offers lifestyle advantages. For example, it is possible to bring children on calls, when necessary, affording them the opportunity to see the parent "in action," taking care of important responsibilities. The opportunity to see the parent/practitioner discuss cases with clients helps teach children valuable lessons about compassion and communication. Setting one's own hours to fit one's schedule, especially the ability to shift hours around as children grow, makes it possible to attend concerts or school plays or to watch or coach baseball games and soccer matches. In equine ambulatory practice, patient scheduling is largely under the control of the practitioner. Thus, one can schedule vacations, attend conferences, or take a day off, as desired. In addition, in ambulatory practice, one's "downtime" is one's own; when practice is slow, or during gaps in the day, one can run errands or finish personal agendas, things that may be more difficult to do when one is on "company time."

One last significant advantage of 1- to 3-person practices is that they tend to produce strong doctor-client bonds. Being appreciated for the medicine one practices is an emotional bonus that is earned from consistent, caring interactions with clients. Emotionally satisfaction with practice is one of the keys to avoiding "burnout," helps in coping with practice demands and pressures, and directly influences one's general psychological well-being.

Equine ambulatory practitioners may be often considered "throw-backs," the equivalent of the old human family practice doctors, and, over time, they may help their clients through a variety of emotionally taxing situations, including ones that may not only involve horses. The intensity of the one-on-one doctor-client-patient relationships is enjoyable to many practitioners. In general, clients want a sense of ownership of their doctor; they want to see their own veterinarian, not a substitute; in equine ambulatory practice, the veterinarian they call is the one they get. For equine ambulatory practitioners, over the years, clients become friends, and their horses become familiar companions, which deepens the joy of caring for both of them (anyone who does not understand that a significant portion of ambulatory practice involves caring for the horse *owner* is likely to find ambulatory practice quite frustrating).

DISADVANTAGES OF AMBULATORY PRACTICE

The disadvantages of solo equine practice are also very real; one major issue is call coverage when one decides to take some time off. In equine ambulatory practice, one must be constantly available for emergency calls. Constant availability may be comforting to clients, but it can also be draining to practitioners, who may find that trying to take a weekend off is stressful, or that even a modest vacation requires some significant concessions. Further compounding the problem is that if one is constantly available, it tends to lead to an illusion of indispensability, as if the patients, and the practice, could not survive with even a few days off. Of course, days off come at the expense of no pay; the opportunity cost of time spent away from one's practice is significant, not only for the ambulatory veterinarian but for everyone who is self-employed.

The perceived expense of opening an ambulatory practice may be daunting to some. Still, careful planning can help—the chapters by Drs Baus and Magnus in this issue of *Veterinary Clinics* provide much detail on decisions such as equipment purchase, fee setting, and accounts management, as well as inventory control. Maintaining an ambulatory practice need not be expensive, and practicing high-quality medicine in an ambulatory setting is a very achievable goal.

Solo practice veterinarians lack advantages offered by internal economies of scale. In ordering drugs, supplies, and equipment, large veterinary practices can often take advantage of decreased cost per unit of product ordered. For equine ambulatory practitioners, this can make overhead more burdensome. Of course, the cost savings offered to larger practices can be offset if ambulatory practitioners keep inventory to a minimum; conversely, ambulatory practitioners generally do not have to offset the considerable overhead costs carried by larger practices.

Billings and collections offer significant challenges for equine ambulatory practitioners. While, over time, building a stable clientele can provide some assurance of a continuing cash flow, even ambulatory practitioners must pay rent, retain an assistant, bookkeeper, or an accountant, and pay for billing systems, computers, or new equipment. Fixed costs of equipment and facilities can be difficult for solo practitioners to maintain, particularly when clients may have other priorities besides paying their veterinarian. Larger practices, with sophisticated billing systems and full-time personnel dedicated to financial management of the practices, seem to offer a comforting alternative to having to make sure that the bills are collected and paid. But the economy affects all equine practitioners; the current economic slowdown is making matters more difficult for veterinarians. Veterinary revenues nationwide are falling as clients who have lost their jobs or homes have difficulty affording horses; as costs of feed and boarding rise, horse owners may start skipping appointments, or stop paying their bills altogether. As people tighten their belts, they may defer things that they think are not absolutely necessary, or stop paying for them altogether.

One other issue that may keep veterinarians away from ambulatory practice is the perceived professional isolation. When in veterinary school or in a large practice setting, veterinarians are often surrounded by eager students, colleagues in residency training, and older practitioners with a wealth of experience. Journal clubs, conference, and patient rounds provide ample opportunities for bouncing questions off peers. This is not just a theoretical problem; studies in human medicine have shown that solo and nonurban practice, nonmembership in a professional group, and aging are all associated with underperformance and may be indicators of professional isolation.[1] While cutting oneself off from the intellectual support of colleagues may increase professional isolation, the problem is not insurmountable, and many of the advantages of equine ambulatory practice may be significant enough to make taking the chance worthwhile.

CHALLENGES AND SOLUTIONS
The Doctor-Client Bond

It's important that anyone considering equine ambulatory practice have the answer to one question: "What am I trying to do?" Certainly, one wants to make a living and be able to enjoy some measure of career success, but success is measured in different ways.

One huge benefit in equine ambulatory practice is the opportunity to interact meaningfully with clients. This is not only emotionally fulfilling but also an important way to build client loyalty and a successful practice. Exploring veterinary decisions together with the client, listening to stories about horse show triumphs, training successes, or just fun trail rides, and addressing all of the horse health issues that arise during veterinary visits is not only good practice but also creates a strong and lasting bond. In addition to providing one-on-one service, ambulatory clinicians have other opportunities to personalize their services in ways that cannot be offered by large equine clinics.

For example, ambulatory clinicians can easily and quickly respond to requests for prescriptions, filling out forms, and answering messages. Clients love the response, "Sure, no problem, I can take care of that right away." Computerized record keeping and internet access allows rapid and complete access to data that has been collected, which practitioners can also use to show outcomes in similar cases, with other clients. Computers also allow ambulatory practitioners to spend less and less time doing paperwork, which frees up more time for both practice and personal activities. A good ambulatory practice is lean and efficient, with a good business plan that is efficiently implemented. It treats its clients as a valuable asset. This goal is ideal practice, for the veterinarian and the client, as well as the horse.

When it comes to forming a strong doctor-client bond, equine ambulatory practitioners should consider striving for several goals:

1. Eliminate barriers between the client and the doctor. In the author's experience, many practitioners fear that giving clients ready access to them would destroy any vestige of privacy: that may not be the case. By making cellular and home telephone numbers and e-mail address widely available and asking patients to use their best judgment regarding after-hours calls, clients feel that they have access to the practitioner but rarely abuse it. Creating a practice website that answers common questions and provides links to information about health and welfare issues also helps clients get answers that they are looking for, with no need to call the practitioner. In the author's experience, true and unfettered access by clients to their veterinarian results in *less* needless work. The calls that an ambulatory practitioner receives are almost always about horses the veterinarian knows personally; thus, calls tend to be shorter. Almost without exception, clients do not abuse their direct access to their veterinarian; to the contrary, they take their access as a personal responsibility, and treat it with respect and consideration. In the human field, when barriers to access are removed and patients are given direct access to their personal physician, their health care experience is enriched, the connection between physician and patient is strengthened, the understanding of patient's needs is deepened, and the work becomes easier. Such is the case in equine ambulatory medicine, where access to the veterinarian and understanding of the problem for which the horse/patient is being treated fosters trust and confidence in the client.

2. Always try to offer same-day appointments, regardless of whether they are emergencies or not.[2] It has been shown that when physicians reduce barriers to access and offer same-day care, it improves the odds of patients seeing their own physicians and also increases patient satisfaction. In so doing, patients begin to trust the doctor's ability to provide care in a timely fashion, and, in return, they actually request fewer visits. Fewer visits means longer visits, where horses can be inspected more carefully, and problems not initially recognized can be identified and treated. Fewer visits per person also allows for managing a larger population of patients, if the veterinarian chooses to do so.

3. Handle their own after-hours calls. If clients know that the veterinarian is available for after-hours calls, patients actually tend to be *more* respectful of the veterinarian's time.
4. Take the time to make each visit meaningful. Ambulatory clinicians have unique advantages, by virtue of their lower overhead. By paying for facilities, staff, insurance, etc, ambulatory practitioners can run a more profitable business, while still seeing fewer horses per day than their large clinic- or hospital-based colleagues. Fewer client visits means more time per client, allowing for more meaningful visits. Meaningful interaction is the foundation of excellent health care and builds client loyalty. Clients love it when they are allowed to speak without interruption and when they can share stories about their horses. This kind of interaction is rewarding, both personally and professionally. The goal of the practitioner should be more than meeting the expectations of a good visit; it should be to exceed expectations.
5. Invest in technology, especially technology that makes scientific and patient information readily available to both the veterinarian and the client. The human medical Institute for Heathcare Improvement[3] asserts that by so doing, a practice (in this case, a human medical practice, but it would be the same for veterinary practice) attains "reliability"; that is, it can be assured that it is delivering the care that is most likely to be effective. Ambulatory clinicians are not infallible, and veterinary medicine is rapidly changing; it is unreasonable to expect oneself to make all of the correct recommendations for all of the cases all of the time. Attempting to stay current by reading more or by going to continuing education events may not be not enough for ambulatory practitioners; having access to a computer helps veterinarians read about and provide current care, gives clients assurance that the best care is being provided, and can be used to help track the progress of cases.
6. Stay vital, lean, and fresh. A good ambulatory practice has a happy owner, satisfied employees (if there are any), and an innovative spirit and is financially viable. Large offices are burdened by policies, procedures, and lots of staff, which adds more expense and requires ever-increasing numbers of patients or procedures to financially support the practice. Without a burdensome overhead, equine ambulatory practitioners are able to eliminate unnecessary expenses and focus on providing better value for their clients. The practice qualities that clients value most are access, communication, and high-quality care. If ambulatory veterinarians focus on those three things, they may recognize that a great deal of what they do is not perceived by the client as added value. By using technology and creating lean systems, nonveterinary tasks can be handled with minimal hassle, while at the same time increasing the time spent with clients.

Call Coverage

By offering unfettered access, the author finds that his clients seem to make *fewer* telephone calls. Perhaps the increased access produces an increase in trust and respect. Clients often apologize for calling on an emergency basis and appear to respect after-hours and emergency time.

At its core, equine ambulatory practice is a local, very personal process. When veterinarians are available to their clients when their clients need them, when veterinarians treat each interaction with a client as if the client is the only one, and when veterinarians treat each patient interaction with concern and caring, veterinarians are also able to more easily convey their understanding of the most current veterinary knowledge to the individual patient. This is what the "art" of medicine is really all about.

Ambulatory practitioners may worry about who takes care of patients when they are out of town. This worry may be 2-fold: worrying about the lack of available care and worrying about losing clients to competitors. When the author is out of town, he leaves a message on his telephone that simply says, "I'm out of town. Please leave a message. I'll be checking my messages regularly and will call you back. If you have an urgent need, please call me on my cell phone at 555-5555." If a client calls needs an appointment that cannot wait, it is usually not difficult to put the patient in touch with colleagues who can take the case in my absence; providing an alternative when the practitioner is unavailable is another way of showing care and concern for one's clients.

Keep Costs Down

Equine ambulatory practitioners are much better suited than are large practices to keep costs of operation at a reasonable level. By keeping inventory to a minimum and ordering what is needed, when it is needed, avoiding the fixed costs of a large facility, by using cell phones for communication, and by using computers for invoicing and data management, the ambulatory practitioner can weather turbulent economic times. For those times when no one calls, there's no money to be made, but there's also no money going out: no "daily nut" for utilities and staff.

Economies of Scale and Growth

While economies of scale may offer some advantages to larger practices ("More buying power!"), and ambulatory practitioners may be tempted to buy in larger quantities to take advantage of per unit cost savings, other, more important advantages may be available to equine ambulatory practitioners. Since overhead costs are much lower than in larger practices, even though a relatively higher cost per unit may be paid for inventory, the ambulatory practitioner does not have the added expense of maintaining that inventory (higher overhead); in fact, the difference in cost of product is negligible.

The goal of an equine ambulatory practice does not need to be about getting larger. Growing a practice may be a long-held dream, thought of as the way to wealth, or may be considered as a way to create more opportunities for loyal staff: in a capitalistic society, it seems only "natural," and desirable. However, the desire to get larger—a goal for some practitioners—comes at a cost. Growth is a double-edged sword, and while growing one's business as rapidly as possible may seem desirable—such growth can be exhilarating: even patriotic, in a time when more jobs are needed—growing a business may not make much sense for a small ambulatory practice. Ambulatory practices also can be used to provide creative options to help practitioners balance work and family; in an environment where approximately 80% of veterinary school graduates are women who may also want to have a family, group ambulatory practice can allow for several practitioners to work part-time and allow the individual practitioner to more easily balance practice and family obligations.

At its foundation, the decision to grow and to take advantages of economies of scale comes down to individual priorities. Growth means taking on risk. Important questions have to be answered. In order to grow a practice, does an individual practitioner want to take on more debt in the form of outside capital? Does the practitioner want to take on partners, which cuts into autonomy? Is growth worth the responsibilities of more employees, or the stress and aggravation of additional responsibilities? Growth is complicated. Just because something can be done, doesn't mean it *should* be done. The most important word when considering whether to try to grow a small practice could conceivably be, "No."

The successful equine ambulatory practitioner need not answer to anyone other than customers, employees, and, most importantly, family. Solicitations for more and better equipment may not result in more business. New equipment may simply bring in more expenses, and more aggravation.

Business is not just about growth; it is also about making a profit., which many companies seem to forget as they grow themselves out of business. A successful business also needs to be prepared to weather economic storms, lawsuits, competitors, and natural disasters, as well as manmade disasters such as burgeoning accounts receivables. An overextended business is one that is in danger of failure. Sometimes, *not* growing is the safer and more prudent course of action.

Ultimately, the equine ambulatory practitioner should remember one word, when it comes to economies of scale, and growth: Why? Why should an ambulatory practitioner take on more risk? While there is a carrot of more money, there is also the possibility of *losing* money. Furthermore, financial success and growth may come at any additional cost: to family, to health, and to peace of mind. Ultimately, while one must determine one's own priorities, one must also recognize one's limitations.

Billing and Collections

Billing and collections can be problematic for the ambulatory practitioner. Simply stated, one can work all one wants, but if the money is not coming in, the business can't run. Further, the pursuit of revenue eventually adds unpleasant and uncomfortable drudgery to the primary work of equine practice and cuts into the time needed to build trusting relationships with clients. This, then, erodes the sense of joy that the practitioner obtains from his or her work; the performance of a meaningful service in caring for horses becomes merely an exercise in going through the motions to get a paycheck.

In a typical office, the doctor is expected to do the doctoring. That's true: to a point. Completely delegating billing brings extra expense, and also carries some risk of losing track of one's accounts receivable. There's no reason to continue to work for a client who is not also interested in paying their bill. Many ambulatory practices do their own billing, but even when billing is outsourced to an accountant or bookkeeper, it is incumbent on the practitioner to keep a finger in the pie.

There are several things that the ambulatory practitioner can do to keep good cash flow and improve the bottom line. Here are 6:

1. Make sure that the client is clear on terms of payment prior to performing any service or procedure. New patients should be told that they are expected to pay at the time that services are rendered BEFORE any service is rendered.
2. Collect ample and accurate information from the client. Get the client's full name, date of birth, address, work, home and cell phone numbers, as well as their work information. The more information that the veterinarian can collect, the better. Even getting a Social Security number or a driver's license number (if possible) is a good idea; it's useful in the event that an account has to be turned over to a collection agency.
3. Verify equine mortality and major medical insurance coverage, if any.
4. Make sure that the clients sign invoices and that the invoices include written information detailing their responsibility to pay. Information regarding interest charged to carry accounts should be included, as well as language stating that in the event the account is turned over to a collection agency for nonpayment, that

the patient will be responsible for collection costs (check with an attorney: state laws may vary).

5. Payment arrangements should be an available option, especially for people who have financial difficulties. Accept credit cards, and absorb the fees: it's better to give up a small percentage in order to get paid. Making reasonable payment arrangements helps generate positive cash flow.

6. Know when it's time to turn delinquent accounts over to a debt collection agency or to pursue legal action for collection. While most people are honest and pay their debts, there are other people who are less responsible, and some who have no intention of paying. The longer an account goes unpaid, the less chance there is of getting paid. At the most, an account should be slated for some form of collection action after 120 days of no payment (some would say 90 days). Ambulatory practitioners increase the chance of getting paid if accounts that are not paying get sent to collection earlier rather than later.

Some practitioners may also consider boosting their incomes by offering other products for sale, such as various nutritional supplements. While the evidence base for such products is essentially nonexistent, the fact is that many horse owners purchase them for their horses based on the hope or belief that they do some good, and some practitioners may respond to those hopes and beliefs, accordingly. However, selling products may not be a particularly good way to boost income; indeed, it is difficult for a small practice to compete with feed stores and Internet-based companies. The best and most unique thing that the ambulatory clinician has to sell is his or her services.

Sadly, if economic circumstances dictate, no practice model can succeed if clients do not have the money to pay for services rendered. As a result of such circumstances, some veterinarians have abandoned certain areas of practice altogether; as a result, there are those who assert that there is a shortage of rural veterinarians.[4] Even strategies such as loan forgiveness for the veterinarian are unlikely to be effective in resolving the shortage if rural clients are unwilling or unable to pay.

Professional Isolation

The equine ambulatory practitioner has two valuable tools to help combat isolation: the Internet and the telephone. Both of them are increasingly valuable to both help increase professional knowledge and to give a sense that one is not alone.

Whenever there is a question in ambulatory practice about a patient, the proper dose of a drug, the appropriate laboratory test for a particular presentation or condition, or the ideal technique for a necessary procedure, there's one ready solution: pick up that phone! Referral hospitals are in business, too. Answering questions and giving suggestions are part of good business on their part. Suggestions for case management generally also include information about when it might be best to refer the patient; in fact, if referral institutions are unwilling to help, that's usually just an indication that the ambulatory clinician should seek a new referral institution. In addition, the return letters from referral institution frequently serve as a valuable source of continuing education. Over time, consulting with colleagues in referral settings helps gives the equine practitioner confidence in his or her ability to make good diagnoses or, alternatively, to know when to quickly and confidently refer cases that are beyond the practitioner's scope of practice. In addition, telephone conversations can start now friendships; conversations that were once exclusively devoted to the details of body temperature, pain assessment, and signalment turn into opportunities for small talk and sharing personal news. The respect that one has for a more highly trained colleague ultimately becomes mutual.

The Internet offers other valuable opportunities to relieve ambulatory practitioners from their relative isolation. The American Association of Equine Practitioners maintains a listserv for discussion of a wide range of topics, including equine medicine and surgery[5]; recent governance changes will result in "AAEP Rounds," a large number of membership forums, that will operate on a moderated electronic listserv during the year, ending with a face-to-face meeting at the Annual Convention (eg, Dentistry Rounds, Welfare Rounds, Podiatry Rounds).[6] The Equine Clinician's Network, hosted by Washington State University, gives another opportunity for interactions with other equine practitioners.[7] These networks give the solo ambulatory practitioner the ability to consult with other clinicians on particularly problematic cases, as well as gain new ideas and practice tips from colleagues.

SUMMARY

Current economic conditions make the practice of equine medicine challenging, to say the least. The downward trend in the US economy has had a huge impact on horse owners and equine veterinarians alike. Horses are expensive to keep; as such, economics are the driving factor in the problem of the unwanted horse.[8]

Under these conditions, efficient equine ambulatory practices are well-suited to weather the economic storm. As contributors to this issue of *Veterinary Clinics of North America* note, one can practice high-quality medicine and surgery without the overhead and expense of a large clinic. Ambulatory practitioners certainly face formidable challenges, but they also have opportunities to establish and secure a good future.

REFERENCES

1. St George IM. Professional isolation and performance assessment in New Zealand. J Contin Educ Health Prof 2006;26:216–21.
2. Murray M, Tantau C. Same-day appointments: Exploding the access paradigm. Available at: http://www.aafp.org/fpm/2000/0900/p45.html. Accessed January 12, 2012.
3. Institute for Healthcare Improvement. Available at: http://www.ihi.org/Pages/default. aspx. Accessed December 5, 2011.
4. Whitcomb R. Rural veterinary shortage caused by retention issues, not attraction. Veterinary News, DVM360.com. June 1, 2010. Available at: http://veterinarynews.dvm360. com/dvm/Veterinary+Food+Animal/Hard-times-in-the-heartland/ArticleStandard/ Article/detail/672673. Accessed December 5, 2011.
5. AAEP General Discussion List. Available at: www.aaep.org. Accessed December 4, 2011.
6. AAEP Rounds. Available at: www.aaep.org. Accessed December 4, 2011.
7. Equine Clinician's Network. Available at: http://www.vetmed.wsu.edu/orgecn/index. asp. Accessed December 4, 2011.
8. Unwanted Horse Coalition. Available at: http://www.unwantedhorsecoalition.org/. Accessed December 6, 2011.

Ambulatory Equine Practice Management

Mark R. Baus, DVM

KEYWORDS

- Ambulatory practice • Practice management
- Equine practice • Inventory • Accounting

The practice of veterinary medicine is part art and part science, especially in an ambulatory setting, where medicine is often performed in front of clients and other interested spectators. Irrespective of art and science, an ambulatory veterinary practice is also a business; without attention to sound practice management practices, the ambulatory practitioner will ultimately not be able to practice, or will not be able to practice and enjoy the financial rewards that can come from a job well done.

FEE SETTING

To remain competitive with other veterinary practices on services and medications, veterinarians have historically set their fees too low. Even without competitive forces, equine veterinarians have undervalued their professional time and services. However, equine veterinary practice takes years of experience to achieve success and it requires significant investments in technology compared to other professions. A fee structure that recognizes the expertise of the equine practitioner not only rewards the doctor, it supports the quality of care sought by the horse owner. Another challenge to a fair and reasonable fee structure has been a tendency in equine practice to sell drugs and supplies at inflated prices while keeping the fees for professional services too low. In the past, it was not uncommon for 50% of a practice's profit margin to come from the sales of pharmaceuticals, a figure that was possible because horse owners were not aware of the costs of the products themselves. Now that medications are readily available from Internet-based pharmacies, horse owners are able to quickly find the lowest price possible. These prices are typically lower than most equine practices can offer and may even be available to horse owners at costs below what the veterinarian has to pay.

Partially assisted by equine practice management groups, the trend to undervalue professional services and "make it up" by selling pharmaceuticals is changing. However, when the economy was affected by the recession, it became increasingly

The author has nothing to disclose.

Grand Prix Equine, 434 Main Street South, Bridgewater, CT 06752, USA

E-mail address: mbaus@grandprixequine.com

Vet Clin Equine 28 (2012) 11–23
doi:10.1016/j.cveq.2012.02.003
0749-0739/12/$ – see front matter © 2012 Elsevier Inc. All rights reserved.

challenging to maintain fees at a level that would support a reasonable profit margin based on such a model.

Determining the ideal fee structure for an equine practice is particularly difficult for many reasons. To help overcome such difficulties, there are 3 pricing strategies that can be adapted to most goods and services.[1]

- Price professional services based on value
- Price highly shopped services and medications competitively
- Price medications based on cost.

Fees for Professional Services

It may be particularly complicated for equine practitioners to establish fees for professional services. The profit margin on medications continues to shrink year by year so it is essential that the fees for an equine practitioner's service reflect their expertise. Unfortunately, reasonable fees for professional services are often higher than the industry is currently willing to support.

In the past, the veterinarian's examination was virtually complementary: performed in an effort to sell other goods and services. For example, a lameness exam might have been offered at no cost to recoup profit from subsequent joint injections. Even the joint injections might have been offered for free just to sell the medications injected into the joints. This model does not work; in fairness to both horse owners and practice owners, it is essential that every fee charged stands on its own merit.

The foundation for determining professional fees is the hourly rate. The concept of an hourly rate is well known in the legal and accounting world but is largely foreign to the equine veterinary world. Obviously the hourly rate will vary depending on the region of the country where a veterinarian practices, but as a starting point, consider a rate of $250 per hour for a professional exam.

In this example, if the average examination requires 20 minutes to complete, the basic examination would therefore be one third the hourly rate, or approximately $85. In reality, this is only part of the necessary time to complete the examination. Although the *exam* requires 20 minutes, the veterinarian will spend considerably more time communicating the findings with the horse owner or the stable manager. Even more time is necessary to complete the medical records. Because of the time spent communicating with the horse owner and caretaker, it is essential that the fees for professional services are set at a level that also recognizes the hidden time spent providing a valuable service.

Basing an examination on a set period of time deserves further scrutiny. The ambulatory veterinarian spends a great deal of time driving from one stable to the next. Although the logical solution would be to bill the same professional hourly rate for the travel time, most horse owners do not consider the stable call as having the same value as the professional service. Indeed, the stable call may be viewed as an unreasonable expense, rather than a necessary one. Therefore, if an ambulatory practice spends excessive time driving from stable to stable, the professional service fees must be set at a higher rate than usual, because recouping driving costs by increasing call fees can be met with considerable resistance from the client.

Fees for Imaging Services

A digital radiography system often represents the largest investment an equine ambulatory veterinarian will make. It is crucial that the fee for this service is competitive with the local market and also provides the practice owner with a reasonable return on investment. Fees for providing radiographic and ultrasound services are based not only on time but also on the cost of the equipment. Other fixed costs include the interest on the loan, the maintenance agreement, property taxes, and insurance.

Before calculating the fee for digital radiographs, it is necessary to estimate the number of radiographic images that will be taken in a year. Using a formula developed by Andrew Clark, DVM, MBA,[2] it can be determined how many views will need to be billed yearly for a specific fee in order to obtain a specific return on investment. Here's how this formula works in practice, starting with the following assumptions:

- DR system and x-ray generator depreciated or paid for over 5 years: $70,000
- Maintenance agreement: $7500 per year
- Taxes and equipment insurance: $1200 per year
- Veterinarian commission and technician cost: $10.54 per view.

At $40 per view and with no return on investment, the DR system would need to bill 795 views in a year. To achieve a 20% return on investment, 1077 views would need to be taken. If the fee is $45 per view, 705 views would need to be taken to break even and 954 views would support a return on investment of 20%.

In order to make these calculations work, it is important that a reasonable estimate is made for the number of images that will be generated. It is also important to know what the local equine market expects to pay for this service before determining the best fee for a given practice. Other facts may also need to be considered. For example, in an established practice, more images are likely to be billed and at a higher fee; thus, a higher return on investment is ensured. Conversely, in a developing practice with no guarantee of the views taken per year or with a fee that is too low, the owner of the DR system would be at risk for losing significant revenue on his or her investment.

Charging for setting up imaging equipment and for archiving the images is an accepted and recommended fee for imaging studies. This charge mitigates the difference in revenue between setting-up equipment to take 1 or 2 views versus taking a large number of views for a purchase exam; the amount of effort to set up the equipment is identical, even though the revenue obtained from the procedure itself may not be. A typical setup fee is between $30 and $50 for radiographic studies and $20 to $40 for ultrasound studies.

Highly Shopped Services and Medications

This category of fee items includes goods and services that horse owners can easily compare from practice to practice or, more likely, from a veterinary practice to an Internet pharmacy. It will include medications that are costly and may be used on an ongoing basis. GastroGard (Merial, LLC; Duluth, GA, USA), Regumate (Intervet Inc; Millsboro, DE, USA), Legend (Bayer Healthcare, LLC; Shawnee Mission, KS, USA), and Adequan (Luitpold Pharmaceuticals, Inc, Animal Health Division; Shirley, NY, USA) are typical examples. Whether the appropriate charges for such items occur in a discussion between fellow veterinarians or with horse owners, the cost of highly shopped veterinary goods and services will likely generate more dissent than agreement. Nevertheless, highly shopped medications and services will generally provide the least margin of profit for all billed items so they must be managed carefully.

The most commonly compared service that the ambulatory practitioner offers is the stable call. Although the equine practitioner is offering the horse owner nearly every aspect of a fully equipped equine hospital at their stable, he or she often cannot appreciate why the stable call from one practice should be any different from another practice. Although one practitioner's vehicle might be newer, cleaner, and more fully equipped than that of a nearby colleague, for competitive reasons, the profit margin for a stable call fee must typically match the charge by nearby veterinary practices for driving from stable to stable.

Another highly shopped service is wellness care. Although most horse owners would prefer to not administer their own inoculations, they are able to compare fees because the price of the vaccine is readily available online or from the many periodicals they receive. Horse owners also cannot easily recognize the value of one practice's wellness program over another. One suggestion for pricing vaccinations is to set a markup for each dose of the vaccine (see later) and bundle this fee item with an intramuscular injection fee. This will allow for a reasonable profit margin while allowing the fee to change with the cost of the vaccine.

Pricing Medications Based on Cost

For the sake of fee setting, pharmaceutical items can be categorized into one of the following groups.

1. Food and Drug Administration (FDA) approved and readily available from an online pharmacy
2. FDA approved and not prescribed on a routine basis
3. Controlled drugs
4. Compounded medications
5. Vaccines.

The single greatest challenge to effectively managing the inventory in the equine ambulatory practice is shrinkage. Shrinkage is defined as "the loss of products between. . .purchase from supplier and point of sale."[3] Equine practice owners lose the value of products prior to the final sale for many reasons:

- Medication was dispensed to the horse owner but not billed, due to forgetfulness of the veterinarian, or as a courtesy
- Expired or outdated product (wastage)
- Damaged medication or container
- Theft.

In setting the fee for drugs in each of these categories, it is also important to consider the overhead charge. The overhead charge (usually 10%–25%) is necessary to account for the cost of ordering, stocking, and handling medication. It must also take into account the anticipated shrinkage that will occur from maintaining any inventory. Although this would appear to be an unnecessary step for managing a pharmacy, it is important to understand the cost of stocking each medication before a discount is given or before any profit is realized from its sale. The additional overhead charge should be added to the direct cost of the medication before a markup is determined and it should not be considered for a doctor's commission if a production-based formula is used to determine the salary for associate veterinarians.

The markup for medications that are dispensed in the event of illness or injury should be set with a higher markup than those items that are discretionary and readily available by prescription from an online pharmacy. One example of this is eye ointments. Since eye ointments are needed immediately at the time of service and because it is common for them to go out-of-date before dispensing, their markup should be considerably higher than that for a medication that is used on an ongoing basis.

Because controlled drugs require specialized handling and licensing, their markup should also be higher than regular medications. Controlled drugs require a DEA (Drug Enforcement Agency) number, must be stored within 2 locked containers, and represent a significant threat of theft for the practice. As such, the minimum markup, with or without an added overhead charge, should be at least 150% of the purchase price.

Compounded medications are commonly, albeit somewhat controversially, used in equine practice. Because they are not manufactured with the stringent requirements of an FDA-approved medication,[4] there is added risk with their use. Also, since compounded drugs cannot establish an official expiration date for their products (the FDA establishes expiration dates for approved medications), most compounding pharmacies set a recommended "use by" date that is usually much shorter than their counterparts from the FDA. This contributes significantly to wastage and should therefore increase the margin or markup of compounded medications.

Wastage is also an important consideration in pricing vaccines. Vaccines, although occasionally shopped by the horse owner, should carry additional markup to compensate for the refrigeration that is required for storage as well as the wastage of unused vaccine.

Laboratory Services

The fee for laboratory services should be at least 250% of the cost of the test (150% markup). For example, if a complete blood count costs $16, the fee charged should be at least $40. In addition to the cost of the test itself, additional charges should be considered for processing and submitting the sample, as well as the professional fees added for interpreting and reporting the results. Coggins tests, as well as other tests mandated for the shipment of horses, are also deserving of a higher markup beyond their cost based on the added time to complete the form, as well as the fact that federal accreditation is required to perform this test.

CHART OF ACCOUNTS AND FINANCIAL STATEMENTS

Why bother keeping accurate accountings of practice expenses, revenues, assets, and liabilities, much less practice equity? There are 3 main reasons:

- An accurate set of books is required for tax purposes.
- Banks require financial data before approving a loan.
- Critical management decisions require a close study of the financial health of the practice.

A comprehensive review of the chart of accounts and financial statements for equine practice was written and compiled by Marsha Heinke, DVM, EA, CPA, CVPM.[5] The Equine Practice Chart of Accounts should be referenced for specific and detailed information concerning the accounting needs of the equine veterinary practice. Dr Heinke's book is an invaluable resource for the practice owner prior to or even after establishing a chart of accounts.

The chart of accounts is a list of the assets, liabilities, equity, revenue, and expenses that form the foundation of the bookkeeping system for the equine practice. In order to discuss these 5 categories, some definitions are required of the various terms and financial statements that are used to manage an ambulatory equine practice.

- Assets are things that, tangible or intangible, are owned to produce value for the practice and can be converted into cash. The equine practice vehicle is an asset.

- Liabilities are obligations that the practice owes to another entity. These are usually loans, such as a vehicle loan, due to a lending institute.
- Equity is, in simplest terms, the difference between the assets of a practice minus its liabilities.
- Revenue is income that the practice receives from its normal business activities.
- Expenses are funds paid by the practice for goods and services that support day-to-day operations. This category would include drugs and supplies, vehicle expenses (including interest on the loan), and salaries.
- Cash versus accrual methods of accounting. The difference between these 2 methods is mostly a question of timing.
  - The cash method records expenses or revenue when they are paid or received respectively.
  - The accrual method records expenses or revenue when they are incurred or earned respectively.
  - The accrual method is preferred for management purposes for practices generating more than $1,000,000 yearly but is required for tax purposes for all businesses with more than $5,000,000 in gross receipts.
  - The cash method of accounting is adequate for both management purposes and for tax purposes in the small practice.
- The profit and loss statement (income statement) is a list of all revenue and expenses for a stated period of time. This financial statement provides the best analysis of profit (or loss) for the business over time. The profit and loss statement can be stated on either a cash basis or an accrual basis depending on its use as management tool or for tax purposes.
- The balance sheet is a summary of practice assets, liabilities, and equity on a specific date. While the profit and loss statement is for a stated period of time, the balance sheet marks a specific point in time.

Maintaining the chart of accounts will never be one of the more fascinating duties of an equine practitioner. However, the security of knowing that the books are in top shape will allow the practitioner to offer undistracted focus to the rest if his or her job. Traditionally, the chart of accounts is set up in a customary order that allows the practice to generate all necessary financial statements. These financial statements (profit and loss statement; balance sheet) are useful for managing the practice efficiently and are essential for preparing tax returns.

Within the asset and the liability accounts, each account is listed from the most liquid to the least liquid. Liquidity describes how quickly an asset can be converted to cash or how quickly a liability is coming due. Using the Equine Veterinary Practice Chart of Accounts as a guide, each ledger entry is assigned a 5-digit number. Although only a fraction of the available numbers will be assigned a ledger entry, this system allows for additional ledger entries as a practice grows in size and complexity.

- 10000 through 29999 represent asset classes starting with cash accounts and ending with fixed assets.
- 30000 through 39999 represent liability accounts starting with short-term liabilities.
- 40000 through 49999 represent owner equity accounts.
- 50000 through 59999 represent the revenue that an equine practice generates.
- 60000 through 89999 represent the expenses incurred, most importantly, the cost of professional services such as drugs and supplies. This group would also include the cost of practice employees.

Accounting Programs

Three commercially available accounting programs are most commonly used by equine practices to maintain the chart of accounts:

- Quicken (http://quicken.intuit.com): Useful for home and small business accounting needs
- QuickBooks (http://quickbooks.com): A more robust accounting program that is appropriate for most equine practices
- Sage Peachtree (http://peachtree.com): Comparable to QuickBooks.

Most accounting programs, including these 3, offer the equine practitioner the ability to generate invoices and medical records within the program. This offers the benefit of managing the practice with one program. It merges the revenue side of the practice (billing the clients) with the expense side of the practice in a way that makes year-end calculations more easily performed.

As a practice grows and develops, simple accounting programs are no able to offer the flexibility and reporting that a proprietary practice management program is designed to do. Most of the commercially available programs for practice management offer a practice the ability to maintain accurate invoices and detailed medical records at the time a service is performed. Furthermore, allowing the veterinarian to view the client's account and the patient's medical records at the stable is invaluable.

Although there are significant advantages to practice management programs, they are unable to manage accounts payable, fixed assets, and payroll expenses. Therefore, despite the affordability and ease of maintaining one program to run all aspects of a practice, it is most likely that one program will be necessary to run the expense-side of the practice (the accounting program) and another program will be necessary to run the revenue-side of the practice (practice management program).

Assisting the Bookkeeper and Accountant to Maintain the Chart of Accounts

The bookkeeper and the accountant require the input of the practice owner when assigning expenses to the proper account. Never is the difference between a bookkeeper and equine veterinarian more apparent than when a bookkeeper is trying to assign a specific expense to its correct category!

It is essential that whenever an expense is incurred, an accurate record is kept to describe the purpose of the expense. In the event of a tax audit, an accurate accounting of each expense will be necessary. For management purposes, it is important to know if an expense was incurred for a specific service to a patient or if it was simply an office supply. If it is a dinner with a colleague, it is helpful to the bookkeeper and the accountant to know who the dinner was with and the purpose of the meeting. If it is a credit card expense at an office supply store, a notation on the receipt designating software from a general office supply item is helpful. While in a 1-person equine ambulatory practice it may not be necessary to fill out an expense report for each expense as is required in a large company, even a simple notation on the credit card receipt can be quite helpful to maintain an accurate chart of accounts.

The Value of a Well-Structured Chart of Accounts

Other than completing tax returns or applying for a bank loan, why would an equine practice owner bother with developing an accurate chart of accounts?

Furthermore, what is the purpose of analyzing profit and loss reports or a balance sheet?

By providing information about cash flow (the movement of money in and out of the practice) and profitability, the practice owner can accurately answer any of a number of questions about the health and growth of the practice:

- Should an associate veterinarian be hired?
- Would it be worth hiring a technician?
- Can a new piece of equipment be purchased?
- Is it time to raise fees?
- Can benefits packages be expanded?
- How much can be contributed to a retirement fund?

As the standard of care in equine medicine and surgery rises, and as an equine practice grows and develops, decisions will need to be made to support the increasing demands on the practice. With careful attention to the financial data generated by a well-organized chart of accounts, the decisions on how and when to develop a practice become easier and more accurate.

INVENTORY CONTROL

Although the principles of maintaining an efficient pharmacy pertain to the mobile equine practitioner, stocking a practice vehicle in a manner that is both functional and profitable is particularly challenging. Limited space and extreme temperatures can make the task of stocking a vehicle with the necessary supplies quite difficult. It is important to maintain an inventory in an ambulatory equine practice that provides a valuable service to the patient but is also profitable to the practice.

Any inventory should be regarded in the same manner as cash. Since the best use of cash is not to be sitting on the shelves or in the practice vehicle, a profitable inventory is one that requires minimum quantity while still providing whatever medication is necessary for the daily practice. Equine veterinary practitioners are notorious for overstocking their vehicles with drugs and supplies; this can significantly impact the bottom line.

Prioritizing Inventory Items

Using the principals of ABC (Activity Based Costing) Analysis,[6] a system that suggests that not all items of inventory are of equal importance, inventory can be divided into three categories. "A" items are stocked and sold in larger quantities than other items, are tracked carefully from purchase to sale, and are those for which accurate records are necessary; they are among the most important items to manage in the practice. "B" items are ordered in smaller quantities and are less tightly controlled than "A" items; "C" items require the simplest controls and are stocked in the smallest quantity possible.

For this exercise, assume that an ambulatory equine practice stocks 50 drugs in their vehicle. As a starting point, the 10 most commonly dispensed products from a practice vehicle should be identified. These medications are the "A" category of drugs. In most practices, the class "A" drugs would account for 50% to 70% of total inventory sales and must, therefore, be managed carefully. It is essential to an equine practice that class "A" drugs are stocked at levels so they are always available for use. It is important to track class "A" drugs from the initial ordering until they are dispensed and invoiced to the client. Although wastage is expected in class "C" medications, it should not be tolerated with class "A" medications.

The "B" group of drugs, although essential, are stocked in low numbers and monitored carefully. As a rule of thumb, the "B" group of drugs would be stocked at twice the number that is necessary for a single treatment. Stocking levels are also determined by the turnover rate which is discussed later. Although they may comprise 50% of the number of items in the pharmacy, the "C" group of drugs are dispensed only occasionally and are stocked in minimum quantities.

Maintaining the correct amount of each of category of drugs is based on 2 calculations. First, how much is sold on an annual basis? Second, how rapid is the turnover rate of each product?

The turnover rate is important to understand when it comes to inventory control. By definition, the turnover rate is the number of times a supply of drugs is sold in a year and can be calculated for each drug or for the entire inventory. The ideal turnover rate is as high as possible and is usually between 5 and 12 times per year. Consequently, each drug is ideally ordered once a month to maintain a useful supply. As such, if 48 bottles of phenylbutazone tablets were sold in 1 year, and the practice wanted to turn over the supply on a monthly basis, it would stock 4 bottles at time. However, if phenylbutazone tablets were a Class A drug, the practice might choose to stock 6 bottles to avoid running out of this necessary drug.

In order to keep the inventory as lean and profitable as possible, it is important to consider alternate methods for providing medication that does not involve stocking it in the practice pharmacy. One such method is the drop shipment. Most distributors of medication and supplies offer this service at little or no added expense depending on the value of the order. The drop shipment allows the veterinarian to fulfill a medication need by placing the order with the distributor. The veterinarian places the order and the distributor ships the product directly to the client, usually within 1 or 2 days of ordering. Importantly, the veterinarian should request that the packing slip not include an invoice showing the veterinarian's cost of the medication. The veterinarian then bills the medication at the usual rate without having to receive and stock the medication.

Another means of dispensing medication without stocking it is to collaborate with a third-party online pharmacy. This online service can be embedded into the veterinarian's website, allowing the client to order the product directly while the veterinarian still determines the cost of each item. Several companies offer this service including VetCentric (http://www.vetcentric.com), VetStreet (http://www.vetstreet.com), and ProxyRX (http://www.proxyrx.com). Although the third-party company will add their own fee to this service, this collaboration allows the veterinarian a reasonable profit margin without adding to their existing pharmacy.

Providing prescriptions for medication is a service that is highly appreciated by many horse owners and is usually required by states' practice acts. This allows the client to shop for the least expensive medication and most online pharmacies ship their product promptly. Although the veterinarian realizes no profit from writing prescriptions, it develops goodwill with the horse owner when they realize that the veterinarian's recommendation for any medication is not predicated on selling it. Prescriptions records should be noted in the patient's history file for future reference. Each online or catalogue pharmacy has its own protocol for fulfilling a prescription. Some will fax or email their own prescription form to be completed by the veterinarian, while other pharmacies will fulfill a prescription with a telephone call to the veterinarian. Most pharmacies will not accept the veterinarian's own written prescription sent by fax or email since the client could fill the order several times with different pharmacies.

DEVELOPING A TEAM

Depending on the size, type, and growth rate of the practice, equine ambulatory practitioners may employ 1 or more staff, including a veterinary assistant. The role of the assistant to the ambulatory equine practitioner has changed immensely in the past few years. At one time, this person was referred to simply as a "rider," and only employed during the busiest times of year to handle horses and perform the most basic services for the veterinarian. While incorporating an assistant into a practice is an additional expense, in many circumstances, this person has the potential to significantly improve the standard of care for the practice, as well as to enhance revenue.

Within each practice, there are numerous responsibilities that can be assumed by the veterinary assistant. In many cases, the assistant can take over responsibilities that were previously performed by office-based personnel or by the veterinarian. But consider: Who is in a better position to manage an ambulatory practice than the person working alongside the veterinarian day by day?

Many, if not most, ambulatory practitioners choose to work without an assistant. This is understandable for 2 primary reasons. First, a qualified veterinary assistant can easily cost a practitioner 10% of their gross revenue. Second, veterinarians who work without an assistant enjoy the autonomy of coming and going as they wish. Nevertheless, in certain circumstances, the extra expense and the loss of freedom are offset by the many benefits of employing a veterinary assistant in the ambulatory practice. With the necessary training, the responsibilities of a veterinary assistant can be expanded well beyond the traditional expectations of a veterinary technician.

The veterinary assistant can perform services for the veterinarian that allow the veterinarian to concentrate on the veterinary medical services for which he or she was awarded a professional license. This not only enhances the level of care to the horse, but it also supports the client's expectations. The basic responsibilities of the equine ambulatory technician traditionally include:

- Horse handling and restraint experience
- Preparing for all common medical and surgical procedures
- Understanding sterile technique
- Obtaining lab samples and submitting them for appropriate testing
- Presenting a neat and tidy appearance
- Providing excellent client relations
- Maintaining client/patient confidentiality
- Computer skills
- Restocking the practice vehicle at the end of each work day.

In exchange for meeting these expectations the veterinarian/employer should offer the following:

- A clear definition of the job responsibilities (job description)
- A payroll system that provides a regular paycheck with the proper deduction of payroll and withholding taxes
- Benefits, sick leave, maternity leave, and vacation time as outlined at the outset of employment
- Adherence to all requirements of labor law
- Opportunity for job and career development.

Expanded Responsibilities for the Ambulatory Equine Assistant

The ambulatory equine assistant has a unique role compared to other veterinary technicians. Since every element of equine ambulatory practice is brought to the stable, the assistant is in a position to "wear many hats" as it regards the needs of the veterinarian and the practice.

Scheduling

With the use of call forwarding or a virtual phone service, the assistant can be the first person to answer a client's call. With the assistant's proximity to the veterinarian, questions can be answered immediately. With a mobile computing system that allows access to all records and scheduling programs, the client can arrange an appointment immediately and much sooner than if a call back were required. At the time the appointment is scheduled, the technician can gather background information and history concerning the case that is essential to the veterinarian prior to the examination.

Lab technician

The veterinary assistant technician can play an important role in obtaining, processing, and submitting lab samples.

- All necessary forms can be completed and submitted (or mailed) to the lab with the samples.
- When lab results are returned, they can be entered into the practice management program and submitted to the doctor.
- The assistant can also ensure that the horse owner or caretaker is contacted with the results.
- A cross check of the management program can ensure that the service was properly billed.

Imaging technician

Setting up equipment and preparing the patient is an important time-saver for the veterinarian in providing this valuable service. The technician can also contribute to this process in the following ways:

- Archive all studies and send studies to colleagues and owners as necessary.
- Maintain equipment service contracts.
- Ensure that all imaging services are billed to the client.

Inventory management

The greatest expense for most equine practices is its inventory of drugs and supplies. Although too little inventory will compromise the quality of care, too much inventory represents a significant loss of revenue for the practice owner. Because the assistant is present when medication and supplies are dispensed, he or she is the most qualified person to maintain a well-stocked vehicle and to oversee the practice inventory.

A practice vehicle that is overstocked can represent a significant loss of revenue. If overstocked, medications may become out of date before they can be dispensed. Also, medication containers tend to become damaged as they remain too long in the vehicle. A properly stocked vehicle can carry a minimum amount of inventory, which also allows the practitioner to choose a vehicle that is smaller and more economical to maintain.

A practice management program with an inventory management module allows the assistant to generate purchase orders and purchase receipts, in addition to placing the order with the necessary vendor. This allows the veterinarian to oversee the purchasing process and helps ensure that the proper amount of medication is ordered and that the prices are adjusted according to their fluctuation.

Invoicing and record keeping

Missed charges can represent a significant loss of revenue for the equine practitioner. Despite confidence in their extraordinary memory, many services and medications may be forgotten by the veterinarian before they are finally entered into the practice record-keeping system. Working closely with their veterinarian, the assistant can play a critical role in capturing all services and dispensed medications. Initiating the invoice at the time of the call will ensure that all work is billed and that the medical records are accurately entered. Of course, the veterinarian should ultimately recheck each invoice and complete the medical record for accuracy, but with 2 sets of eyes on each invoice, missed charges will be significantly reduced.

Maintaining autonomy

To a large extent, ambulatory equine veterinarians enjoy the autonomy of coming and going as they wish. If the veterinarian has a family function in the middle of the day, a practitioner who chooses not to employ an assistant can attend the function between appointments without further ado. However, employing an assistant does not also mean that the veterinarian must relinquish his or her autonomy.

To support the ideals of autonomy (for both the veterinarian and the technician), it is important to develop responsibilities that allow the technician to function while the veterinarian is not working. In the author's experience, this can be done by assigning the assistant additional responsibilities and providing them with their own computer. This enables the assistant to fulfill his or her duties at any time of day.

Autonomy and flexibility for the veterinarian are also enhanced by compensating the assistant with a weekly salary, as opposed to an hourly wage. This allows the veterinarian and the technician to work together when it is necessary and to work apart when it is not without tracking the exact amount of time the technician is working. However, a decision to provide a weekly salary should not be motivated by an effort to avoid overtime pay.

SUMMARY

The horse owner not only expects outstanding care for their horse; they also recognize and appreciate a well-run equine practice. They expect their veterinarian to show up on time for appointments; they expect to receive decipherable invoices and statements on a regular basis and they appreciate an assistant who enhances the services that their veterinarian provides.

A well-managed ambulatory equine practice supports the ideals of both high standards of care *and* mobility. In fact, a poorly managed practice will ultimately impact the care that an equine veterinarian attempts to provide the horses in his or her care. Without careful attention to profitability and efficiency, the practice's ability to grow and develop with emerging therapies and technologies is impossible. Furthermore, a poorly managed practice will significantly contribute to the frustration that an equine veterinarian feels after working long hours and receiving only nominal pay.

REFERENCES

1. Denise T. CPA; Top 3 ways to price products and services. Veterinary Economics 2011;52(9):36.
2. Andrew Clark, DVM, MBA; Available at: http://www.dvmmba.com. Accessed January 6, 2012.

3. Shrinkage. Available at: http://en.wikipedia.org/wiki/Shrinkage_(accounting). Accessed October, 2011.
4. Drug Compounding. AAEP Member login. Available at: http://www.aaep.org/drug_compounding_practitioner.htm. Accessed March 18, 2012.
5. Equine Veterinary Practice Chart of Accounts; Marsha Heinke, DVM, EA, CPA, CVPM; AAEP and Milburn Equine; 2006.
6. ABC Analysis. Available at: http://en.wikipedia.org/wiki/ABC_analysis. Accessed December 21, 2011.

3. Shrinkage en. Available at: http://en.wikipedia.org/wiki/Shrinkage_(accounting). Accessed October, 2011.

4. Drug Compounding. AAEP Member login. Available at: http://www.aaep.org/drug compounding_practitioners.htm. Accessed March 18, 2012.

5. Equine Veterinary Practice Chart of Accounts. Marsha Heinke, DVM, EA, CPA, CVPM. AAEP and Milburn Equine, 2008.

6. ABC Analysis. Available at: http://en.wikipedia.org/wiki/ABC_analysis. Accessed December 21, 2011.

Technology and the Ambulatory Equine Practitioner: Implementing and Affording the 21st Century

Mark R. Baus, DVM[a], Robert P. Magnus, DVM, MBA[b],*

KEYWORDS

- Information technology • Cloud computing
- Paperless office • DICOM • Capital investments
- Negotiating • Financing

The mobile equine practitioner faces many challenges day by day. Providing horses with high levels of care while serving the needs of the horse owner, trainer, and caregiver and, at the same time, managing the intricate needs of a business and a balanced home life can be overwhelming. Horse owners expect immediate and high-quality care from their equine veterinarian, all of it provided while he or she is driving from stable to stable away from the central office.

Technological advances in the past several decades have provided many useful tools to help ambulatory equine veterinarians overcome these challenges. For example, cellular telephones have provided a communication system that allows an instant connection between the veterinarian and horse owner or caregiver. Of equal importance, networked computers allows for digitized medical records to be shared freely among veterinarians, horse owners, and any of the key personnel involved in the care of the horse.

Information technology offers the mobile equine veterinarian opportunities to provide uncompromising levels of care, maintain an open line of communication with his or her clients and colleagues, produce sophisticated images of any part of the horse's body, and create detailed medical records, while, at the same time, generating an invoice that captures all fees incurred at the time of service. All of this can be achieved at the stable allowing for practice to be conducted with a high

The authors have nothing to disclose.
^a Grand Prix Equine, 434 Main Street South, Bridgewater, CT 06752, USA
^b 39151 Delafield Road, Oconomowoc, WI 53066, USA
* Corresponding author.
E-mail address: bmagnus@wiequine.com

Vet Clin Equine 28 (2012) 25–38
doi:10.1016/j.cveq.2012.02.004
0749-0739/12/$ – see front matter © 2012 Elsevier Inc. All rights reserved.

level of professionalism, while simultaneously freeing time for the veterinarian to pursue other aspects of life.

THE PAPERLESS PRACTICE

Virtually every piece of paper in the mobile equine practice can be replaced by its digital form. Not only can this information be stored on a computer, it can be stored online with the help of cloud computing further enhancing its security and accessibility. Cloud computing is a method of processing and storing information that relies on software and data storage centers that are accessed by the Internet.

A paperless work environment offers advantages beyond saving large amounts of paper. Among those advantages are:

- Information is stored in computers or servers that are both onsite and online, eliminating the risk of losing documents.
- Medical records, documents, and contact information are readily available to the practice through a computer network or an online connection.
- During an examination, a horse's past medical history can be reviewed while the new medical record is being generated.
- All documents, including radiographic and ultrasound images, can be easily shared with clients and colleagues.
- As information is made available in a digital form, the need for a central office becomes less and less important. This reduces the fixed costs of managing a practice such as floor space for filing cabinets as well as staffing.
- Every aspect of operating an equine practice can be managed from any location with a laptop computer and an internet connection.

Hardware for the Paperless Practice

Developing an efficient office system for the ambulatory equine practice requires several pieces of hardware along with a few software programs. Hardware needs in a fully digitized practice include the following:

- *Laptop computer.*
  This is the core of the paperless office. It will allow the equine practitioner to transition from working in the office to working in the field. To further enhance its usefulness, the laptop can be networked to an office-based server or, preferably, an online server.
- *Scanner.*
  This device is a critical piece of hardware for the paperless office. There are many choices of scanners but an ideal scanner accepts multipage document ts, scans in color and scans on both sides of a sheet. The scanner should also be able to convert all documents into a Portable Document Format (PDF) that can be renamed and filed into the appropriate folder on the practice's computer or server (NeatDesk Scanner; neat.com). (The Neat Company, Philadelphia, PA, USA)
- *Wireless router and cable modem.*
  These devices connect all computers in the workplace and home to the Internet without a wired connection.
- *Docking station for your laptop computer.*
  This allows for a quick and easy connection to the power supply, desktop monitor, as well as peripheral devices such as the printer and scanner while working in the office.

- *Printer.*
  Although the goal is a paperless office, many documents still need to be printed because they require pen and ink completion. Also, many clients still count on printed documents and statements.
- *Desktop monitor.*
  In a paperless office, most documents and medical images are viewed on a monitor instead of paper or film; thus, a large, high-quality monitor is essential. The monitor of the laptop can function as a secondary monitor to extend the desktop over a larger area.
- *USB hub.*
  A 6- to 8-port USB hub allows for numerous peripheral devices (phone, printer, scanner, camera, MP3 players) to connect to the laptop or docking station with 1 plug.

In the paperless practice, the veterinarian's vehicle becomes the doctor's secondary office. Many aspects of managing the practice can be conducted from the vehicle. This includes entering records from the last stable call, answering e-mail messages, and sending a text message to the next stable to let them know the practitioner is on the way. If an assistant is employed by the practitioner, such tasks can even be performed while on the road!

The following is a list of hardware items recommended for maximizing the efficiency of the mobile office.

- A *laptop mount* is essential for mobile computing (Jotto Desk Laptop Mounts; www.jottodesk.net; 2724 Otter Creek Ct. #101; Las Vegas, NV 89117). For safety purposes, the laptop mount should not interfere with the function of the airbag system while the vehicle is in motion.
- *Power inverter.* Inverts of 1000 W are necessary to operate a laptop and other peripheral devices. The inverter should be hardwired to the vehicle's electrical system, preferably to a second battery to avoid draining the vehicle's primary battery.
- *Broadband card.* This is a USB device connected to the laptop or, preferably, to a mobile wireless router installed in the vehicle and provides a connection to the Internet through a cellular carrier.
- *Mobile wireless router.* A mobile wireless router is a network device that combines a router, switch, and Wi-Fi access point (Wi-Fi base station) in 1 box (CradlePoint Mobile Router; www.cradlepoint.com; 805 W. Franklin Street; Boise, ID 83702). Wireless routers provide a convenient way to connect a small number of wired and any number of wireless computers to the internet simultaneously. For example, by using a mobile wireless router, while radiographs are taken nearby, the images can be immediately and automatically uploaded to the archiving system. The mobile wireless router also adds to the convenience of connecting to the internet, freeing the practitioner from plugging the broadband card into the laptop each time it us carried in and out of the vehicle (picture archiving and communication system, or PACS).

SOFTWARE PROGRAMS FOR THE MOBILE EQUINE PRACTICE
Practice Management Software

The principal software for operating a paperless equine practice is the practice management program. These programs allow the practitioner full access to patient and client information in the field. They also allow the practitioner to generate new invoices and medical records while they are out of the office. As each of these programs collaborate with archiving systems and diagnostic labs, the electronic patient file will include access to all lab results and all images generated for each patient.

For some practices, existing accounting programs such as Sage Peachtree (Sage North America, Irvine, CA, USA) and QuickBooks (Intuit Inc., Mountain View, CA, USA) may be able to perform the basic functions of a practice management program adequately but they are more difficult to operate in the field and are more difficult to manage as the practice hires additional veterinarians and staff members.

Medical records are more accurate and thorough if they are entered while the service is provided. Furthermore, invoices created at the time of the examination will capture more fees. In order to fully capitalize on the advantages of immediate input, certain features from a management program are desirable. These features allow a practitioner to perform the following tasks away from the central office:

- Create medical records from an existing template or in a SOAP (Subjective, Objective, Assessment, Plan) format.
- Generate invoices simultaneously with the medical record.
- Print or e-mail invoices and medical records as soon as they are finalized.
- Have immediate access to existing records as well as client and patient information.
- Add new clients and patients.
- Access and modify the schedule.

In addition to the version that operates in the field, most practice management programs offer a more complete version that operates in the veterinarian's central office. This centralized version will generate the client's bills at regular intervals, track inventory, and provide the necessary reports to manage the practice.

The programs currently available for managing equine practices include:

- IDEXX Cornerstone (Idexx Laboratories, Inc., Westbrook, ME, USA)
- DVM Manager (ImproMed, Oshkosh, WI, USA)
- DVMAX (Sneakers Software Inc./DVMAX, New York, NY, USA)
- HVMS (Business Infusions, Inc., Calgary, AB, Canada)
- ImproMed Infinity (ImproMed, Oshkosh, WI, USA)
- ImproMed Advantage+ Equine (previously known as Vetech) (ImproMed, Oshkosh, WI, USA)
- ImproMed Triple Crown (ImproMed, Oshkosh, WI, USA)
- Rx Works (Rx Works, Las Vegas, NV, USA)
- VIA Elinc (VIA Information Systems, Frisco, TX, USA).

Smartphone applications for practice management programs are available on a limited basis and although they have limited functionality, they allow access to the doctor's schedule as well as client and patient information.

Archiving Program

If the most important program for running an ambulatory practice is the management program, the second most important program is PACS. PACS breaks down the physical and time barriers associated with traditional film-based systems. PACS also ensures that the image is permanently stored with recovery in the event of an onsite disaster.

PACS consists of 4 basic components: an imaging modality such as radiography or ultrasound, a network for transferring the image to the archive, a workstation for viewing the images, and a server that stores the images electronically. As with all forms of data storage, it is critical that all image storage has an online backup in the event of a natural disaster or equipment failure.

The most universally accepted format for image storage and retrieval is DICOM (Digital Imaging and Communications in Medicine). The DICOM format enables studies from various imaging devices to integrate into the PACS. Because of its broad acceptance in the human imaging world, DICOM storage and viewing is favored over other formats. However, image can also be stored and viewed in JPEG (Joint Photographic Experts Group).

Ideally, all images generated for each horse should be accessible from anywhere and can be readily transferable to colleagues and owners. Even though the most common modalities used in the field are radiography and ultrasound, the complete file for any equine athlete could also include magnetic resonance imaging, nuclear bone scans, computed tomography scans, and thermal images.

In the past, the only method for sharing images was to mail radiographic films to colleagues; however, copies were rarely made to protect the original films. A more recent practice is to copy images to a CD or DVD and send the disc in the mail or by overnight express. The current standard for sharing all forms of imaging is to send a link to the sender's PACS via e-mail so the images can be downloaded into the recipient's PACS for viewing on their own workstation (www.asteris.biz).

Portable Document Format (PDF)

- PDF is an open standard that is widely used for exchanging documents. The original document used to create a PDF could come from a variety of sources including Microsoft Word or Excel (Redmond, WA, USA) or anything that is scanned. The advantage of a PDF file is that once created, a document is easily transferred, filed, or printed. Furthermore, once created the document cannot be altered from its original form.
- To read PDF documents, a free download for Adobe Reader is available from www.adobe.com (Adobe Systems Incorporated, San Jose, CA, USA).
- Many of the documents used by equine practitioners, such as consent forms and client agreement forms, can be converted into PDF and readily transmitted to clients from the field.

Many programs are available to convert documents from their original source into a PDF document. Most scanners do this automatically but occasionally a document from various sources will need to be converted into PDF. A search of the internet for PDF conversion programs will yield many choices (Docudesk.com).

Voice to Text Programs

Widely used in the human medical field, real-time speech recognition allows the veterinarian to record their findings into a recording device or laptop computer for transcription into text. The most popular version of this software for healthcare practices is Dragon Medical (Nuance.com). Although other voice recognition systems are available, Dragon Medical is recommended for use by veterinarians to recognize the necessary medical terminology.

With a laptop and a headset in the practice vehicle, invoices and medical records can be recorded by voice, converted to text, and entered into the medical records program for rapid and accurate record keeping.

Communications Programs

In the past, the conventional method of connecting the horse owner with the veterinarian was by landline telephone. The ambulatory equine veterinarian is now able to communicate with clients, colleagues, the diagnostic laboratory, equine insurance companies, and stable managers with devices such as a smartphone, tablet, or laptop computer. With various programs or apps (applications or software programs widely available from the Internet), the landline phone and fax machine are quickly becoming obsolete, in favor of wireless and cellular networks.

Listed are a few of the advances that are readily available for handling all forms of communication:

1. *Virtual phone system.* A virtual phone system allows the veterinarian to use their existing practice phone number (or a new toll-free number can be provided) to unify all forms of voice and fax communications. These services offer a nearly infinite number of choices for handling incoming calls and faxes. Calls can be immediately routed to a designated phone number (landline or cellular) or the caller can be greeted with a message allowing them to select the appropriate extension.
    ○ This service is available through several companies including Grasshopper (grasshopper.com), Ring Central (Ringcentral.com), Google Voice (www.google.com/voice), and Onebox (www.new.onebox.com).
    ○ One phone number can function for voice and fax.
    ○ Voice messages can be sent to an e-mail address for notification and some services will transcribe the voice message into text.
2. Fax–to–e-mail and e-mail–to–fax services. This service can be bundled with a virtual phone service and eliminates the need for a fax machine. It allows:
    ■ Faxes to be received as PDF files and routed to 1 or more e-mail addresses.
    ■ Lab results to be reviewed, filed, and shared without printing a copy.
    ■ Insurance forms to be printed, completed, scanned, and then returned to the insurance company using available e-mail–to–fax services.
3. E-mail programs
    ○ Web-based e-mail (Webmail) is by far the most popular form of e-mail service. The most common providers for this service include AOL, Gmail, Yahoo! and Hotmail, but many more are available. Webmail is usually a free service and offers its users most of the features associated with e-mail systems such as:
        ■ Sending digital messages to recipients
        ■ Attaching documents and images
        ■ Managing and storing contact information
        ■ Maintaining a schedule with an advanced calendar system
    ○ Exchange-based e-mail programs allow all of the options of the Web-based e-mail but the e-mail address is based on the practice Web site. For example, if your practice Web site is excellentequine.com, your e-mail address will be yourname@excellentequine.com. Although the hosted e-mail program provides an address that is specific to your practice, it is a much more technical program to maintain without professional help and may not be desirable for small practices.
    ○ Whichever type of e-mail service is chosen, managing e-mail through a software program such as Microsoft Outlook or Entourage allows the user several advantages:
        ■ Several e-mail accounts can be used without separate logins.
        ■ The program is functional when an Internet connection is not available. E-mail messages can be created or answered and they will be delivered when an Internet connection is restored.

- Contacts can be managed and synced with a mobile device.
- The calendar feature also allows for scheduling and syncing with mobile devices.
- Add-on programs to Outlook, such as Xobni, allow for easy access to all e-mail addresses that have been used in Outlook and allows for the easy retrieval of all prior e-mail messages and attachments.

4. Online file-sharing programs. These programs are an efficient way to store and share documents, photographs, and any form of digital information that would be difficult to send as an e-mail attachment. Although these online programs had a nefarious beginning when music and other digital content were inappropriately shared, many legitimate file-sharing programs are available for little or no cost. The author has used Dropbox (dropbox.com) for more than 1 a year and it has proved to be reliable and easily accessible by the selected recipient.

TECHNICAL ASSISTANCE

Integrating a fully computerized and paperless practice usually requires the assistance of a qualified computer technician to configure the necessary technology and equipment. While the services of a local technician are important, the vast majority of software installations and repair, including computer repairs, can be performed remotely with online support.

Proprietary practice management programs and image archiving programs offer extensive support that is usually provided by remote access to the practice network as well as the veterinarian's computer.

Once the practice is fully paperless, the reliability of software and hardware is essential. Although computers are more stable than in the past, the highest level of computer service contract offered provides the practitioner the most security. A high-level computer service contract would include online support, onsite service, and overnight delivery for more involved computer problems.

Although computer and software reliability is the greatest concern in digitizing every component of an ambulatory equine practice, there are several steps that mitigate this risk. In a fully digitized workplace, a catastrophic loss of all physical property related to an equine practice, including all records and computers, does not necessarily mean that any useful information will ever be lost.

First, a backup laptop computer is helpful. A second computer could also be the computer used by the veterinarian's assistant or office manager. Second, all data and software should be backed up to an external hard drive and online backup systems. This is an important component of the practice management software and a necessary component of the archiving system. All data not backed up in the archiving and practice management program can be automatically backed up online with programs such as Crash Plan, Carbonite or Mozy.

IMPLEMENTATION

Converting an ambulatory equine practice to a fully digitized workplace can begin with a few easy steps. The first step is to bring the laptop computer into the practice vehicle. This will require a laptop stand and a power source. Once the laptop is functioning in the vehicle, it will be necessary to incorporate the numerous programs that the practice already has in place.

With voice recognition software and a headset, case-by-case information can be quickly and easily entered into the laptop for eventual invoicing and medical record keeping.

If the practice is using an accounting program (such as QuickBooks) for invoicing and medical records, upgrading to the online version (QuickBooks Online) will allow access to the program wherever there is an Internet connection. Using a smartphone as a wireless hot spot, the laptop can be connected to the internet while traveling. If the ambulatory vehicle is outfitted with a digital or computed radiography system or an ultrasound machine, images from either device can be transferred to the laptop for viewing and archiving.

For the practitioner's office, a scanning device will convert paper documents into a PDF format, stored on the laptop and ultimately to an online program. This will include completed equine insurance forms, lab results, referral documents, and client agreement forms. Using a scanner to its fullest potential, the contents of conventional filing cabinets will shrink significantly.

MOVING FORWARD

One might reasonably ask, "How does a digitized practice benefit the equine veterinarian who is providing care to horses at the stable or the show grounds?" In fact, a digitized practice offers the veterinarian many advantages. A horse's history will be available during an examination. This allows the owner to play an immediate role in decision making, even if he or she is not present for the exam. For optimum accuracy, medical records and invoices are generated as the service is performed. Furthermore, all of this information is stored in remote data centers that will offer absolute security and immediate accessibility. The vast amount of information currently stored on paper in filing cabinets, and therefore inaccessible in the field, will become immediately available to the equine practitioner no matter where he or she is located.

How does this benefit the care of the horse? The accessibility and accuracy of digitized medical records and digital images can provide the caregiver with vital information about the horse's medical history much sooner than relying on paper records or conventional film. This allows the practitioner to review previous medical records, for example, in order to accurately continue previous treatments or to review previous diagnostic findings. In addition, today's horse is very mobile; a horse may be in one section of the country for a horse show one weekend and in an entirely different part of the country on the next weekend. Even when they are living in one location, several veterinarians or veterinary practices may be providing care at different times. Digitized medical records can be easily shared allowing for continuity of care, thereby reducing redundant and unnecessary treatments.

The equine practitioner who is taking full advantage of the technological opportunities available is also able to seek the advice of colleagues and specialists at the time of the examination and provide them with up-to-the-moment images and records, which further enhance the standard of care that horse owners expect.

Considering the advances in technology in the past decade, it is not difficult to see how technology will affect equine practice in the coming years. Computing devices will continue to get smaller while at the same time increasing their computing power. Internet access will be readily available in more locations including the stable. Digitized information will be not be stored exclusively on local servers and computers but in online data centers. Cloud computing will become the standard by which all information is stored and retrieved.

The equine practitioner can accomplish the lion's share of developing a fully digitized business with minimal expense. Although it is difficult to calculate the cost of converting the equine practice to a paperless workplace, it is easy to predict that the cost of technology goes down year by year. In the author's practice, the cost of maintaining a paperless practice is approximately 2% of gross revenue. However, the gains in efficiency and communication offer tangible, albeit significant, benefits toward the operation of a practice with lower fixed costs. The most significant impediment to developing a digitized practice is not so much the cost as it is the discipline necessary to regard all forms of information in an entirely new way.

Technology plays an increasingly important role in the care of the horse. The development of a fully digitized practice has been, in the author's experience, extremely gratifying. With the help of qualified technicians working remotely in Canada, Texas, Colorado, and New York, his practice's technology needs have been fully met. Clients appreciate the ability to have quick access to all aspects of their horse's health. Technology also enhances the professional fulfillment of the equine practitioner. It is no longer a matter of whether technology will be implemented into ambulatory practice; it is a question of when and how quickly.

CAPITAL INVESTMENT CONSIDERATIONS FOR EQUINE AMBULATORY PRACTICE

While numerous persuasive arguments can be advanced as to the reasons for integrating new technology into the veterinary practice, equine ambulatory practitioners are also faced with the reality that such equipment must be paid for. The decision to acquire new technology must be made with a firm grasp of the financial consequences. It does a practitioner no good to upgrade to the latest available technology if, in so doing, the practitioner is subsequently financially hamstrung by repayment obligations.

Thus, when faced with the opportunity or need to acquire a new or used piece of equipment, the tendency of practitioners may be to regard the purchase in one dimension: "it's all about the money." In fact, the purchase of new or used equipment has both emotional and financial components that should be addressed as part of the analysis and decision-making process. The most important consideration in buying a new asset is to have all of the facts and details gathered so as to better understand what this type of transaction means to the practice owner. Investigating the true cost of equipment is a question of balancing the veterinarian's intellect, on the business side, with the passion to acquire "toys," on the personal side. It is easy to get caught in the trap of the latest-and-greatest-I-gotta-have-it-to-succeed-as-a-veterinarian equipment purchase dilemma. Veterinarians are tempted by what other practices are doing and by the equipment featured in journals and displayed at trade shows. Ultimately the decision to buy or not to buy comes down to a simple question of what the practice owner "needs" versus what he or she "wants."

Capital investments include many purchased items (assets) including the laptop in the ambulatory vehicle, the vehicle itself, and the diagnostic equipment necessary to provide care for horses. The analysis process is the same for a solo ambulatory practitioner as it is for a larger ambulatory practice with multiple veterinarians, but the decision to invest may be different.

Equine practitioners have a propensity for buying new, shiny objects or toys that is driven by a passion to have the best tools available to help horses. The purchasing decision often does not include an analysis of core business principles when it is time to actually spend the money. Using the example of purchasing diagnostic equipment, this article will apply accepted business strategies to assist in the decision-making process for making sizable equipment investments. At the end of this article is information for worksheet resources accessible via an Internet link. This Web site provides access to templates and easy-to-understand examples to assist in the decision-making process. Getting a handle on how to approach this process is just as

> **Box 1**
> **Practice scenario**
>
> The neighboring practitioner down the road just purchased an awesome, state-of-the-art DR system. The practice's x-ray system is an older plain film system. Both systems produce quality diagnostic images with one major difference—the DR system allows the user to immediately process the image onsite, whereas the plain film technology requires the practitioner to return to the office to process and view the images. A few clients have commented on this new DR system, stating that they wished the practice had one so they did not have to pay another call fee to treat the horse after the images were viewed. The clients were very impressed to see the pictures right away because it allowed the vet to diagnosis the problem and treat the hocks on the spot.

important as plugging the numbers into a spreadsheet and finding a numeric answer. Numbers are best interpreted if the user fully understands the methodology used to create the information that helps equine practitioners arrive at a sound business management decision.

CAPITAL INVESTMENT CONSIDERATIONS
The Value of Money

Today's dollar does not have the same purchasing value that it had 20 years ago, nor will it have the same purchasing ability 20 years from now. Many factors affect the value of currency and the purchasing power of the dollar. The term *net present value* is a calculation that forecasts financial decisions and provides a better understanding of the true cost of money. This calculation helps determine whether buying a new ultrasound or digital radiography (DR) system is a good deal. In most cases, the value of money decreases over time. For example, the purchasing power of $10.00 in 1991 has a relative value of $16.00 in 2011 (this value is obtained by multiplying the $10.00 by the percentage increase in the Consumer Price Index [CPI] from 1991 to 2010). During the investigation of a purchase decision, the changes in monetary value or purchasing power need to be taken into consideration in the overall analysis.

The Analysis

The analysis begins with an assessment of the goals of the practice. What are the short-term and long-term growth strategies? Does purchasing a new ultrasound unit or radiography system make sense considering where the practice is today, and also considering the practice owner's goals? Simply put, is the capital purchase "want" in alignment with the practice's "needs?" An investigation of 4 important influences, along with a real-life scenario, will help answer these questions (**Box 1**).

Marketing and competitive forces

The example in **Box 1** illustrates many of the marketing pressures and emotions that enter the picture with new technology and services. The horse owner expects, and even demands, immediate answers. Will the equine practitioner lose market share (clients) because he or she is not able to give an immediate answer? The DR system might be very desirable but is it truly necessary and is it a smart business decision? The numbers will tell the financial story, but the client should also be considered in the decision making process. The client's buying or purchasing behavior is complicated and differs by geographic location. Knowing what is important to the customer is just as important as the financial analysis when projecting future sales.

Projections

Detailed analysis of the projected costs (not just the purchase price) and revenue growth (current and new potential sales) is at the heart of all purchase decisions. This is described in more detail below and best understood using worksheet templates to analyze each individual purchase.

Costs are defined as the expenses associated with the activity of performing a service such as taking radiographs. This includes the cost of the equipment, the financing costs, labor, disposable items, and more. Some of these expenses are *variable costs*, that is, costs that change in proportion to the activity or behavior of the service. For example, the number of views taken with a new DR system along with the time, assistant help, veterinary compensation, and wear and tear are variable costs built into using this new equipment. *Fixed costs* are incurred whether or not the equipment is used to generate revenue. Examples of fixed costs include acquisition costs of the equipment, service contracts, insurance taxes, and support. The *contribution margin* is the marginal profit per unit of sale and plays a role in the overall cost to the practice. There are many hidden costs to consider in the final analysis.

Growth is a business goal to increase revenue and profitability using the new diagnostic equipment. Pricing and volume are the 2 major contributing factors to revenue growth. While assessing the pricing structure and projections of future growth for a specific service like DR, the financial impact will become clearer. What is left at the end of the day, the "net" profit, is really the key driver in the decision process. Another consideration is the marketing costs to make clients aware of the new diagnostic capabilities.

To determine the value of an expensive asset, an analysis of projected usage and expense allocation, otherwise referred to as *activity-based cost analysis,* will assist the practice owner in understanding the value of purchasing an expensive piece of equipment such as a DR system. This type of analysis also provides valuable information on ways to improve efficiency and profitability.

Breakeven is a calculation to examine the unique, practice-specific breakeven point in the analysis of a particular service. The breakeven analysis considers all expenses and all potential revenue changes in the calculation of how long it will take to pay off the initial investment. Several methods are available to calculate this estimated time frame—examples are available in the resource area at the end of this article. A word of caution, however; sales representatives will create this analysis without truly understanding the unique attributes of a practice or the true cost of doing business. In most businesses, the breakeven timeline is less than 2 years on a capital investment in diagnostic equipment.

Several important questions will need to be answered before making the final decision. What is the goal for paying off the equipment and how long will that equipment last before it must be replaced? Is there a significant annual cost to maintain or service the purchase? These questions and more will help to make an informed decision on a new purchase.

Financing

Whether paying cash for the new DR system, financing it as a loan with a bank or leasing it from another vendor; the purchasing decision affects available cash (*cash flow*) and the cost of money in the purchase analysis. Tax planning should also play a role in how the asset is financed. The practice owner is advised to contact their tax advisor to strategically expense this new purchase in a manner that makes sense for tax purposes. Tax rules changes may have a significant impact on net profit at the end of the year.

Service attributes

It is exciting to buy a new DR, but how does it affect profitability for a service that is already offered? Some capital investments are made to offer completely new services to clients; other investments do not afford dramatically different services than those that are already provided. The DR versus plain film dilemma is a great example of the cost of doing business to maintain high-quality services and add new service attributes. It sounds great, but it comes at a cost. The practice's current system is probably paid off and the true profit from that service is high. The practice will increase expenses by buying a new machine (new costs), which will reduce profit on the bottom line. The profit per radiographic view may be reduced by several dollars per shot. By multiplying that difference by the volume of radiographs taken, the effect on profitability can be quantified. Will the volume of this service increase enough to offset the profit loss? Can the marketplace accept a fee increase per view taken to offset this net loss? The cost may be too much or it may be of great value depending on pricing and volume changes. It is crucial that the profitability of current services is compared to the same services with a new piece of equipment.

There are also intangible factors to consider when making an asset purchase such as a DR system. Though it should never drive the entire decision making process when acquiring a new piece of equipment, take in to consideration the brand image to the practice and what this acquisition will mean to the clients. When communicating the decision to purchase (or not purchase) new technology to the practice's clients, it is important that they understand the difficulty of providing the best diagnostic capabilities while also keeping the costs of services as low as possible. At best, it is difficult to accurately predict client behavior but it is wise to carefully consider the proper response to questions that might arise. Clients are quick to wonder what this purchase might do to their "bottom line" as well! Their perception is their reality.

Warranty, Service Contracts, and Insurance

The excitement generated by the consideration of a new purchase may quickly dissipate when discussing the warranty and service contracts with the salesperson. It is common for the warranty and service coverage portion of the contract to be in small print, full of legal jargon, and difficult to interpret. What must be remembered is that there is a cost of ownership. It is therefore important to think about the following when considering the service contract: down time, insurance, periodic maintenance, software updates, future enhancements, coverage details (labor, parts, shipping, preventive maintenance), service loaner policy, and warranty value. All of these factors play a role in the ability to generate revenue while using the machine and the expenses that are incurred when the machine is out of service. In addition, these aspects of asset investment affect the residual value of the asset and the fair market value when the used equipment is sold. In the end, it comes down to a cost versus benefit assessment and the willingness to accept a level of risk. Prior to signing on the dotted line, it is up to the buyer to be fully aware. Dig into the details and incorporate these costs in the analysis of purchase, including cost estimates once the service contracts expire or are renewed. The time to negotiate a better deal or an extended warranty is as a buyer not as an owner.

Negotiation

Retail price, wholesale price, discounts, rebates, service, warranty options, and support all play a role in the eventual cost for a piece of equipment or an automobile. Negotiation is an art and there are many tools to learn to get the best overall deal. To gain a greater understanding of the art of negotiation, it may be advisable to enroll in a negotiation training seminar at a local business school. The investment in this training will pay for itself time and time again. The goal in negotiations is to understand both sides of the equation: what are the seller's needs and wants, what does the buyer need and want from this activity? It might even be necessary to walk away from the deal if a reasonable balance cannot be made between the needs of the seller and the buyer. Identifying the details and facts that surround each buying decision based on product information and services enables the practice owner to be more informed when it comes down to final pricing, delayed billing options, and trade-in value. Ethical negotiation training is one more tool to advance the business career of the equine veterinarian.

SUMMARY

Purchasing new or used capital assets involves both emotional and financial components in the decision making process. In addition, there are intangible factors such as client perceptions and expectations that fit into the equation. Identify the facts from a business perspective and then define whether this investment (expense) is good for the practice and fits with the short- and long-term growth strategies. Ask the tough questions, analyze the numbers, understand the clients' needs, and tie this together with the practice brand and strategic objectives. The informed and prepared buyer is usually successful in making the right decision.

QUESTIONS TO CONSIDER

Divide a blank paper into 2 columns and on one side write down the "pros" and the other side the "cons" before making a major capital investment. Scan this paper and look at both the big picture and details for your business. Another exercise to do is to ask questions like the group below before signing on the dotted line:

- Do you "want" it or do you "need it?"
- Is this purchase part of my strategic business plan?
- Will the cost be paid for in 2 years? Is a longer payoff okay?
- Will this investment increase my "net" profitability now, later, or not at all?
- Am I losing clients because of a lack of proper equipment?
- What will price of the service after the purchase? Can it be increased?
- What type of volume change do I expect in the next 12 to 24 months?
- Is the money I tie up in the new purchase better spent somewhere else in the company?
- How long will this asset serve the business?
- What types of costs are involved on an annual basis?
- Will this purchase significantly increase my insurance costs?
- What type of risks am I willing to take with regard to service and down time?
- How will I tell my customers about this new service?
- How will this purchase affect associate compensation?
- Can I negotiate a better overall structure to the purchase?
- What is my walk away number for this deal?

RESOURCES: ANALYSIS TEMPLATES AND EXAMPLES

Templates for equipment and ambulatory vehicle analysis are available on the resource page of the Web site www.equinebusinessmanagement.com to help gather all the facts and analyze the numbers for potential capital investments for an equine ambulatory practice. These are designed to be modified to suit the individual needs of each practice. It's a great place to start the process of being more informed when making a sizable capital investment.

DEFINITIONS

Activity based cost analysis—method of allocating or assigning the costs to a specific service activity or product to ascertain the value or profitability for the activity.

Assets and equity—assets are any resource tangible (like equipment, vehicles, cash, etc. . .) or intangible (goodwill, blue sky, reputation) that is owned or controlled to produce value. Equity is the claim by an owner on those assets.

Capital investment—financial contribution in an asset with the expectation of a gain.

Cash flow—flow of money in and out of a practice during a specified period of time.

Contribution margin—portion of revenue (sales) that contributes to the offset of fixed costs.

Deductions—tax deductions are variable tax dollars that are subtracted from your gross income based on local and federal tax rules.

Depreciation—decrease in the perceived value of an asset based on initial cost that is recognized as an expense by businesses for financial reporting and tax purposes. This is a non-cash activity, rather an accounting entry for reporting.

Fixed costs—expenses that are not dependent on the goods and services produced by the practice or business.

Goodwill—intangible asset defined as the difference the purchase price and the fair market value of the net assets of a business. Common considerations include the value of the business reputation or brand equity that are part of the value over and above the identifiable business assets.

Net present value (NPV)—calculation of the sequence of cash flows taking into consideration purchase price, future cash flows, and rate of return (discount rate). The calculation is represented below:

$$\text{NPV} = \frac{R_t}{(1 + i)^t}$$

t = the time of the cash flow
i = the discount rate
Rt = the net cash flow at time

Variable costs—expenses that change in proportion with the level of activity for services and products produced by the practice or business.

Walk away number—point in negotiations where either the price or the benefits of the deal are not beneficial to the company. This is an objective assessment defined before negotiations on purchasing an asset begin to enable the buyer to reduce the emotional impulse to buy unfavorable terms.

Do You Know Your Equine Practice Clients?

Philippe Moreau, DVM, MS

KEYWORDS

- Equine practice • Equine veterinarian • Clients
- Expectation • Management • Client satisfaction

In the language of practice management, horse owners are clients. Skills in the art and science of equine medicine are only one way that clients evaluate their equine ambulatory veterinarian. Many other factors besides the practice of veterinary medicine are important for a veterinarian to be perceived as having done a good job and to be rewarded with client loyalty.

What is it that clients expect from the veterinarian, and how can he or she meet and exceed these expectations? How should the veterinarian organize the practice, run a clinic, and work—alone or as a team—to satisfy the clients? How does a veterinarian learn to communicate with these clients, and with staff? How do veterinarians obtain a sufficient degree of client loyalty? A veterinarian should always be prepared to answer these questions, and keep in mind that while one could be the best veterinarian, if one is not in phase with some elementary aspects related to a client's needs and expectations, the chances are that the veterinarian will not be successful. Success, in terms of communicating with owners, leads to improved compliance but also leads to client loyalty. All these crucial features also influence job satisfaction from the veterinary health team and ultimately will also impact the financial results of the veterinary enterprise.

VALUE

When dealing with horses, as is the case with companion animals, in addition to the actual medical problem, veterinarians are often dealing with emotions and affection. Horse owners are, for the most part, passionate and often highly demanding when it comes to horse care. People refer to the "sentimental value" of the animal; as a consequence, there may be no limitation to the cost of the care that horse owners are willing to provide. For example, some horse owners will keep a horse in a field, all expenses included, even when the animal can no longer be used for riding.

As is often the case with any profession, background, education, and culture all influence professional behavior. This includes the attitude of some veterinarians when

The author has nothing to disclose.
Medi-Productions, SAS, 5, rue Sainte Claire, 87000 Limoges, France
E-mail address: pmoreau@mediproductions.com

Vet Clin Equine 28 (2012) 39–49
doi:10.1016/j.cveq.2012.01.006
0749-0739/12/$ – see front matter © 2012 Published by Elsevier Inc.

facing the cost of care. Some veterinarians may look at the animal's "market value," as opposed to the "sentimental value," and therefore advise their clients that a treatment may not be justified. Under such circumstances, some practitioners might suggest that euthanasia should be considered because the expense of treatment is not "worth the economical value of the animal," and particularly in difficult economic times.

The horse, however, once merely a working animal, is now also a sport animal and considered by many as a "companion animal." As such, advice based on the economic value of an animal is often not what the clients are expecting! Some veterinarians may not be mentally prepared to make medical recommendations based on economics, because it was not part of their culture, their background, their education, and even their initial motivation when they joined the profession. On the other hand, a veterinarian's different personal philosophy and background (eg, being raised with horses as stock animals in agricultural production) may be partially responsible for a completely different attitude. Under any circumstances, it is important to explain to the owner the realities of the case (ie, the chances of a cure, subsequent life expectancy, ongoing pain, the cost of medical care, etc) and then let him or her decide how to proceed. Deciding for the client may not work well in many circumstances.

MANAGEMENT OF THE PRACTICE

In the current, more selective, and challenging professional environment, veterinarians have started to look closely at the management and marketing of their practices, clinics, and hospitals. The era when veterinarians were financially successful from day one, simply by placing their name and title on their door, no longer exists. Today, competition is stronger and the number of veterinarians is increasing, even as the total number of animals is stationary in most countries. However, farm animal veterinary activities have dropped significantly; decrease in horse ownership is a well-documented fact in the United States.

Owners, breeders, and trainers are now well educated and expect high-quality service, for horses as well as small animal pets. In this consumer environment, client pressure and demand for better quality and more efficient services have increased the pressure on veterinarians to comply with their needs, as well as those of their animals. Competition from other veterinarians and, possibly more significant, from other professions working with animals is another reason why veterinarians must excel in their professional veterinary services, not only in their execution but also in their delivery.

To practice veterinary medicine today, it is no longer sufficient to be only a good clinician and surgeon. It could even be said that it is more important that the veterinarian be a good administrator, a good communicator, and a person who is always available, concerned at all times with the patients' needs and the owners' requests. This new and additional "science of communication" is often not covered in the veterinary school curriculum. It is, however, a true science based on technical knowledge and theory, and one for which numerous practical examples and applications exist. In this new competitive veterinary market, the use of good practice management and proper veterinary marketing techniques allows veterinarians to develop their business and become successful entrepreneurs. As such, one can affirm that *good practice management is good veterinary medicine.*

Effective practice skills for the equine ambulatory practitioner are concerned with adapting methods to better fit the new environment of the future and making daily work a more profitable venture for all: the veterinarians, the veterinary profession, and

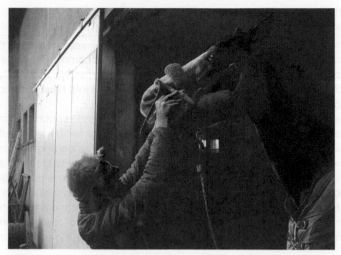

Fig. 1. Ambulatory veterinarians are expected to offer a wide range of services, including radiography.

the clients and their animals. Practice management is no longer the "icing on the cake"; it is an essential ingredient in a recipe for success! Today veterinarians are running small businesses and need to be aware and knowledgeable about the management aspects of the profession in order to succeed.

A FULL SERVICE ENVIRONMENT

Veterinary practices offer both medical services and also product sales (**Fig. 1**). While the latter have been mainly medications, the past 20 years has seen the development of paramedical product sales by veterinary practices. The development of preventative medicine, no longer limited to vaccinations and deworming, is a key element of the modern veterinary profession. Veterinarians are no longer limited to the care of the sick and injured animal, but they are actively involved in the management of the healthy animal. Some now refer to "wellness" medicine as an additional component to complete care, as opposed to its longstanding counterpart, "illness" medicine, whereby practitioners respond to examine sick animals; a good example of this concept is the sending of reminders for the annual medical check-ups.

Today, clients "consume" the services and products of veterinary practices, and therefore react with a consumer's attitude. They compare prices. They want full service. They like a "one-stop shop." They attach importance to the value of the services, which should not be confused with the cost of the services. They look for convenience and for treatments that are easy to administer. They are also concerned about protection of the environment and safety of the products they buy and use, and of possible unwanted effects on their family, themselves, and other animals. Finally, they want "peace of mind" and rely on the veterinarians to prevent problems with their animal(s) and to reassure them about their animal's well-being. It is important to keep these general expectations in mind when offering to manage and check on a healthy animal.

CLIENTS: WHO ARE THEY AND WHAT DO THEY EXPECT?
Who Are the Clients?

Clients of modern practices are mobile and choose their veterinarian on the basis of their personal circumstances and preferences. In smaller communities, the majority of a veterinarian's clients may come from the local community, especially when the practice is the only one in the area, but in most cases clients have a choice and take advantage of it.

A clientele develops over time, based on the image and reputation that the clinic has with the clients. This is a long-term process and cannot be changed overnight. The modern client base is characterized by factors such as demographics, lifestyles, (higher) expectations, more vocal attitude, being more knowledgeable, and placing great attention to personal experience. A veterinarian's clientele is ultimately based on the total package of services provided and products sold, as well as the location of the clinic (if there is one), the operating hours, and the culture and atmosphere created by the veterinarian and staff. While price might be a reason for clients to prefer certain practices, in general, quality of care (perceived value) is far more important than the price.

Who Is My Veterinarian?

How do clients choose their veterinarian? Location, visibility (both of the premises as well as in the media), and word of mouth are the key drivers for the first visit. The next important criterion is the initial and overall impression made during the first visit. It's been said that, "Clients do not care how much you know, until they know how much you care." As such, the ambulatory clinician or clinic staff have to communicate the message that they care about a client and the client's horses. Knowledge and skills alone are not sufficient to be successful (**Fig. 2**). Care is communicated by everything the clinician or clinic does and does not do, including the design of the building (eg, in a mixed practice, separate pet and horse areas). Other ways to communicate or "market" the services and care would include communication tools such as practice

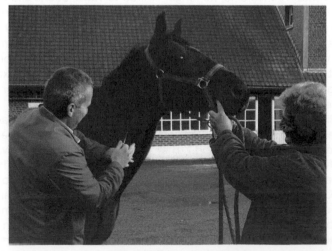

Fig. 2. Careful palpation skills may be essential to good diagnosis, but are not the primary means by which clients select their veterinarian.

brochures, leaflets, digital signage, practice website, and presence on social networks such as Facebook and Twitter.

The most important demonstration of caring is in the attitude of the veterinarian(s) and staff. Good client relations are achieved by showing kindness and demonstrating active listening skills, genuine personal interest, and empathy. When the veterinarian and staff are able to impress the horse owners with care to a level exceeding the clients' expectations, the likelihood that they will come back and become loyal clients is much increased. When the perceived value provided by the practice during the visit exceeds the expected value, the client will be satisfied. Satisfied happy clients play a very important role in generating new business. It has been proved over and over again that unhappy clients tell more than 10 others about their negative experience, whereas happy clients only tell an average of 3 others. Positive recommendations are a very powerful driver of new business.

CLIENT EXPECTATIONS

Clients typically have high expectations. However, in the word "expected" one can perceive the possibility of dissatisfaction if an expectation is not, or is no longer, fulfilled. In other words, clients may be initially impressed because a service was beyond their expectations, but the ongoing challenge is that once the bar is raised, this level of service must be sustained on subsequent visits. A lower standard will no longer be tolerated. For example, it was not long ago that when one called a veterinary clinic, or any other consumer service–oriented business, one received a typical welcome such as, "Good morning!" Today a more appropriate welcome would be something like this; "Welcome to the Upson Downs Equine Clinic, Jenny speaking. How may I help you?" It has even reached the point that when people do not receive this type of personal greeting, they wonder if they have dialed the wrong number!

There are several kinds of expectations. Those that are expressed are called "explicit" expectations. Those that are not expressed by the customers are called "implicit" expectations. It is quite important to know what a client's implicit expectations are since, by definition, these will not be mentioned by them. A perfect example is the fact that (almost without exception) people expect the personnel and staff in a veterinary clinic to have a "professional appearance" (white or a medical style of clothes). If that is not the case, people may be surprised or even upset. They will not mention it because the expectation is implicit for them, but they will be disappointed nonetheless. Veterinarians need to have a good understanding of these types of expectations.

Some other classic consumers' implicit expectations include:

- *Availability:* prompt service, flexible hours, easy access and parking to a facility (if available), sufficient stock, etc
- *Transparency:* prices should be clearly labeled, invoices should be itemized, etc
- Choice: various products & services, "freedom of choice," etc.
- *Environment:* facilities should be comfortable, neat, clean, odorless, friendly, modern, etc. Practice vehicles should be clean and well-organized.
- *Clarity of the offer:* prices should be detailed, estimates accurate, badges should identify personnel, etc
- *Services:* services offered should be adapted to various owners' needs.

Clients cannot easily judge the level of medical and surgical care a veterinarian gives, but they can and do judge the level of service they receive (read: perceive). In the clients' eyes, the level of service that a client receives is the only major factor that

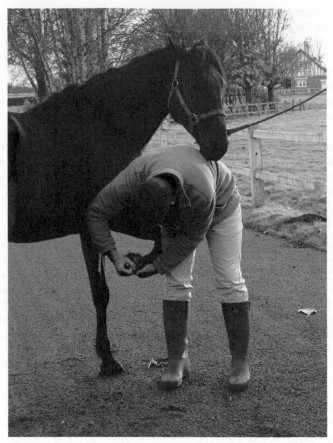

Fig. 3. The skill and kindness with which a veterinarian gives an injection may help reinforce his or her expertise in the eyes of the client.

distinguishes a veterinarian, and makes the veterinarian unique from other practices. Striving for excellence in client services is therefore essential.

Surveys have shown that *what clients are looking for in a veterinarian*, in order of importance are:

1. Kindness (**Fig. 3**)
2. Availability
3. Capacity to listen
4. Competency.

Clients rank competency only after these initial basic abilities! Why does competency only rank in fourth position? Simply because all veterinarians have the same diploma and, therefore (in the clients' eyes), all have the same level of competency to treat their horse's common medical problems. People react the same way in dealing with their family doctors. While the situation is somewhat different when dealing with specialists, and, in such a situation the lack of "client orientation" will usually be somewhat tolerated, competition is also present among specialists and, at the end, clients will choose those who also fulfill the basic client needs.

A survey conducted by the American Veterinary Medical Association (AVMA) revealed the factors that influenced people's choice in selecting their small animal veterinarian:

- Proximity (65%)
- Recommendation (42%)
- Prices (39%)
- Hours and availability (31%)
- Road signs (7%)
- Others.

What is quite remarkable in this study is the fact that while proximity is the major factor, recommendation also has a very strong influence. Veterinarians tend to believe that pricing is always a sensitive issue in whatever part of the world they work. However, one should also take note of the paramount importance of "recommendation." This is a veterinarian's best marketing tool. Everyone knows that there are good and bad recommendations. Both are very powerful.

CLIENT SATISFACTION

Client satisfaction does not follow mathematical rules. It is associated with emotions, perception, and personal opinion. An individual horse owner's priority is to have "peace of mind," live a happy life with their animal, and avoid "problems." Even large breeding, racing, or training operations may have the same concerns. Therefore, veterinarians and their staff should focus on and attempt to ensure client satisfaction as the number one priority. This is also why preventive medicine, along with nutrition advice and wellness plans, is very important (**Fig. 4**). Veterinarians should not only be involved with medical and surgical procedures to treat the sick and the injured animal; they should also see well patients, and focus on keeping them that way.

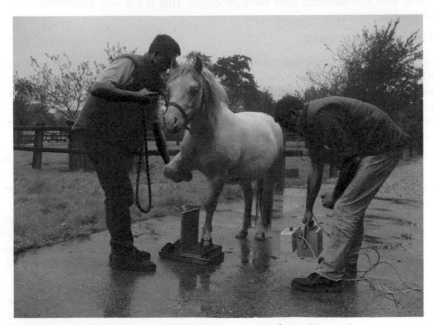

Fig. 4. Regular oral examinations are an important part of a wellness plan.

Satisfaction in the veterinary practice among clients follows a bell-shaped curve. Most veterinarians can report from personal experience that some clients were unhappy, are unhappy, and will always be unhappy. Nothing can go right with these people; they can be classified as "unreasonably unhappy." For these clients, everything the veterinarian does is wrong. The good news is that the practice also has a group of "unreasonably happy" clients. Whatever the veterinarian does, these clients are fans, and will always be fans, and remain loyal to the veterinarian and to the clinic. While everybody needs a "fan club," the input from unreasonably happy clients does not provide direction and should be enjoyed but not taken more seriously than the comments by "unreasonably unhappy" clients. Of more importance is to identify the median satisfaction level for the products and services provided by the practice. Otherwise stated: What is the perception of the majority of a veterinarian's clients?

Attention to client satisfaction can help maintain a more stable, satisfied client base. Satisfaction is often a measure of the client's perception of quality. The highly satisfied client will feel he or she has received a high-quality service, whereas the dissatisfied client will be disappointed by the (perceived) lack of quality of service. Client service is the ability to meet client requirements and to exceed their expectations. Services are "experienced" by the client, and veterinarians, as service providers, should be as concerned in managing the client's experience as they are in providing technical expertise.

The first law of services concept, as summarized by Wyckoff and Maister in their 1984 book, *The Laws of Service Businesses*, is: *Satisfaction = Perception − Expectation.* In other words, if the client perceives services as better than expected, the client will be satisfied, and the experience will be positive. If perception is greater than expectation, satisfaction will always be the end result; the greater the gap, the higher is the level of satisfaction. This is, in fact, the way all consumers analyze the services that are provided to them. The aim of an ambulatory practitioner, or veterinary team, should be that every client who comes to the practice goes away satisfied with the services they have received. This is the way veterinarians should build their businesses.

IN TOUCH WITH CLIENTS

For a practitioner and practice to understand the existing clientele, and to service their needs optimally and develop new services, it is important to be in touch with them. Obviously it is important to read the literature and observe trends in the markets at home and abroad, but the best way to know what clients want and how they would react to new initiatives is to ask them and to test them using a selected group of clients. There are different ways to do this. Each way comes with advantages and disadvantages:

1. The veterinarian (or another staff member) can ask individual clients ad hoc during a consultation.
2. The veterinarian can install an "input box" (a real one in the clinic and/or a virtual one on your web site) and invite and encourage people to use this.
3. The veterinarian can hand out a survey to all clients visiting the hospital during a certain time period, or throughout the year on a fixed day of the week or month.
4. The veterinarian can create a client panel of trusted owners and meet with them to obtain ideas, comments, and feedback on existing procedures and programs as well as on new initiatives.

Client feedback should be part of the regular strategic planning and evaluation processes. For example, clients can be invited to join a "focus group" and be confronted with ideas and asked for feedback. These groups can even be conducted by outside professionals, in order to avoid personal bias. Finally, clients can be part of a "representative" group of owners who are part of the practice management and meet regularly with the veterinarian and/or practice staff to discuss customer-related issues. Creating an atmosphere in which staff also informs the veterinarian of information they have actively received or passively picked up (conversation in the reception and waiting area) also guarantees valuable input. Clients often share comments and opinion with the support staff that they do not communicate to veterinarians.

Special attention should be given to those loyal customers who bring in the bulk of the business. A rule of thumb is that for any business, a minority of good clients (25%) bring in the majority of the business (up to 80%). These numbers might not be fully applicable to veterinary practices—according to recent studies, it may be more like 45% to 50%—but the general principle that a minority bring in most of the revenue holds true. Obviously this group is of utmost importance to the practice. They deserve special attention and should be treated as VIPs.

Existing clients can also help to convince potential clients of the good value of the services provided by sharing their experience. A veterinary practice that provides top of the market, highly priced diagnostic and surgical procedures may consider asking some satisfied clients if they will consider sharing their feelings of satisfaction and act as "experts-by-experience," sharing testimonials on the website and answering questions from concerned new owners. Quality training of these ambassadors by the staff is essential to turn this project into a success.

HOW TO CREATE A LOYAL CLIENT BASE?

Celebrity veterinarian Dr Marty Becker has stated: "In the face of unprecedented competition veterinarians and their teams must fight back with better skills, increased attention to detail, and a commitment to exceed client expectations." Loyal clients are those horse owners who, when they think of animal health, products, care, service, and advice, think of "their veterinarian" and not any other provider (pharmacist, drugstore, supermarket, pet or feed store, horse trainer, etc). There will always be people who will use other sources for certain services and products; this is normal. However, in modern society, people's time is so valuable that many customers are looking for a one-stop purchase (no need to travel somewhere else to get quality reliable food or insect repellent). Also, clients are often looking for specialized and customized services and high-quality products. This is again the reason why they select premium products and services provided by a health care professional (ie, by their family veterinarian). This is also a fundamental principle basis for establishing a loyal and faithful clientele. The ideal clientele will use the practice services not only for the sick and injured horse but even more so for the healthy one. A new word, "wellness," has been added to the veterinarian's dictionary to cover this all-inclusive concept.

To establish loyal clients, veterinarians and their teams need to do everything that is required to make people happy and to incite them to call the veterinarian as frequently possible. This requires more than matching client expectations. It requires exceeding client expectations.

The AVMA-KPMG survey on the future of veterinary medicine has shown that the loyal client of a veterinary practice visits the clinic about 2.8 times and spends about $144 each year (excluding food). Loyalty certainly has a direct economic impact, but it also has an emotional one since it is rewarding and motivating to work with clients who follow your suggestions. This is an important reward in our busy work life. The statement by Walt Disney—"We will do what we do so well, that the people who see it will want to see it again, and bring their friends"—is an excellent way to summarize what veterinarians should achieve when creating a loyal client base.

CLIENT COMPLAINTS

Perhaps equally as important as cultivating a loyal client base is understanding reasons why clients may complain. By understanding why clients complain, veterinarians can attempt to avoid conflicts, and thereby build a more satisfied client base. Some of the common complaints from clients that are visiting veterinarians are:

- Long waiting time
- Delayed appointments
- Too much information
- Not enough information
- Veterinarians and staff in a hurry
- Lack of listening
- Dirty premises
- Unpleasant and unfriendly staff
- Lack of concern and compassion
- Roughness and brutality with their animal
- Lack of courtesy
- Giving back a dirty or smelly animal if the horse has been hospitalized
- Not knowing the animal's name or sex
- Failure to take care of an emergency immediately
- Ignoring a client's concerns.

Addressing most of these factors requires little more than awareness and attention to detail. Veterinarians who address these issues *before* they become client concerns are more likely to be rewarded with a loyal clientele.

REFERRING CLIENTS

Clients are well aware and happy to accept the principle of referral. The fact that not all services are available in the first-line clinic and that the general practitioner (GP) veterinarian occasionally advises clients to consult a specialist are not limitations to the ambulatory veterinarian; on the contrary, these are well appreciated. People understand the referral process from their experience in human medicine and appreciate the fact that their veterinarian refers cases where he or she knows that better care will be available from a specialty hospital. Referral is not perceived by the owner as poor quality veterinary care; rather, it is highly appreciated when the veterinarian indicates the limits of general practice compared with the specialist facilities. In the referral clinic, a team of specialists (including board-certified diplomates of various specialist colleges in the United States and/or Europe) and their staff will make sure the best diagnostic and therapeutic health care is suggested and given to the owner whose horse needs specialist care. Surveys have shown that owners indicate that they want, and many can afford specialist-level equine health care when it is needed. There is generally little reason for concern from loss of business due to referral; after providing treatments, the specialist usually informs the referring veterinarian of any necessary follow-up treatment and this postreferral care, together with future every day and preventive health care (so-called first-line or basic care) continues to be maintained by the referring veterinarian. As such, there should be no competition between the 2 levels of veterinary care (generalist and specialist); rather, they are complementary and together provide a synergy of optimal care. This cooperation is exactly what most clients expect from the veterinary profession.

SUMMARY

A healthy group of loyal clients is of the utmost importance for a healthy practice. Knowing the clients' expectations and making every effort to exceed them when clients meet with the veterinarian or visit the clinic will result in continued client satisfaction. Clients will show loyalty to a veterinarian when they perceive that the care provided to them suits them and their animal and exceeds their expectations.

ADDITIONAL READING

- Bailey R (1995). *How to Empower People at Work.* Management Books 2000 Ltd (UK). ISBN 10: 1-852-52235-6; ISBN 13: 978-1-85252-235-3
- Bower J, Gripper J, Gripper P, Gunn D (2001). *Veterinary Practice Management* (3rd edition). Wiley-Blackwell ISBN 10: 0-632-05745-9; ISBN 13: 978-0-63205-745-0
- Covey SR (2004). *The 8th Habit: From Effectiveness to Greatness.* Free Press, New York. ISBN 10: 0-743-28793-2; ISBN 13: 978-0-74328-793-7
- Jevring-Bäck C and Bäck E (2006). *Managing a Veterinary Practice* (2nd edition). Saunders Elsevier. ISBN 10: 0-702-02820-7; ISBN 13: 978-0-70202-820-5
- Kaplan L and Kovan TR (2006). *The Power of Nice: How to Conquer the Business World with Kindness.* Broadway Business. ISBN 10: 0-385-51892-7; ISBN 13: 978-0-38551-892-5
- Lee DE, editor (2006). *Veterinary Clinics of North America, Small Animal Practice.* 36(2): Saunders Elsevier, Philadelphia. ISBN 10: 1-4160-3582-6; ISBN 13: 978-1-41603-582-4/ISSN 0195-5616
- Mercader P (2011). *Management Solutions for Veterinary Practices.* Grupo Asis Biomedia, S.L. editors. ISBN 978-84-92569-58-8
- Moreau P and Nap R (2010). *Essentials of Veterinary Practice: an introduction to the science of practice management.* Henston editors. ISBN: 978-1-85054-159-2
- Shilcock M and Stutchfield G (2008). *Veterinary Practice Management: A Practical Guide* (2nd edition). Saunders Elsevier. ISBN 10: 0-702-02920-3; ISBN 13: 978-0-70202-920-2
- Wayner CJ and Heinke ML (2006). Compliance: Crafting Quality Care. In: Lee DE (ed), *Veterinary Clinics of North America, Small Animal Practice.* 36 (2): 419-436.

USEFUL RELATED WEBSITES

AAHA (2003). The path to high quality care compliance. Compliance: taking quality care to the next level/Executive summary:
www.aahanet.org/protected/ComplianceExecutiveSummary0309.pdf

Australian Veterinary Practice Management Association
www.avpma.com.au

AVMA KPMG survey on the future of veterinary medicine
www.avma.org/reference/mega715c.pdf

Stephen Covey
www.stephencovey.com

Mission to Learn
www.missiontolearn.com

Veterinary Business Management Association
www.vbma.biz

Veterinary Hospital Managers Association
www.vhma.org

Veterinary Practice Management Association
www.vpma.co.uk

Ambulatory Medicine in Equine Practice

Susan S. Gillen, DVM

KEYWORDS

- Equine medicine • Colic • Respiratory disease
- Physical examination • Esophageal obstruction
- Medical disorders • Toxicosis • Liver • Kidney
- Neurologic • Enterocentesis • Enteral fluids

The diagnosis and treatment of equine medical disorders in the field can present exceptional challenges to the ambulatory practitioner. While medical conditions themselves may present their own challenges, the situations that the equine ambulatory practitioner may find himself or herself in are often chaotic and unpredictable. Field conditions vary greatly, and instead of a controlled and sterile clinic environment, the equine ambulatory practitioner may find himself or herself treating a sick horse in less than ideal circumstances (eg, in someone's backyard, in the middle of the night, illuminated by flashlight, and in the pouring rain). Add to these factors a lack of readily available and trained personnel and a sometimes hysterical owner, it is no wonder that some veterinarians may be leery of ambulatory practice.

Nevertheless, there is a definite need for ambulatory veterinarians who practice good medicine. Many horses, especially in rural areas, will never see the inside of an equine veterinary hospital for a variety of reasons, including (1) a lack of available hospital facilities, (2) the owner's inability to transport the horse to a hospital for treatment, and/or (3) the cost of hospitalization. However, these owners may be willing to perform whatever treatment they can for their horse at home. As such, the equine ambulatory practitioner is often the equivalent of the "primary care physician" or "triage doctor." Thus, it is important for the equine ambulatory practitioner to be able to determine whether his patient can be safely and successfully treated in the field, should be referred to a hospital facility for further diagnostics or care, or perhaps should even be euthanized for the good of all involved.

THE EXAMINATION

As in all clinical situations, the physical examination and history are of paramount importance in working up an equine medical case. As opposed to equine veterinarians working in a clinic setting, the ambulatory practitioner must perform a thorough

The author has nothing to disclose.

Gillen Equine Veterinary Clinic, 7314 Pleasant Grove Road, Pleasant Grove, CA 95668, USA

E-mail address: susangillen@succeed.net

exam in the field and gather as much information as possible in a single visit; an exam followed by hospitalization and an endless battery of tests is typically not an option. However, equine ambulatory clinicians may have an advantage over hospital-based personnel in seeing the horse in its natural surroundings; environmental contribution(s) to the horse's condition may not be discovered in a distant hospital setting. For example, the cause of the oozing sores on the distal limbs becomes more apparent when it is noted that the pasture is choked with yellow star thistle. Ornamental oleander noted along the fence line may explain the gastrointestinal and cardiac signs exhibited by the patient or a recent sudden death. Therefore, in addition to the actual physical exam, equine ambulatory clinicians should thoroughly explore a horse's environment for the presence of noxious or toxic weeds, trees, or shrubs to assist in reaching a diagnosis, in addition to examining hay, feedstuffs, and water sources for contaminants.

Toxicoses commonly observed in horses are varied. Knowledge of the common poisons and toxic plants in the practice area helps the practitioner to narrow the range of poisons from which a diagnosis may be made. While signs of poisoning are typically nonspecific, it is helpful to know how different organ systems are primarily affected. For instance, rodenticides, insecticides, fumonisin, larkspur, locoweed, lupine, black locust, and selenium-containing plants produce primarily central nervous system signs, while gastrointestinal signs characterized by colic and diarrhea may develop from plants such as castor bean, oleander, and bracken fern. Pyrrolizidine alkaloids cause primarily liver problems, while ingestion of wild onions or red maple may result in hemolytic anemia and hemoglobinuria. Consumption or exposure to black walnut shavings can cause colic and laminitis.

A history of the problem or condition should be taken, and any changes in animal husbandry, feed, or physical activity should be noted. The quantity of feed consumed and amount of water consumption should be determined if possible. Any and all supplements that the animal is receiving should be noted. Clients often neglect to mention the feeding of vitamin and mineral supplements or substances that they consider to be "natural." If uneaten feed is present in the stall or paddock, it should be examined as well. Consistency and quantity of feces should be noted, and the client should be questioned if there is any change in defecation or urination habits. The duration of illness or clinical signs should be elicited from the owner, and care should be taken to ascertain if the owner has given any form of drug or treatment, or if the horse has been treated or examined by another professional or "paraprofessional." Vaccination and deworming history should be obtained in addition to any history of previous illness. Proximity to other horses at the same facility or at neighboring ranches, history of a new contact or addition to the herd, and any recent history of travel to horse shows or events and/or exposure to other horse populations are noted. The type of stabling should be noted, whether stalled or pastured; the adequacy of ventilation and potential exposure to dust, molds, and other allergens is also surveyed.

PHYSICAL EXAMINATION

The ambulatory veterinarian has the advantage of viewing the horse in his own surroundings, without the undue stress of an intimidating hospital environment. In an unfamiliar environment, nervousness or changes in demeanor may falsely elevate heart rate and respiratory rate, and mask otherwise subtle disease signs. Prior to any hands-on physical exam, the overall appearance of the horse should be assessed. Does the horse appear calm and quiet, bright and alert, stressed, painful, or obtunded? Is he severely depressed, struggling to breathe, ataxic, sweating, showing signs of severe abdominal pain, or recumbent? Obviously, a horse exhibiting signs of an emergency medical condition will require a different workup than an otherwise calm and quiet animal, and efforts to stabilize the horse will take precedence over other examinations.

If the initial assessment of the horse's demeanor and appearance does not indicate a critical life-threatening situation, the ambulatory practitioner should continue with the normal physical examination. Temperature, pulses, heart rate, and respiratory rate are taken; references on normal ranges are readily available. Mucous membranes should be assessed for color, moistness, and capillary refill; changes in mucous membranes most commonly reflect dehydration, sepsis, or shock. Any icterus of the mucous membranes or sclera should be noted, and can occur with liver disease, hemolytic anemia, or prolonged inappetance.

The presence of excessive salivation or ulcerations of the lips and mouth should elicit further exploration of the oral cavity. Sharp grass awns (*Setaria* spp) or plants with sharp burs such as cocklebur (*Xanthium* sp) may cause injury to the mucous membranes, resulting in excessive salivation and anorexia. Dysphagia may accompany the presence of foreign bodies in the oral cavity, dental abnormalities, or injuries to the tongue and mucous membranes but may also be seen in conditions such as rabies, yellow star thistle poisoning, or even botulism.[1,2] Any abnormal odor emanating from the mouth or nostrils should be noted and explored. A foul odor accompanying a nasal discharge may indicate a sinus infection or abscessed tooth, while an abnormal odor emanating from the mouth may indicate oral infection, foreign body, injury, or abscessation of the oral mucous membranes or tongue. Horses with colic that are not eating or drinking often have a "stale" smell to their mouth and breath. The practitioner should note if the nasal discharge is present in one or both nostrils; discharge from one nostril may indicate a problem relating to a tooth, sinus, or guttural pouch, whereas discharge from both nostrils may indicate involvement of the lower parts of the respiratory tract. Endoscopy can be performed in the field to determine the source of the discharge if indicated. The character of the discharge and the presence of any saliva or feed material emanating from the nostrils should be noted. Blood from the nostrils could indicate head or nasal injury, neoplasia, ethmoid hematoma, exercise induced pulmonary hemorrhage (EIPH), or guttural pouch mycosis; feed material mixed with saliva may indicate esophageal obstruction.[3] A cursory examination of the head should note any swellings, lymph node enlargements, or possible cranial nerve deficits.

Clients usually recognize skin abnormalities and readily point these out to their practitioner. A complaint of bumps or swelling with or without any overlying skin abnormality would indicate that a thorough examination of the integumentary system is in order, looking for evidence of injury, urticaria, edema, vasculitis, lymphangitis, cellulitis, or local abscessation. *Corynebacterium pseudotuberculosis* commonly causes lymphangitis and abscessation along lymphatic channels, and may be presented by the client as a "wound," an injury, a localized swelling, ventral edema, or a swollen leg. In an endemic area, the presentation of a firm and painful pectoral swelling is more likely to indicate a developing *C pseudotuberculosis* abscess than neoplasia of the prescapular lymph nodes. Since some diseases are endemic to certain areas, practitioners should be aware of common presentations for regional diseases (eg, *Anaplasma*, Potomac horse fever, *C pseudotuberculosis*).[4–6]

Unusual swellings usually merit deeper investigations. Ultrasound examination is easy to perform in the field, and even a rectal probe normally used for reproductive examinations can be used to identify abscesses or soft tissue masses. A needle aspiration may be performed on any identified mass or abscess.[7]

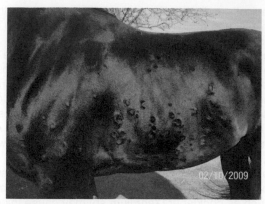

Fig. 1. This horse exhibits the edematous wheals typical of urticarial lesions.

If urticaria and ventral edema are present, the visible mucous membranes should be examined for hemorrhages that may point to purpura hemorrhagica[8] (**Fig. 1**). If hirsutism is present, the owner should be questioned about the normal shedding pattern of the horse. Many owners mistakenly assume that old horses routinely exhibit hirsutism; however, hirsutism in older horses is almost pathognomonic for pituitary pars intermedia dysfunction (PPID or equine Cushing syndrome),[9] a condition that is usually quite amenable to treatment, despite some owners' misconceptions.[10]

A client complaint of lameness, reluctance to move, or trembling may direct the practitioner toward a thorough examination of the musculoskeletal system. There may be some overlap between medical and musculoskeletal problems. Medical conditions such as enteritis may be accompanied by laminitis; a horse with exertional myopathy may prompt an owner to call with a complaint of colic or lameness. Similarly, polysaccharide storage myopathy (PSSM) and hyperkalemic periodic paralysis (HYPP) may be presented to the veterinarian as a colic with muscle fasciculations or as a horse that had been found down and unable to rise.[11,12]

In cases exhibiting severe myopathy, owners should be questioned about HYPP or PSSM status and any recent viral or bacterial infections possibly triggering an immune-mediated myositis.[13] Evaluation of serum muscle enzymes should be performed in the patient with clinical signs of myopathy and dark or tea-colored urine. Tetanus should be suspected in horses with a questionable vaccination history that exhibit stiffness of gait and third eyelid prolapse, with or without a history of injury[14] (**Fig. 2**).

Some horses that present with a complaint of depression, anorexia, or mild colic signs may actually be exhibiting neurologic signs, and a neurologic examination should be performed.[15] The horse should be examined for reluctance to move, obtunded mental status, neurologic deficits, ataxia, muscle tremors, fever, and/or weakness; such signs can indicate West Nile virus infection or equine encephalomyelitis. In the horse with neurologic signs, the possibility of head injury should be explored, and blood from the mouth, ears, or nostrils may be indicative of a skull fracture. Neurologic signs accompanied by icterus may indicate hepatoencephalopathy from liver disease; a blood panel can confirm elevated serum liver enzymes. Fever, weakness, ataxia, depression, dependent edema, and mild to moderate icterus may also indicate infection with *Anaplasma phagocytophilia* (formerly *Ehrlichia equi*), especially in a horse that has recently been exposed to ticks.

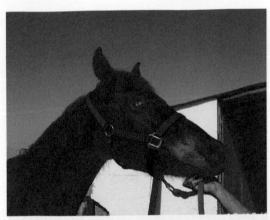

Fig. 2. A horse exhibiting signs of tetanus with stiffness of the muscles of the head and neck, rigidity of the facial expression, and prolapse of the third eyelid. This horse did not have a history of injury and was unvaccinated.

Evaluation and diagnosis of neurologic conditions in the field can be difficult, as subtle neurologic deficits can be hidden or disguised by musculoskeletal disease or serious systemic illness. As well, for most neurologic conditions, there is no specific treatment, and supportive or symptomatic therapies frequently produce little or no significant improvement. Many neurologic diseases are only definitively diagnosed by postmortem examination. While the ambulatory practitioner should be familiar with basic evaluation and examination of the neurologic system, hospital referral for further diagnostics should be considered in all cases without an obvious diagnosis. Trauma to the brain or spinal cord may be amenable to treatment in the field if the deficits are not severe (**Fig. 3**). Some infectious causes of neurologic diseases may respond to symptomatic and supportive treatment in the field (West Nile virus, equine encephalomyelitis). Properly diagnosed cases of equine protozoal myeloencephalopathy (EPM) may improve with antiprotozoal treatment. Degenerative conditions of the brain and spinal cord are generally not satisfactorily treated. Young horses with weakness, ataxia, and spasticity of all 4 limbs should be suspect for cervical vertebral stenotic myelopathy (CSM), and radiographs may confirm the diagnosis. However, clinical signs of equine degenerative myeloencephalopathy (EDM) and neuroaxonal dystrophy (NAD) are generally indistinguishable from CSM and also are seen in young horses. The ingestion of various toxins and toxic plants can produce neurologic signs; prompt diagnosis and treatment may be imperative to recovery. Thus, referral of difficult neurologic cases may be the best course of action for most ambulatory veterinarians. Practitioners should also be aware of reportable diseases that manifest with neurologic signs, such as rabies, West Nile virus, equine encephalomyelitis, and equine herpes myeloencephalopathy, and know the proper reporting procedure for suspect cases.

The respiratory exam should begin with an evaluation of respiratory effort and rate and character of breathing; flared nostrils, abdominal respiratory effort, and uneven airflow between nostrils are noted. Volume and type of any nasal discharge and the presence of a cough are noted. A cough may easily be elicited in a horse with tracheitis by deep tracheal or laryngeal palpation; a cough to tracheal palpation in the absence of other signs of infection may indicate that irritation of the respiratory tract (eg, dust, allergy) is the underlying problem. In the field, the practitioner may

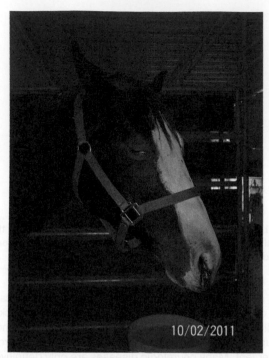

10/02/2011

Fig. 3. A horse exhibiting neurological signs due to skull fracture and brain trauma. Note the obtunded mental status, swelling around the eyes, abrasions on the head, and blood from the right nostril. The horse had vestibular disease as well as optic and oculomotor nerve deficits.

encounter difficulty in auscultating the lung because of background noise or wind. Auscultation of respiratory sounds may be enhanced with the use of a rebreathing bag held loosely over the nares.[16] This simple technique results in much deeper respiratory movements than normal and accentuates sounds. Alternatively, the horse may be encouraged to take a few deep breaths by first occluding his nostrils for a short time. Moist or dry rales, friction rubs, and the presence of quiet or consolidated areas or pleural fluid lines are noted.

A complaint of abdominal pain (pawing, looking at flanks, getting up and down, and rolling) should begin with evaluation of the nature, severity, and frequency of clinical signs.[17] Nature, character, and quantity of feces passed should be ascertained, and determination should be made of when the last feces were passed. Contrary to the beliefs of some owners, the passage of feces is not necessarily a good prognostic sign, especially early in the onset of the condition, as horses will commonly evacuate their rectum, even while the problem lies proximally. All areas of the abdomen should be carefully auscultated, including the ventral abdomen at the xiphoid region for sand accumulation.[18] The characteristic roaring sound that can be described as waves washing over a beach is diagnostic of sand accumulation in the colon; however, lack of these sounds does not preclude the existence of accumulated sand. A rectal examination is warranted in most cases of abdominal pain.

In the emergency situation with a horse in severe distress, no matter the cause, immediate assessment and stabilization of the animal are necessary. Whenever possible, vital signs should be taken and a basic assessment of condition should be made prior to the administration of any drugs or medications. However, the safety of the handlers and the practitioner should be a priority; a horse that is rolling and thrashing due to uncontrolled abdominal pain may require short-term sedation or analgesics in order to safely perform a physical exam.

While excellent medicine can be practiced in the field, the ambulatory practitioner should maintain a good working relationship with referral clinics and hospitals. Although some owners prefer not to hospitalize cases due to financial considerations, horses that require constant monitoring and management may not receive proper and adequate treatment at home. Owner compliance is imperative in critical care, and many owners find themselves unable to fulfill the demands of 24-hour nursing care. A horse that requires around-the-clock intravenous fluids or constant monitoring is best referred to a facility that is equipped to handle such cases. Patients that may require surgery or advanced diagnostic procedures benefit from early referral.

EVALUATION AND TREATMENT OF COMMONLY ENCOUNTERED CONDITIONS OF THE EQUINE PATIENT IN THE FIELD

The initial clinical signs and findings will direct further diagnostics and treatment. For instance, if a depressed and anorexic horse is found to have a high fever, the horse is far more likely to have an infectious agent than a colonic impaction or torsion, and the practitioner will direct his/her examination as indicated. A depressed, anorexic, and febrile horse, exhibiting signs of cough and nasal discharge, will warrant further examination of the respiratory tract.

In the nonfebrile horse, signs of anorexia and abdominal discomfort will generally be worked up as a colic case. An anorexic horse showing signs of colic and distress, with saliva and food emanating from the nostrils and mouth, is more likely to be suffering from esophageal obstruction, and initial assessment should obviously include passage of a nasogastric tube.

Colic

Colic is one of the most common medical emergencies that the practitioner will experience in the field. Sometimes the horse has been treated by the owner prior to calling the veterinarian; the practitioner should always inquire as to the duration of clinical signs and inquire if any drugs or treatments have been given prior to his/her arrival. If the horse is very painful, making examination difficult, short-term sedation with alpha-2 agonists may offer necessary pain relief to safely examine and evaluate the patient in the field. The use of xylazine (Anased) or detomidine (Dormosedan) does not appear to interfere with the practitioner's ability to properly assess the patient. Rather, the short-term pain relief and sedation gained from the use of low doses of these drugs assist the practitioner in making a proper diagnosis by allowing a more thorough exam. Any mild bradycardia or secondary heart block caused from the administration of alpha-2 agonists appears to be insignificant in evaluating a colic case. On the other hand, the failure of these agents to temporarily control colic pain may indicate a more severe etiology that will require surgery for resolution.

The ambulatory practitioner must quickly determine whether the horse can safely and effectively be treated medically in the field, or whether hospitalization or surgery will be necessary to correct the abdominal crisis; in cases where the practitioner may not be able to immediately determine if a horse requires colic surgery, referral to a surgical center may be a good conservative option that allows the horse more immediate access to necessary treatment and eliminates concerns about waiting too long before surgical intervention. Heart rate, respiratory rate, capillary refill time, color of the mucous membranes, degree of pain, and gastrointestinal sounds are important in the evaluation of the colic case. Any horse with unrelenting pain and a sustained heart rate of greater than 70–80 bpm is likely to need surgical or hospital referral, and fever and diarrhea are more likely to accompany a case of enteritis, colitis, or peritonitis. The intensity of pain is often reflective of the severity of the problem.[19] Lack of response to treatment or the resumption of pain after analgesic administration should be considered an indication of the need for surgery. Horses with unrelenting pain that do not respond to analgesics or horses that respond initially to medical treatment but relapse with pain several hours later are best referred to a surgical facility if surgery is an option for the owner. Geriatric horses commonly appear more stoic than their younger counterparts, and the owner may mistakenly assume that the horse is improving although vital signs are deteriorating.

The vast majority of colic cases that the ambulatory practitioner encounters will respond to medical treatment. However, early referral of cases without an obvious diagnosis is a conservative approach that is more likely to have a positive outcome for the horse, regardless of diagnosis. The ambulatory clinician should always offer a surgical referral regardless of the impression of the value of the animal or the client's ability to pay. Since many owners do not have the ability to transport their horse, the ambulatory practitioner may provide a service to his clients by keeping a list of potential emergency haulers. Unfortunately, the costs of abdominal surgery and hospitalization are beyond the reach of many owners. Therefore, owners should be warned that in the event of nonsurgical treatment failure, there may be no humane alternative for these patients other than euthanasia.

A full exam should be performed in an attempt to determine the cause of abdominal pain. Blood work is not practical on a colic patient in the field, as the results will not be readily available. A rectal exam is warranted in all but the mildest of cases. While a dry rectum and a feed impaction at the pelvic flexure may be obvious signs of a large colon impaction, dilated loops of small intestine may indicate a small intestinal obstruction, enteritis, or, in a geriatric horse, a strangulating lipoma. Enteroliths are not commonly palpated, but the distended and painful colon of a large colon volvulus can usually be identified.

Rectal exams can be safely performed in the field with the use of proper restraint. While most horses can be restrained with only a twitch, field rectal exams on more fractious horses can often be safely performed in a horse trailer or by positioning the horse's hips in the doorway of a stall. Patients are sometimes more compliant and exhibit better rectal relaxation if the base of the tail is grasped and elevated straight over the patient's back. Another useful technique is to grasp and lift the base of the tail with the free hand, applying mild to moderate rearward pressure on the tail as the other arm is inserted into the rectum. Copious lubricant should be used while evacuating the rectum. Safety is of paramount importance; sedation can be performed to facilitate a rectal exam on the fractious horse, and N-butylscopolammonium bromide (Buscopan) can be used in the patient that is straining.

Primary treatment of the nonsurgical colic case is directed at treating dehydration, stimulating intestinal motility, decreasing intestinal inflammation, decompressing the gastrointestinal tract, and relieving pain. Feed should be withheld until there is evidence of resolution of the colic, but water consumption should be encouraged.

Nonsteroidal anti-inflammatory drugs (NSAIDs) are commonly used for relief of pain associated with colic. Although not without controversy, flunixin meglumine (Banamine) is commonly considered to be the most effective of the NSAIDs used to treat colic pain in horses and may be helpful in diminishing the detrimental effects of endotoxin release. While indiscriminate dosing of the drug is certainly unwise, flunixin alone is unlikely to significantly alter visceral pain except in the case of an uncomplicated medical colic, and the concern that its use may delay surgical referral is largely unwarranted. Intense visceral pain can be treated with potent opioid analgesics, and butorphanol tartrate (Torbugesic; Dolorex) appears to provide the best pain relief with the least adverse side effects, although it can reduce small intestinal motility. Butorphanol can also be used in combination with xylazine (Anased) or detomidine (Dormosedan), which are themselves potent analgesics that cause muscle relaxation and sedation. Spasmolytic drugs can relieve pain indirectly by reducing spasms of the intestine but may also contribute to intestinal ileus and abdominal stasis. The spasmolytic drug N-butylscopolammonium bromide (Buscopan) may facilitate a rectal examination due to the drug's relaxation effect on the rectal wall.

Passage of a nasogastric tube has both diagnostic and therapeutic indications. A nasogastric tube can usually be passed in the unsedated horse with the use of a twitch, enabling the practitioner to check for gastric reflux or administer fluids. While the administration of sedatives may make the horse more compliant for passage of the nasogastric tube, sedation may decrease the horse's swallow reflex. An attempt to start a siphon should be made in all cases by filling the tube with water and then lowering the end of the tube below the level of the stomach, as stomach pressure may not force fluid through the tube even with extreme stomach distention. Significant reflux from the nasogastric tube can indicate small intestinal or gastric obstruction, small intestinal ileus, or enteritis.

In horses without stomach distention and reflux, impactions in various anatomical locations can be treated by the administration of water via nasogastric tube. Horses with pain from mild intestinal ileus and distention often respond immediately to fluid administration. Up to 10 L of water can be administered per hour without problem, although theoretically, prolonged treatment may result in alterations of serum electrolytes. Enteral administration of a balanced electrolyte solution is effective in hydrating colon contents without altering serum electrolyte values.[20,21] A balanced electrolyte solution can be administered through a feeding tube at the rate of 5 to 10 L/h as long as care is taken not to overload the stomach.[22] A balanced electrolyte solution for enteral administration can be made in the field using readily available and inexpensive ingredients. A total of 3 teaspoons of table salt, 1 teaspoon of Litesalt, and 4 teaspoons of baking soda added to 5 L of water will provide a solution approximating 5.37 g NaCl, 0.37 g KCl, and 3.78 g $NaHCO_3$ per liter and is effective in softening colonic impactions and providing systemic hydration.

Mineral oil is often used to treat colic cases in the field. While some hypothesize that mineral oil may provide a degree of softening and lubrication for impacted food masses, there is evidence that the administration of intravenous or enteral fluids is more effective in relieving intestinal impactions.[23] However, mineral oil can be a good marker and indicator of intestinal transit. In addition, it may be helpful, along with psyllium, in removing accumulated sand from the colon and in reducing the rapid pH drop in the large intestine by acting as a laxative and a binding agent for the undigested starches in cases of grain overload.

Enteral fluids should not be administered, or administered only with care, in the horse with gastrointestinal distention and ileus. Horses with suspected gastric or small intestinal distention should be decompressed via a nasogastric tube, and the creation of a siphon should be attempted to relieve reflux due to small intestinal obstruction or ileus. The nasogastric tube can be taped in place for passive decompression of horses with continuing gastric distention and reflux and for horses that are being shipped to a referral hospital.

A severely dehydrated horse is probably best referred to a hospital for intravenous fluid therapy, but many mildly dehydrated horses can be adequately managed in the field with owner assistance. Isotonic fluids can be safely administered to the tractable horse in the field via the placement of a jugular catheter, and owners can be taught how to change bags of fluids in the absence of the treating veterinarian. Short-term catheters are typically not left in place over 24 to 48 hours, and the client can be instructed on how to care for and remove the catheter when intravenous fluids are no longer necessary.

One disadvantage in the field is the inability to determine electrolyte and acid-base status. However, in any horse other than an HYPP case, lactated Ringer's solution is generally safe for administration in the nonhospital setting and can be administered at double or triple maintenance levels. The intractable horse may present a challenge for owners in maintaining the intravenous lines, but even these cases can be bolused with fluids periodically while under mild sedation. When a bolus of fluids is administered, 10 to 20 L can be administered over a 2-hour period. The administration of fluids is helpful in softening impacted food masses and relieving fecal obstructions.

In the horse with cecal distention, enterocentesis can be performed in the field to relieve primary cecal tympany or gas accumulated from a large or small colon obstruction. The cecum can be decompressed by placing a 5- to 6-inch 14- to 16-gauge catheter over needle through the surgically prepped right paralumbar fossa, midway between the last rib and the ventral prominence of the tuber coxae. The catheter is advanced into the cecum, and the stylet needle may be removed. Suction may be used to facilitate gas removal, or the practitioner may palpate the cecum per rectum to push gas into the cecal base. After the gas is removed and the cecum is decompressed, an antibiotic and sterile saline solution should be infused through the catheter or needle as it is pulled out of the cecum to prevent pulling contaminated material through the peritoneum. Mild peritonitis may result from cecal enterocentesis, and prophylactic antibiotics are warranted.

Esophageal Obstruction

Horses with esophageal obstruction are often presented by the owner as a case of colic. The signs of choke are variable and may include dysphagia, retching, intermittent flexing and extension of the neck, frequent and ineffective attempts to swallow, collapsing, rolling, and coughing.[24] Most cases of esophageal obstruction will have evidence of regurgitated saliva and feed material around the nostrils and mouth. If the site of obstruction is cervical, focal swelling may be seen and many will exhibit signs of discomfort when the area of obstruction is palpated. Some esophageal obstructions will resolve spontaneously if all foodstuffs and water are removed, so owners should be instructed to place the horse in a stall without feed, water, or bedding. The simplest way to diagnose esophageal obstruction is the inability to pass a nasogastric tube from nostril to stomach. Treatment requires relaxation of the esophageal musculature and lowering of the horse's head to minimize the possibility of aspiration of food and saliva. Most obstructed horses are not cooperative in passing a nasogastric tube; sedation with xylazine or detomidine assists in both patient compliance and lowering of the head. A twitch will assist in controlling the head during passage of the nasogastric tube. When the tube reaches the obstruction, care should be taken not to exert too much pressure, possibly causing a perforation of the esophagus. Gentle flushing with warm water may assist in either flushing the obstruction into the stomach or breaking up the food bolus. Water containing food particles will be seen exiting the nostrils. Oxytocin or *N*-butylscopolammonium bromide may assist in esophageal relaxation.

If gentle lavage is not successful at relieving the obstruction, more vigorous lavage can be accomplished by passing a cuffed endotracheal tube nasally to the site of obstruction and inflating the cuff. A nasogastric tube is then passed through the endotracheal tube to the site of obstruction, allowing a more vigorous lavage with large volumes of water and lessening the chance of aspiration. Most cases of uncomplicated esophageal obstruction can be resolved in the field. In cases where severe mucosal damage is suspected or where hard obstructions cannot be broken up and relieved, hospital referral is recommended.

NSAIDs are recommended to control pain and inflammation and to lessen the chance of esophageal stricture formation. A possible complication of esophageal obstruction is aspiration pneumonia. Most obstructed horses will have aspirated even a small amount of feed material, and fluid may be heard in the trachea. Prophylactic broad-spectrum antibiotics should be considered in all but the simplest cases of esophageal obstruction. Oral fluids should never be allowed until the obstruction has been alleviated. In cases where the obstruction has been long-standing, intravenous fluids may be necessary to treat dehydration. Horses that have had simple obstructions relieved with minimal or no mucosal damage can be fed after 12 to 24 hours, starting with small amounts of softened pelleted gruel or green grass. Hay should not be fed initially. Horses suspected to have sustained more severe mucosal damage should have feed withheld for longer than 24 hours.

Respiratory Diseases

The evaluation of the equine patient with respiratory disease requires careful auscultation and evaluation of the lung fields, and an attempt should be made to find a quiet area away from wind and inclement weather to examine the patient. A sudden high fever and anorexia with a serous nasal discharge with or without a cough usually accompany a respiratory virus, and initial pulmonary sounds may be normal. A more long-standing illness accompanied by a purulent nasal discharge may indicate a bacterial component. A mucopurulent nasal discharge with a concurrent cough and abnormal lower respiratory tract sounds may be indicative of bacterial pneumonia.

Strangles (*Streptococcus equi equi* infection) is usually accompanied by a high fever, dysphagia, swollen intermandibular lymph nodes, and a purulent nasal discharge. Horses with retropharyngeal lymph node involvement will have difficulty swallowing, inspiratory respiratory noise from compression of the dorsal pharyngeal wall, and an extended head and neck. However, milder cases of strangles may present with a mucoid nasal discharge, cough, and mild fever. Signs of strangles are typically confined to the upper respiratory tract, although complicated cases ("bastard strangles") may present with many clinical signs not related to the respiratory system.[25]

Signs of cough, exercise intolerance, and mucous accumulation in the airways, usually in an afebrile horse, may indicate inflammatory airway disease. A horse that presents with fever, cough, anorexia, cyanosis, nostril flare, and a restrictive breathing pattern should be suspected of having pleuropneumonia or interstitial pneumonia. Pulmonary ultrasound examination can be performed in the field with most 5-MHz probes by directing the beam between the ribs and is often diagnostic.[26,27]

In febrile cases where an uncomplicated upper respiratory virus is suspected, treatment should be directed toward reducing the fever and inflammation, as most viral respiratory diseases are self-limiting. Although clients often demand antibiotic treatment, antibiotics should be reserved for bacterial infections. There is no evidence that antibiotic use in influenza or upper respiratory virus cases will prevent secondary bacterial infection. Financial considerations may dictate that bloodwork is not a requirement of treatment. Clients should be counseled about providing a proper and healthy respiratory environment. Many show barns are closed up, especially in cold weather, creating poor air exchange, increased concentrations of ammonia in the air, and an unhealthy environment for the respiratory case.

Cases of pneumonia should always be considered for broad-spectrum antibiotic treatment; the initial choice of an antibiotic may be influenced both by finances and the ability/inability of the owner to administer the treatment. Transtracheal aspiration (TTA) should be performed in severe or unresolving cases of pneumonia. A TTA sample can be easily obtained in the field.[28] In the author's opinion, suckling foals with pneumonia should always have a comprehensive complete blood count performed, since *Rodococcus equi* is both common in this age group and resistant to many commonly used antibiotics. *R equi* infection is usually accompanied by very high white blood cell values and elevated fibrinogen levels.[29]

Pleuropneumonia should be suspected in any horse that has been transported a significant distance and shows signs of fever, lethargy, and increased respiratory effort.[30] Blood work typically shows a hyperfibrinongenemia, with variable leukocytosis. Ultrasonagraphy can be used as a guide to sample or drain pleural fluid for analysis and culture. While pleural drainage and lavage can be performed in the field, hospital referral is preferred.[31]

Recurrent airway obstruction (RAO), or heaves, describes episodes of lower airway obstruction typically triggered by exposure to mold, dust, and allergens that result in severe airway inflammation. Inflammatory airway disease (IAD) may include infectious and noninfectious problems of the lower airways—that is, bronchitis or bronchiolitis. Coughing and exercise intolerance are common signs of RAO and IAD, often with a historical lack of response to antimicrobials.

Coughing is a normal mechanism by which the respiratory tract clears mucus and can arise from exposure to dust and molds in an arena environment. A cough that becomes chronic, occurs in the stable or during feeding times, or persists during a workout is more likely to reflect IAD. In the absence of pulmonary bacterial infection, the affected horse may benefit from rest, increased turnout, reducing dust, and a change of diet away from hay. If coughing continues despite a change of environment and rest, further diagnostics such as TTA or bronchoalveolar lavage (BAL) may be indicated.

The treatment of RAO (heaves) is aimed at preventing further inhalation of dust, especially in hay, decreasing inflammation in the lower airways, and providing relief of airway obstruction. Systemic or inhaled corticosteroids, bronchodilators, expectorants, and mucolytic agents are commonly used along with environmental changes. Environmental management is critical in the treatment of RAO, as environmental changes alone may alleviate clinical signs in many horses without the concurrent use of drugs. Client education and compliance are crucial for the successful management of these cases.

The Down Horse

The recumbent horse that is unable to rise may present a diagnostic and therapeutic challenge to the equine ambulatory veterinarian. Often the patient is a geriatric or arthritic individual, the majority of whom may be able to rise unassisted, or with minimal assistance, after they are rolled to the opposite side. However, other cases are not as easily managed. The ambulatory practitioner may encounter a recumbent emaciated horse that is unable to rise due to a lack of sufficient muscle mass to support its body weight. Although these horses may also be bright and alert and eating, management of a recumbent horse in the field is difficult. Younger horses that are suffering from starvation due to "benign neglect" are best rehabilitated in a hospital setting. However, severely cachectic geriatric horses may also be suffering from malnutrition due to poor dentition and disease, and euthanasia of the emaciated down individual may be the most humane option. In any event, the severely emaciated horse that is incapable of supporting its own body weight is best referred for hospital care and treatment or euthanized in the field.

The evaluation of the recumbent horse that is otherwise of healthy body weight is directed toward determining the cause of recumbency. The horse should be examined for catastrophic fractures, as these typically necessitate euthanasia. Neurologic causes of recumbency should be differentiated as to infectious and noninfectious causes.[32] Eastern and Western equine encephalomyelitis, West Nile virus, and equine herpes myeloencephalopathy can cause recumbency that may be recoverable with treatment and supportive care in the field; recumbency caused by neuraxonal dystrophy, equine degenerative myelopathy, vertebral stenosis, leukoencephalomalacia, and rabies are generally not treatable.[33–36] Treatment of the long-term recumbent neurologic case is extremely difficult in the field, and if hospital referral is not an option, euthanasia should be considered.

Horses with HYPP may be found recumbent without the owner having noted any preceding clinical signs. Generally, if the horse has been recumbent for a limited amount of time, treatment in the field can provide immediate improvement.[37] However, longer-term recumbency usually results in severe and continuing degenerative myopathy that would be better treated in a hospital setting. Severe rhabdomyolysis can also result in recumbency, and the cause may be genetically based or immune mediated. Serum aspirate transaminase and creatine kinase values are typically very high in these cases.[38,39] Since recumbency results in further muscle damage, efforts should be directed toward treating the inflammation and getting the horse to its feet. Many of these horses can support their own weight and walk if they are lifted to a standing position. A lift can be fashioned from soft ropes and straps, or a ready-made emergency sling can be utilized (UC Davis Large Animal Lift; Andersen Sling Support Device); a tractor or forklift can be used to lift the horse in the sling.[40] Some of these horses can be successfully treated in the field if hospitalization is not an option, although the practitioner should expect that the horse may need to be lifted to its feet multiple times.[41]

ADR (Ain't Doin' Right)

When a complete physical exam cannot determine the cause of the horse's clinical signs, blood work and other laboratory testing can be invaluable in identifying an underlying disease process. Many times, nonspecific physical findings can be explained by laboratory data, and further diagnostics can be directed toward that organ system.

Liver disease may be first diagnosed by elevated serum gamma glutamyl transferase (GGT) levels in the horse without evidence of clinical icterus, as bilirubin levels may be normal in chronic hepatic disease. Signs of liver disease can include fever, depression, anorexia, weight loss, icterus, photosensitization, edema, hepatoencephalopathy, and abnormal hemorrhage. The most useful serum diagnostic tests for evaluating hepatic disease in horses is quantitation of sorbitol dehydrogenase (SDH), GGT, and serum bile acids. Abnormal laboratory findings should be followed up by ultrasonography and liver biopsy. Causes of liver failure are varied; common etiologies include Theiler's Disease, toxic hepatopathies, acute biliary obstruction, and pyrrolizidine

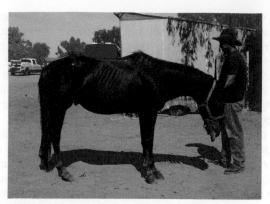

Fig. 4. A horse exhibiting hepatoencephalopathy due to idiopathic severe chronic hepatopathy. The horse showed clinical signs of blindness, ataxia, head pressing, dementia, and paralysis of CN XII. Prior to the exhibition of recent neurologic signs, the owner had noted only weight loss as a possible problem.

alkaloid toxicity (*Senecio, Amsinckia, Crotalaria*) (**Fig. 4**). Liver biopsy may help to determine the etiology of the disease as well as offer a prognosis and can be performed in the field after adequate training. Complications include hemorrhage, pneumothorax, peritonitis, and colon or abscess puncture.[42]

Hyperlipidemia and hepatic lipidosis occur primarily in ponies and miniature horses. Affected ponies are typically obese, have recent history of stress or weight loss, and are in late gestation or early lactation. Onset of signs is typically acute and includes icterus, anorexia, weakness, fever, severe depression, ataxia, mild colic, and recumbency.

Clinical signs of acute renal failure are often nonspecific and include dehydration, depression, and anorexia. Renal compromise is reflected as azotemia, evidenced by elevations in serum blood urea nitrogen and creatinine. The prognosis of acute renal failure depends upon the underlying cause and the duration of the disease process.[43] Cases of suspected acute renal failure are best referred to a hospital early on for further diagnostics and treatment.[44] Chronic renal failure is less common, and clinical signs do not become apparent until 65% to 75% of functional neurons have been lost. Clinical signs include lethargy, anorexia, weight loss, polyuria, and polydipsia.[45] In many cases, identifying the precipitating event is not possible. Because of the progressive and irreversible nature of the disease, long-term prognosis is poor.[46]

Leukocytosis and hyperfibrinongenemia in a horse with nonspecific signs of weight loss, intermittent fever, and depression may be an indication of internal abscessation; *S equi equi* and *Corynebacterium pseudotuberculosis* are commonly incriminated pathogens.[47–49] Serum titers for these organisms may identify the microbial agent involved. Abdominal abscesses may be identified by rectal examination or ultrasonography. Thoracic abscesses are more commonly identified by respiratory signs and thoracic radiographs. If the abscess cannot be successfully drained, long-term antibiotic treatment is necessary for successful resolution.

Horses that exhibit chronic lethargy, anemia, cachexia, and progressive weight loss despite adequate consumption of calories may suffer from abdominal neoplasia. Lymphoma, squamous cell carcinoma, and adenocarcinoma are the most commonly encountered neoplasias of the gastrointestinal tract. Diagnosis is challenging, and while blood counts, chemistry panels, and urinalysis may support a diagnosis of neoplasia, they rarely confirm it. Ultrasonography, peritoneal fluid analysis, and rectal examination may or may not be rewarding. Metastatic melanoma should be considered in gray horses.

SUMMARY

The scope of medical problems encountered by the equine ambulatory practitioner is immense; there is a wealth of information available to ambulatory practitioners pertaining to specific medical topics. It is certainly possible to practice high-quality equine medicine in a field setting. However, hospital referral should be offered to clients for conditions not conducive to successful treatment in the field. Prompt referral of difficult cases is a sign that the practitioner wants the best treatment for the patient and is often gladly accepted by the client. When surgical or hospital referral is not an option, it is imperative that the ambulatory practitioner not only offer humane alternatives but also inform and educate horse owners on equine suffering and welfare issues so that clients do not have unreasonable expectations of a positive outcome.

REFERENCES

1. Schmitz DG. Toxicologic Problems: Yellow star thistle. In: Reed SM, Bayly WM, Sellon DC, editors. Equine internal medicine. 2nd edition. Philadelphia: Saunders Elsevier; 2004. p. 1469.
2. Wilkins P. Botulism. In: Sellon D, Long M, editors. Equine infectious diseases. Philadelphia: Saunders Elsevier; 2007. p. 372–6.
3. Davis E. Respiratory infections. In: Sellon D, Long M, editors. Equine infectious diseases. Philadelphia: Saunders Elsevier; 2007. p. 1–20.
4. Pusterla N, Madigan J. Anaplasma phagocytophilia. In: Sellon D, Long M, editors. Equine infectious diseases. Philadelphia: Saunders Elsevier; 2007. p. 354–7.
5. Pusterla N, Madigan J. Neorickettsia risticii. In: Sellon D, Long M, editors. Equine infectious diseases. Philadelphia: Saunders Elsevier; 2007. p. 357–62.
6. Rees C. Disorders of the skin. In: Reed SM, Bayly WM, Sellon DC, editors. Equine internal medicine. 2nd edition. Philadelphia: Saunders Elsevier; 2004. p. 667–719.
7. Leveille R, Biller D. Muscle evaluation, foreign bodies, and miscellaneous swellings. In: Rantanen N, McKinnon A, editors. Equine diagnostic ultrasonography. Baltimore (MD): Williams and Wilkins; 1998. p. 515–21.
8. Sellon D. Purpura hemorrhagica. In: Sellon D, Long M, editors. Equine infectious diseases. Philadelphia: Saunders Elsevier; 2007. p. 249–50.
9. Toribio R. Pars intermedia dysfunction (equine Cushings disease). In: Reed SM, Bayly WM, Sellon DC, editors. Equine internal medicine. 2nd edition. Philadelphia: Saunders Elsevier; 2004. p. 1327–39.
10. Messer N. Diagnosis of pituitary pars intermedia dysfunction: A review of 1999 versus 2008. In: Proceedings of the Annual Convention of the AAEP, vol 54. Lexington (KY): AAEP; 2008. p. 200–3.
11. Valberg S. Polysaccharide storage myopathy. In: Proceedings of the Annual Convention of the AAEP, vol 52. Lexington (KY): AAEP; 2006. p. 373–80.
12. MacLeay J. Diseases of the musculoskeletal system. In: Reed SM, Bayly WM, Sellon DC, editors. Equine internal medicine. 2nd edition. Philadelphia: Saunders Elsevier; 2004. p. 461–522.
13. Lewis S, Valberg S, Nielsen I. Suspected immune-mediated myositis in horses. J Vet Intern Med 2007; 21:495–503.
14. MacKay R. Tetanus. In: Sellon D, Long M, editors. Equine infectious diseases. Philadelphia: Saunders Elsevier; 2007. p. 376–80.

15. Johnson A. How to perform a complete neurologic examination in the field and identify abnormalities. In: Proceedings of the Annual Convention of the AAEP, vol 56. Baltimore (MD): AAEP; 2010. p. 331–7.

16. Rose R, Wright D. Patient evaluation and diagnosis. Examination of the thorax. In: Colahan P, et al, editors. Equine medicine and surgery. 5th edition. St Louis: Mosby; 1999. p. 93.

17. Blikslager A. Critical decisions in colic. In: Proceedings of the Annual Convention of the AAEP, vol 55. Las Vegas (NV): AAEP; 2009. p. 201–6.

18. Ragle C, Meagher D, Schrader J, et al. Abdominal auscultation in the detection of experimentally induced gastrointestinal sand accumulation. J Vet Intern Med 1989; Jan:12–4.

19. Nolen-Walston R, Ramey D. Evidence-based gastrointestinal medicine in horses: It's not about your gut instincts. Vet Clin North Am Equine Pract 2007;45:243–66.

20. Lopes MA, Walker BL, White NA, et al. Treatments to promote colonic hydration: Enteral fluid therapy versus intravenous fluid therapy and magnesium sulphate. Equine Vet J 2002;34:505–9.

21. Lopes MA, White NA, Donaldson L, et al. Effects of enteral and intravenous fluid therapy, magnesium sulfate, and sodium sulfate on colonic contents and feces in horses. Am J Vet Res 2004;65:695–704.

22. White N. Colic treatment and post-colic nutrition. In: Pagan JD, editor. Advances in equine nutrition, vol IV. Nottingham (UK): Nottingham University Press; 2009. p. 327–45.

23. White N, Lopes M. Large colon impaction. In: Robinson E, editor. Current therapy in equine medicine. 5th edition. Philadelphia: WB Saunders; 2003. p. 131–5.

24. Campbell N. Esophageal obstruction (choke). In: Robinson E, editor. Current therapy in equine medicine. 5th edition. Philadelphia: WB Saunders; 2003. p. 90–4.

25. Sweeney C, et al. Streptococcal infections. In: Sellon D, Long M, editors. Equine infectious diseases. Philadelphia: Saunders Elsevier; 2007. p. 244–57.

26. Ainsworth D, Hackett R. Disorders of the respiratory system: Parapneumonic effusions and septic pleuritis. In: Reed S, et al, editors. Equine internal medicine. 2nd edition. Philadelphia: Saunders Elsevier; 2004. p. 324–5.

27. Rantanen R. Thoracic ultrasound. In: Rantanen N, McKinnon A, editors. Equine diagnostic ultrasonography. Baltimore (MD): Williams and Wilkins; 1998. p. 41–6.

28. Sweeney C. Evaluating the lungs. In: Proceedings of the Annual Convention of the AAEP, vol 45. Albuquerque (NM): AAEP; 1999. p. 290–3.

29. Hines M. Rhodococcus equi. In: Sellon D, Long M, editors. Equine infectious diseases. Philadelphia: Saunders Elsevier; 2007. p. 281–95.

30. Beadle R. Diseases of the pleura, mediastinum, diaphragm, and thoracic wall. In: Equine medicine and surgery. 5th edition. St Louis: Mosby; 1999. p. 553–9.

31. Sweeney, C. Pleuropneumonia. In: Robinson E, editor. Current therapy in equine medicine. 5th edition. Philadelphia: WB Saunders; 2003. p. 421–4.

32. Reed S. Neurology is not a euphemism for necropsy: A review of selected neurological diseases affecting horses. In: Proceedings of the Annual Convention of the AAEP, vol 54. Lexington (KY): AAEP; 2008. p. 78–109.

33. Saville W. West Nile virus encephalitis. In: Reed SM, Bayly WM, Sellon DC, editors. Equine internal medicine. 2nd edition. Philadelphia: Saunders Elsevier; 2004. p. 640–3.

34. Sommardahl C. Rabies. In: Reed SM, Bayly WM, Sellon DC, editors. Equine internal medicine. 2nd edition. Philadelphia: Saunders Elsevier; 2004. p. 644–6.

35. Wilson D, Pusterla N. Equine herpesvirus 1 myeloencephalopathy. In: Reed S, , et al, editors. Equine internal medicine. 2nd edition. Philadelphia: Saunders Elsevier; 2004. p. 617–28.
36. Matthews H, Nout Y. Equine degenerative myeloencephalopathy. In: Reed SM, Bayly WM, Sellon DC, editors. Equine internal medicine. 2nd edition. Philadelphia: Saunders Elsevier; 2004. p. 599–604.
37. Spier S. Hyperkalemic periodic paralysis: 14 Years later. In: Proceedings of the Annual Convention of the AAEP, vol 52. Lexington (KY): AAEP; 2006. p. 347–50.
38. Valberg S. Immune mediated myopathies. In: Proceedings of the Annual Convention of the AAEP, vol 52. Lexington (KY): AAEP; 2006. p. 354–8.
39. Valberg S. Diagnostic approach to muscle disorders. In: Proceedings of the Annual Convention of the AAEP, vol 52. Lexington (KY): AAEP; 2006. p. 340–6.
40. Pusterla N, Madigan J. Initial clinical impressions of the U.C. Davis large animal lift and its use in recumbent equine patients. Schweiz Arch Tierheilkd 2006;148:161–6.
41. Pusterla N, Ferraro G, Madigan J. How to lift recumbent equine patients in the field and hospital with the UC Davis large animal lift. In: Proceedings of the Annual Convention of the AAEP, vol 52. Lexington (KY): AAEP; 2006. p. 87–92.
42. Barton M. Disorders of the liver. In: Reed SM, Bayly WM, Sellon DC, editors. Equine internal medicine. 2nd edition. Philadelphia: Saunders Elsevier; 2004. p. 951–94.
43. Geor R. Acute renal failure in horses. Vet Clin North Am Equine Pract 2007;23: 577–91.
44. Bayly W. Acute renal failure. In: Reed SM, Bayly WM, Sellon DC, editors. Equine internal medicine. 2nd edition. Philadelphia: Saunders Elsevier; 2004. p. 1221–9.
45. Schott H. Chronic renal failure in horses. Vet Clin North Am Equine Pract 2007;23: 593–612.
46. Schott H. Chronic renal failure. In: Reed SM, Bayly WM, Sellon DC, editors. Equine internal medicine. 2nd edition. Philadelphia: Saunders Elsevier; 2004. p. 1231–53.
47. Spier S, Whitcomb M. Corynebacterium pseudotuberculosis. In: Sellon D, Long M, editors. Equine infectious diseases. Philadelphia: Saunders Elsevier; 2007. p. 263–9.
48. Sellon D. Streptococcal infections. In: Sellon D, Long M, editors. Equine infectious diseases. Philadelphia: Saunders Elsevier; 2007. p. 244–56.
49. Rumbaugh G, Smith B, Carlson G. Internal abdominal abscesses in horses: A study of 25 cases. J Am Vet Med Assoc 1978;172:304–9.

The Ambulatory Practitioner and the Referral Center: Two Perspectives in Equine Surgery

Mike Graper, DVM[a], A.T. Fischer Jr, DVM[b],*

KEYWORDS

- Equine veterinarian • Ambulatory • Referral • Surgery

SURGERY FOR THE EQUINE AMBULATORY VETERINARIAN

A successful ambulatory equine practice strives for efficiency in all areas, from vehicle fuel economy to inventory overhead. While elective procedures can usually be scheduled with maximum efficiency in mind, horses and their penchant for trouble mean that surgery can add an inherently inefficient component to the practitioner's schedule. Still, surgeries can add a level of challenge and interest to ambulatory practice, and good surgical skills can serve as something that can distinguish the practitioner, and increase his or her reputation in the local and regional equine community.

Equipment

Surgery equipment for the ambulatory practitioner need not be extensive. The author carries 2 sterile full packs (the "spay pack" is adequate) and 2 sterile suture packs for minor lacerations. Most instrument manufacturers produce an instrument package at a price reduced from that of individual instrument purchase. The typical spay pack includes a Snook hook, needle holder, Mayo scissor, Metzenbaum scissor, Adson Brown forceps, knife handle, 4 Backhaus towel forceps, 2 Halstead mosquito hemostats, 2 Kelly hemostats, 2 straight Rochester Carmalts, 2 curved Rochester Carmalts, and an Allis forceps. Most manufacturers will allow substitution of another instrument in place of the Snook hook or other instrument. Additional instruments, such as emasculators, retractors, tenotomy knives, etc, may be individually packaged or wrapped as desired.

The authors have nothing to disclose.
a Private Practice, Cornerstone Equine Services, 2680 Kennedy Road, Rhinelander, WI 54501, USA
b Chino Valley Equine Hospital, 2945 English Place, Chino Hills, CA 91709, USA
* Corresponding author.
E-mail address: t.fischer@att.net

Vet Clin Equine 28 (2012) 69–81
doi:10.1016/j.cveq.2012.03.002
0749-0739/12/$ – see front matter © 2012 Published by Elsevier Inc.

vetequine.theclinics.com

Of course, a variety of suture materials are desirable for the equine ambulatory practitioners, based mostly on the preferences of the veterinarian. Several sizes of nonabsorbable sutures may be needed. For example, thinner material is ideal for surgeries around the eye, while thicker material may be needed to appose the skin of the flank. One or 2 absorbable sizes of absorbable suture material are usually all that are needed. Bandage materials suitable for covering a variety of surgical wounds reflect the preference of the practitioner but should include (1) something to cover the wound (eg, a nonstick pad), (2) something to secure the item covering the wound (eg, self-adherent gauze), (3) material to wrap over and protect the area (eg, a bulky cotton bandage), and (4) something to secure the protecting material (eg, self-adherent or adhesive bandage).

Surgeries

Surgery in equine ambulatory practice may be simplified into 2 categories: elective and emergency. Emergency surgeries are most commonly repairs of various injuries and can occur at any time. Elective procedures can be scheduled at the clinician's convenience, allow the clinician to demonstrate his or her skills, and provide a good deal of professional satisfaction.

Ambulatory equine veterinarians need to give a great deal of thought to what surgical procedures will be undertaken in the field. A remarkable number of procedures can be successfully and safely performed in the field by equine ambulatory clinicians with adequate training; including, but certainly not limited to, umbilical hernia repair, palmar digital neurectomy, inferior check ligament desmotomy, and excisional procedures for various dermatologic conditions. Both owner and veterinarian must be comfortable with the procedure(s) being recommended. After presenting different surgical options, the informed owner may select the one with which he or she feels most comfortable.

Client circumstances may also dictate which surgical procedures can be performed, as well as the setting under which they may be performed. For example, in the case of a puncture wound to the central frog, an ambulatory clinician could offer referral for radiographs, contrast studies, surgical debridement, regional and systemic antibiotics, and hospital plate shoe application. At the other end of the treatment spectrum, if economic circumstances dictate, wound exploration, tetanus prophylaxis, antibiotics, and phenylbutazone might be administered. While it may not be possible for the equine ambulatory clinician to offer surgical services under the conditions as can be offered in a hospital, it does not also mean that quality surgical services cannot be provided by the equine ambulatory clinician.

The "best" treatment option considers the circumstances of both the horse and the client, as well as the ability of the veterinarian providing treatment. For some clients, referral is not an option, but, under any circumstances, it is important to both offer and document the best course of treatment for the patient, and to include any other viable options for consideration. The logistics of provision of aftercare should be heavily considered as well, with respect to the veterinarian's schedule and ultimate cost to the owner.

When cost considerations dictate, ambulatory clinicians may be able to suggest strategies to reduce the cost of care for the client, while still providing effective treatment. For example, many tendon lacerations can be effectively managed on the farm, but for these and other surgeries, it is not unusual for the cost of treatment on the farm to exceed that of treatment at a referral facility once repeated farm calls are factored in; the client should not assume that treatment on the farm will always be less costly. One option to present is transporting the case to a farm closer to the veterinarian's base of operations or where another case is in residence. This can greatly improve the efficiency of the veterinarian's daily schedule and decrease overall costs to the client.

Finally, it is important for the ambulatory clinician to present all options for the surgical case to the owner. This is both good practice, and it limits the clinician's liability exposure. An equine ambulatory veterinarian should consult with his or her liability insurance carrier prior to deciding which of the more complex surgical cases to undertake on the farm, especially when referral has been recommended but declined. The insurance carrier can also guide the veterinarian as to proper record keeping in such cases, including what type of documentation should be acquired.

Castrations

Of all the elective surgical procedures the ambulatory clinician will encounter, castrations are typically the most common. Castration techniques may be broadly divided into standing or recumbent approaches. The surgeon then has several options for the surgical procedure, including open, closed techniques, or open-closed techniques. Other choices include the choice of primary closure or second intention healing, as well as the type of emasculator used.[1] An additional choice of instrument exists; a closed castration technique using torsion of the spermatic cord has also been described.[2]

The "right" castration technique is one the ambulatory clinician is proficient and comfortable with. Hopefully, through the course of his or her education, the surgeon has been exposed to several methods and has been able to select the one he or she prefers. Comfort with a chosen technique allows for more consistent procedures, less anesthesia time, and fewer complications. It behooves the ambulatory surgeon to be familiar with several techniques for castrations; for example, standing castrations are technically difficult in miniatures and small ponies, but a stallion with reduced carpal range of motion due to degenerative joint disease may have more difficulty recovering from general anesthesia and may be a better candidate for the standing procedure.

After a physical exam, including palpation of the scrotum and external inguinal canals to ensure that both testicles have normally descended and that no inguinal hernias are palpable, and after confirming current tetanus prophylaxis, the author prefers to castrate the horse under general anesthesia after sedation with xylazine (1.1 mg/kg IV). Anesthesia is induced using ketamine (2.2 mg/kg IV) once the horse exhibits profound sedation with the muzzle at or below the level of the carpus.[3] For older or more fractious horses, diazepam (0.5–1.0 mg/kg IV) may be added to the ketamine to provide better muscle relaxation; some practitioners assert that the addition of diazepam provides smoother recoveries.

Individual variations among practitioners in the castration procedure include:

1. **Patient positioning.** Dorsal recumbency can be maintained with hay bales at each shoulder or with assistants holding the horse in place. The uppermost hind limb may be tied forward or held to the side with a soft rope. The author prefers not to depend on the presence of assistants and holds the uppermost hindlimb abducted behind his knee (**Fig. 1**). This provides excellent access to the surgical site and affords a barrier for the surgeon's head should the patient move during surgery.
2. **Choice of preoperative preparation solutions.** The author scrubs the scrotum and inguinal area with alternating povidone-iodine surgical scrub and 70% isopropyl alcohol, and uses a total of 3 scrub cycles.
3. **Injection of anesthetic into the testicle or cord.** Mandatory in standing castrations, the author also injects 15 to 30 mL of 2% lidocaine into each testicle to

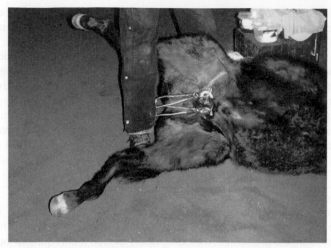

Fig. 1. Patient positioning for castration procedure. The author (Dr Graper) holds the uppermost hindlimb abducted behind his knee. This provides excellent access to the surgical site and affords a barrier for the surgeon's head should the patient move during surgery.

anesthetize the cords and cremaster muscles[4] prior to castration and then performs a final scrub.

4. **Choice of technique.** The author prefers an open technique,[1] using 2 locking emasculators. This technique allows extended crushing time on the cords, improves hemostasis, and makes ligation of the cords unnecessary. The need to transect the cords independent of the emasculators adds an extra step but very little extra time. With this method, in the author's experience, donkeys and mules, typically notorious for excessive bleeding after castration, have no more postsurgical hemorrhage than other equids.

5. **Choice of instrument.** The author prefers a Sands castration clamp, placed on each cord, with the testicles removed with a scalpel. The emasculators are left locked on the cords until the patient begins to be responsive, typically 5 minutes or longer. Numerous other castration instruments exist that both clamp and cut, including Reimer's, Serra, Hausmann, Frank, and White, in addition to the Henderson castration tool.

6. **Preoperative antibiotics.** Research supports the administration of preoperative penicillin to help reduce postoperative inflammation.[5] The surgeon should weigh the advantages of reduced inflammatory processes against exposure of resident microflora to antimicrobials with future resistance in mind. The author does not use perioperative antibiotics with routine castrations.

While the horse is under anesthesia, there may be time to perform other procedures, such as wolf tooth removal. During this time postsurgical management may also be discussed with the client. The author advises that the horse be kept in a stall or small paddock for the first day. Exercise is subsequently encouraged to minimize swelling and promote drainage of the scrotal incisions.

Phenylbutazone (2.2–4.4 mg/kg PO) may be used to prevent swelling and discomfort. In the author's experience, complications such as excessive swelling are uncommon and typically respond to increased exercise.[6]

Castration of cryptorchid horses is best done at a referral facility due to the potential for the need for intra-abdominal exploration. With respect to cryptorchids, if the veterinarian is not prepared to locate the illusive gonad at any point from the internal inguinal ring to its origins at the caudal pole of the ipsilateral kidney, referral should be the first recommendation. Referral should be recommended for these and other surgical cases where a controlled aseptic environment, extended monitoring, or specialized equipment (eg, laparoscopic instrumentation) is needed.

More complex procedures generally require prolonged anesthesia time. General anesthesia time can be extended by administering an additional injection of 50% of the original dose of xylazine and ketamine, combined in the same syringe. For procedures taking longer than the time provided by the xylazine/ketamine/diazepam protocol, a "triple drip" intravenous combination of 1 L of 5% guaifenesin, 1000 mg ketamine, and 500 mg xylazine can be administered via an intravenous catheter. Administration to effect up to 1 mL/kg/hr can be used, for a maximum of 1-hour anesthesia time.[7]

Non-Elective Procedures

Nonelective surgery in ambulatory equine medicine frequently involves lacerations, particularly of the lower limbs. Proper management of these injuries aids in minimizing lost time in the ambulatory schedule and maximizing patient care. Suggestions for efficient management of such conditions include:

1. Using regional anesthesia rather than local wound infiltration. This maintains tissue integrity, and decreases amount of sedation or general anesthesia required. The equine ambulatory clinician should be familiar with areas of the horse's body adequately anesthetized by regional anesthetic techniques.[8,9]
2. For *extensive lacerations or deep punctures of the lower limb or foot,* intravenous regional anesthesia (IVRA, Bier block) provides excellent analgesia and hemostasis.
3. *Regional perfusion of antibiotics* is an invaluable modality when faced with deep infection or synovial structure involvement[10] and can be combined with the Bier block via the same catheter. This combination is ideal for debridement of deep penetrating wounds of the foot. If significant swelling prevents identification of a suitable vein for catheterization, a pressure bandage may be placed and the regional perfusion performed later in the day or the next day, once the swelling has subsided.
4. *Healing of heel bulb and tendon lacerations*, as well as lacerations over joints is aided by the use of casting. For heel bulb lacerations, a foot cast is adequate.[11] For more extensive lacerations, casts should be applied to as to ensure normal phalangeal alignment.
5. For *wounds below the carpus or tarsus* that cannot be closed, or that need repeated debridement or regional antibiotic perfusion, a cast may still be used by applying cast material over the bandage and bivalving the cast. This allows bandage changes as often as needed, while maintaining immobilization.[12] Most clients can manage these changes adequately, minimizing the number of return farm visits.
6. It is helpful for clients to take *digital photographs* and text-message or e-mail them to the veterinarian to aid in monitoring progress and in scheduling further farm visits. A cell phone camera picture can often help the veterinarian on the road decide how to manage the daily schedule, if the wound needs attention that merits an earlier visit than originally planned.

One consistently frustrating aspect of ambulatory surgery is maintenance of a sterile (or more accurately aseptic) field. Wind, flying insects, and farm pets provide ample opportunity for breach of conditions. Sequestering dogs and/or cats in a stall and hanging a box fan near the surgery site to discourage flies are often helpful in maintaining a clean surgical field. If the surgery is elective, scheduling the procedure after dusk can also minimize interference of flying insects. The author carries several separate packs of autoclaved disposable paper cloth drapes, which can be cut to fit most surgical site requirements, or fenestrated as needed.

Referral

Establishing a relationship with a referral facility is an important part of ambulatory equine practice. If there are several facilities within a reasonable distance, becoming familiar with all of them will enable clients to have options with respect to cost, distance, imaging options, surgeon's specialties, etc. If possible, the referring veterinarian should spend some time in the referral facility to be able to answer as many anticipated client questions as possible. A detailed explanation of the referral process, from admission through discharge, can greatly ease the mind of the concerned owner.

While some referral clinics prefer to have as much preparatory work done as possible, in general, in an ambulatory setting, it is often most efficient in emergency referrals to forego some diagnostic or treatment procedures (abdominocentesis, jugular catheter placement, etc) in the interest of getting the horse to the facility without delay (eg, in cases of referral for colic surgery). After the horse is discharged, the ambulatory clinician should request detailed discharge instructions for follow-up examination scheduling, as well as copies of imaging studies for the patient's record.

If referral is not possible, for example, due to the inability to transport the horse or the client's economic circumstances, the clinician may be faced with a situation where adequate care for a significant injury cannot be provided in the field. Under such circumstances, or where the client cannot afford the cost of care, euthanasia should be presented as a humane option.

Summary

Surgery in ambulatory equine practice can be frustrating, due to lack of handlers, lack of client resources, or lack of adequate facilities. However, surgery in the field can be performed successfully despite such limitations, and good surgical skills are an excellent way to build a good reputation in the equine community. Thorough consultation with the client regarding initial care, frequent communication during on-the-farm management and referral, when necessary, can make the daily schedule easier to manage, and allow the equine ambulatory clinician to provide optimum patient care.

THE OTHER SIDE OF THE COIN: FROM THE REFERRAL PERSPECTIVE

Practicing at a referral hospital offers special challenges to the veterinarian. A referral hospital has a different perspective on client relationships. A referral hospital must remember that the number one client of the referral hospital is the referring veterinarian. The referral hospital's job is to provide care to the referred animal and client. The referring veterinarian has trusted the hospital with work that cannot be done in the field or is better done at the referral center. When care is completed on the horse, the referral center should return the client and the horse to the care of the referring veterinarian. While there will be some natural areas of competition between the referring veterinarian and the referral center, the primary job of the referral center is to support the referring veterinarian and not compete with them.

Create Reasonable Expectations

It is important for the referring veterinarian to create reasonable expectations for the client and their visit to the referral hospital. The client should be assured that the horse is being sent to a place that the veterinarian trusts, staffed with people who can help both the client and the horse.

Referring veterinarians should not be too specific in their referral recommendations. For example, one area of potential problems with colic referrals is when the client is told to take their horse to the hospital for abdominal radiographs instead of an examination for colic. The author's clinic frequently sees horses presenting for colic with a heart rate of 80 beats per minute and severe abdominal pain—signs that are more likely to be as a result of a small intestinal incarceration than an enterolith—and then has to convince the owner to allow an abdominal ultrasound instead of abdominal radiographs. Under such circumstances, sometimes, the clinic is almost forced to do the abdominal radiographs first to be able to perform an ultrasound, which results in an unnecessary procedure and charge to the client. If the client had been referred for further evaluation instead of a specific procedure, the diagnosis could have been obtained less expensively and more efficiently.

The same scenario can also occur during lameness evaluation referrals, if the client is told to take the horse to the hospital for an ultrasonographic evaluation or radiography of a specific area without definitive nerve blocks having been previously performed. The referral center is then must explain to the client why a different test or examination is indicated. When expectations of what treatment should be provided conflict with what may be indicated for the horse, this can set up an unnecessary conflict between client, referring veterinarian, and the referral center.

Economics

Clients should be advised of the referral hospital's financial policies in advance of arrival at the hospital to minimize surprises to them, reduce the opportunity for conflicts, and avoid economic hardship. Obtaining cost estimates may be handled in several ways. The referring veterinarian may contact the hospital on the clients' behalf and obtain an estimate of cost for the anticipated services and inform the client. Many hospitals have a place on their website where their financial policies are disclosed; the client can be directed to that site. Alternatively, the horse owner can be put in direct contact with the referral center once the referral is made and the policies and anticipated costs can be discussed with the attending clinician.

The author's clinic prefers that the attending veterinarian at the clinic talk to the client about costs rather than having the task performed by an office staff member. The attending veterinarian can often provide more details and a more accurate estimate of what will be done and what the medical possibilities are. Direct communication with the hospital prior to arrival starts the new client/referral center relationship and provides the client with someone to talk to prior to arrival. In the author's opinion, direct communication with the referral center has the best chance of minimizing confusion regarding costs and policies and keeps the referring veterinarian out of the middle of an already stressful event for the horse owner.

Referral should be a team effort. The referral center should involve the referring veterinarian in the case and may even ask for their assistance with explanation of anticipated treatments or prognosis. The referral clinic expects that if there is something significant in the referring veterinarian's relationship with the client, it is informed in advance. Referral clinics receive clients that range from the great long-term client who does whatever is necessary for their animal, to clients with a known unwillingness to pay for care of their animals, past veterinary litigation, or unwillingness to follow treatment recommendations. It is important that the client realize that the referral center and the ambulatory practitioner are separate entities and different policies will apply.

Avenues of Communication

Communication is almost instant, with access to the Internet, cell phones, and texting (to name a few avenues). The ease of communication provides an opportunity for the referral center to stay in touch with the referring veterinarians and keep them apprised of the status of a case. From the referral hospital side, it is helpful to know how much (or little) contact and information the referring veterinarian wants. The author's clinic sees varying levels of interest and involvement once a case has been referred in. Some veterinarians wish only to have a copy of the discharge summary and not be called as long as things are going well, while other veterinarians are looking for daily or more frequent updates. If the referral center is communicating more or less than what is desired, they should be advised of that fact.

It is also helpful if the referral clinic is aware of the referring veterinarian's preferred method of communication. Is a simple text message enough information, or should a referral letter in a PDF format to be added to your records? Does the referring veterinarian want or expect copies of laboratory results and imaging studies? All of these communication concerns also apply to the referral center's communications with the client and trainers. Finding out what expectations everyone has for communications makes for good relationships.

It is important for the referral center to avoid surprises to the client or referring veterinarian. This is best accomplished by open and frequent communication. Clients need to be kept updated on the status of their horse, changes in care, and charges that are being incurred so they can actively participate in their horse's treatment decisions. Clients do not like to find out that their bill has doubled due to a complication that they did not know about. Complications should be dealt with in a timely fashion and explained as to effects on prognosis and the costs that will be incurred. The author's clinic tries to include a discussion of complications in consent forms, as well as in explanations of the management of the case at the beginning of treatment. Similarly, the status of a case should be updated with the referring veterinarian on a regular basis. The author's clinic generally does not update the referring veterinarian on cases once they are doing well with no complications expected. A discharge summary will be sent at the time of discharge. If complications are occurring or there are conflicts regarding the care of the horse, more frequent communication will occur with the referring veterinarian. It is helpful that the referring veterinarian has knowledge of what is going on so that they can support their client and help them with any decisions that need to be made. If a referring veterinarian believes that more information regarding the case is needed, or more frequent updates are appropriate, he or she should let the referral center know so that these needs can be addressed.

Things Not to Say

Practicing at a referral hospital requires clear communication skills to keep the client informed and the relationship with the referring veterinarian smooth. Unfortunately, sometimes the referral hospital veterinarians may say things that may make the goal of smooth communications more difficult. The following are statements that are best avoided.

"It is too late" This is interpreted by the client to mean that the referral was late and that is why the animal is not going to survive, when what was meant is that the horse has a poor survival prognosis (for whatever reason).

"If only it had been sent in earlier" See above.

"Why would Dr X have done that?" The referral center doesn't know what the referring veterinarian was looking at and what the client was allowing the veterinarian to do. The author's clinic always assumes that the referring veterinarian was doing what he or she thought was in the best interest of the client and horse.

"We don't do it that way." This statement implies that whatever was done was not done properly. For example, while the referral clinic may not use a certain antibiotic in the hospital that is used in the field, it is important for the client to understand that the referral center deals with different population of horses than is in the field, with significantly more stressors. This information should be clearly communicated to the client.

Veterinarians working in referral centers should be aware that some communications difficulties can be caused by the client, and that they are on the same team as the referring veterinarian. Many things that are stated by the client as to what the referring veterinarian has said are simply misunderstandings by the client, or occasionally even fabrications. If there is confusion or concern about information that purportedly came from the referring veterinarian, it is important for the referral center to contact the referring veterinarian and find out exactly what was said, rather than simply accepting what the client represents as fact.

Education

Practicing at a referral center allows for a different perspective on cases and frequently allows the development of more refined techniques for diagnostics. Practitioners in referral centers also generally have access to diagnostic equipment that is not readily available in the field. While many of these technologies can be adapted for field use, or are already in the ambulatory vehicle, they may not be used to the extent that they can be used. An example would be the use of ultrasonography on the thorax or abdomen. Ambulatory practitioners have more opportunities to use ultrasonography on limbs than on any other area and may not be as familiar with use of their machines in other areas. Even so, many ultrasound machines have adjustable frequencies that allow for the deeper penetration necessary for these areas.

Referral hospitals can serve as a good source of continuing education for referring veterinarians. The author's clinic encourages referring veterinarians to use their machines to evaluate these areas on cases that they are referring in for abdominal or thoracic disease. When referring veterinarians express uncertainty about their ability to perform these studies, the author's clinic invites them to the hospital to try it on our patients, with some guidance from hospital staff. Such collaboration benefits horses by improving diagnostic capabilities of veterinarians in the field and improves the relationship between the referring veterinarian and the referral center.

Other areas of education include evaluation of referral radiographs. Referral clinics can provide suggestions for additional images or different evaluation techniques, as well as provide an additional opinion on the case. Field radiography has been immeasurably improved by the dissemination of computed and digital radiography systems allowing immediate review in the field for image quality and positioning.

Some of these exchanges occur face to face but many occur by electronic exchange of images and phone/e-mail/text discussions. It is preferable to make DICOM studies (instead of JPEGs or other lossy types of images) available to the referral center to allow the most accurate data set to be evaluated. When radiographs are available for horses that are being referred, these studies should be provided to the referral center in advance, so that the study is already at the referral center when the horse arrives. The author's clinic frequently must redo studies when the original study was left at the barn by the hauler or trainer, or not mailed in time. Repeating studies unnecessarily increases the client's expense and the staff's exposure to x-rays. In such circumstances, the author's clinic has often discounted the repeat study to avoid antagonizing the owner toward the referring veterinarian.

Continuing education events are frequently hosted by referral centers and have the benefit of providing face to face contact and education. These events are usually subsidized jointly by vendors and the referral centers but do require an investment of time and money by both. The vendors profit from the exposure of their products and representatives to the ambulatory practitioners, which can be hard to obtain due to the ambulatory practitioner's schedule and mobile lifestyle. The author's clinic tries to provide lectures from the staff on topics that are useful to the ambulatory practitioners and solicits input on topics that are of interest. Much of the important contacts occur on the side of the meeting in informal conversations on the side.

Improving the skill set of the referring clinician improves the quality of the referred case and allows both the referral center and referring veterinarian to do a better job. Education is always a 2-way street. Staff at the referral center should have an open mind when communicating with referring veterinarians. Many ambulatory veterinarians have areas of extensive experience and interest and can be coaxed to share their expertise when having a discussion. These discussions turn into both a learning experience for the veterinarian at the referral center and a way to foster the bond between the referral center and the referring veterinarian.

Managing Complications of Others

In the referral hospital, it is not unusual to receive cases that have sustained a complication following a field procedure. Many of these complications are an accepted risk of the procedure, and the client should be made aware of the possibility of such complications prior to the procedure being performed. It is important for the veterinarian who is performing any procedure to clearly communicate possible complications for any procedure to prevent the scenario where the client claims that complications were not properly discussed, leaving open an accusation of improper consent. However, it is also important for the referral center to remind the client that complications may occur, so that the referring veterinarian is not accused of doing something wrong. Most complications are not due to malpractice and the referral center should stress this fact to the client.

Complications are also an opportunity for continuing education for the referring veterinarian if handled appropriately by the referral center. Suggestions for case management can be offered and observations on why the complication might have occurred can be discussed. Prompt referral should be reinforced positively to both the client and referring veterinarian.

Some clients will expect that the referring veterinarian pay for the management of complications. The author's clinic discourages this and points out that the complication is due to the procedure that the client requested and consented to on their horse. Some veterinarians want to pay for the management of the complication to show good faith toward their client, but that should be an individual decision, not an expectation, and certainly not an admission of having done anything wrong. If the referring veterinarian does offer to pay for management of complications, he or she should expect to pay market rate for the veterinary services unless a discount is offered in advance.

Periodically, the author's clinic will see a surge in field procedures that probably should not be done in the field, along with their complications. An example would be abdominal cryptorchid castrations, with complications of not finding the testicle, evisceration, or hemorrhage. These complications have been obviated with the advent of laparoscopic surgery. Fortunately, field implementation of this procedure is becoming less frequent as the referring veterinarian realizes that the procedure is best done in a hospital setting, and that having the procedure done in the hospital obviates client disappointment over complications. Complications offer the opportunity for client education during management of the complication, for example, by explaining the difference between ways of accomplishing procedures. As such, the next time the client has a horse that is a cryptorchid, they may choose the more expensive referral procedure that precludes the complications and the second bill.

When managing complications, it is important for the referral center to not criticize the field attempt at the surgery when a client asks about why a procedure was done in the field but to rather focus on the differences of the procedures and advantages and disadvantages of each. For example, the advantages of field castration are no transportation, and lower costs; however, disadvantages include less equipment and lack of facilities to deal with complications. On the other hand, hospital castration has the disadvantages of increased costs and the necessity to transport the horse, but the advantages of monitored anesthesia, equipment, and facilities to deal with complications and the ability to perform primary closure if desired. Ultimately, the client will choose the procedure and location with the information that has been provided. Clients appreciate the option of referral, and a successful outcome from a referred case only reinforces the client's confidence in the referring veterinarian.

Managing the broken referral center/referring veterinarian relationship
Despite the best intentions of the referral center and the referring veterinarian, situations might occur where a dispute arises between them. These disputes may arise over lack of communication, or from differences of opinion regarding case management, or from poor outcomes. Common sense would dictate a mature discussion over the area of conflict and agreement on a resolution. Disparaging a colleague in front of other colleagues or clients does nothing positive for the profession and only lessens their opinion of the professionalism of the veterinarian doing the disparaging. In some cases, it may be best to just agree to disagree and go separate ways.

Most ambulatory practice areas have multiple referral centers, and the referring veterinarian should use the one that best meets their needs. Referring veterinarians should certainly suggest which referral center that they prefer, but not be too adamant about sending to a specific one. If the client is dissatisfied with their outcome, that dissatisfaction can come back to the referring veterinarian, as well; the client will blame the referring veterinarian for pushing the client to go to clinic x when the client wanted to go to clinic y.

Tips for referring veterinarians
When referring in a horse with colic and nasogastric reflux, it should be sent in with a taped in nasogastric tube. The tube will be returned to you by the referral center or sent back with the owner.

When sending in a horse with an unstable limb (fractures or luxations), the referring veterinarian should contact the referral center regarding what type of splint or cast is appropriate if there are questions.

Please provide a list and chronology of administered drugs and therapies to provide continuity of care and appropriate dosing. This can be communicated verbally, written or electronically.

Avoid high doses of sedatives and analgesics when referring in horses with colic. High doses can obscure the clinical picture and delay therapeutic interventions.

Horses requiring repetitive sedation/analgesic administration with a surgical management option should be referred promptly. Further diagnostics can be performed at the referral center and should not be done in the field if it is going to delay the referral.

It is generally more cost effective for the owner to refer horses with colic after your second visit if the horse is not making significant progress.

SUMMARY

Practicing at a referral center makes one aware of the necessity for consistent clear communication with the referring veterinarians. The referring veterinarian is ultimately the primary client of the referral center and should be respected as such. Once the necessary care has been provided, the client and horse should be returned to the care of the referring veterinarian. It is important that the referring veterinarian stay involved in the case and communicate if they wish for more or less contact with the referral center.

REFERENCES

1. Searle D, Dart AJ, Dart CM, et al. Equine castration: review of anatomy, approaches, techniques and complications in normal, cryptorchid and monorchid horses. Aust Vet J 1999;77:428–34.
2. Reilly MT, Cimetti LJ. How to use the Henderson Castrating Instrument and minimize castration complications. In: Proceedings of the 51st Annual Convention of the American Association of Equine Practitioners. Lexington (KY): American Association of Equine Practitioners; 2005. p. 494–7.
3. Trotter GW. Castration. In: McKinnon AO, Voss JL, editors. Equine reproduction. Philadelphia: Lea & Febiger; 1993. p. 907–14.
4. Galliou M, Tainturier D, Holopherne D. Analgesic efficacy of local infiltration of lidocaine during castration in anesthetized horses. In: Proceedings of the 9th International Congress of World Equine Veterinary Association. Ithaca (NY): International Veterinary Information Service; 2006. p. 249–50.
5. Busk P, Jacobsen S, Martinussen T. Administration of perioperative penicillin reduces postoperative serum amyloid A response in horses being castrated standing. Vet Surg 2010;39:638–43.
6. Getman LM. Review of castration complications: strategies for treatment in the field. In: Proceedings of the 55th Annual Convention of the American Association of Equine Practitioners. Lexington (KY): American Association of Equine Practitioners; 2009. p. 374–8.
7. Hubbell JAE. Options for field anesthesia in the horse. In: Proceedings of the 45th Annual Convention of the American Association of Equine Practitioners. Lexington (KY): American Association of Equine Practitioners; 1999. p. 120–1.
8. Archer M. Regional anesthesia of the equine head and body. In: Proceedings of the American College of Veterinary Surgeons Veterinary Symposium. Malden (MA): Wiley-Blackwell, John Wiley & Sons, Inc; 2011. p. 5880–4.

9. Moyer W, Schumacher J, Schumacher J. A guide to equine joint injection and regional anesthesia. Yardley, PA: Veterinary Learning Systems; 2007.
10. Palmer SE, Hogan PM. How to perform regional limb perfusion in the standing horse. In: Proceedings of the 45th Annual Convention of the American Association of Equine Practitioners. Lexington (KY): American Association of Equine Practitioners; 1999. p. 124–7.
11. Fitzgerald BW, Honnas CM, Plummer AE, et al. How to apply a hindlimb phalangeal cast in the standing patient and minimize complications. In: Proceedings Of the 52nd Annual Convention of the American Association of Equine Practitioners. Lexington (KY): American Association of Equine Practitioners; 2006. p. 631–5.
12. Hogan PM. How to make a bandage cast and indications for its use. In: Proceedings of the 46th Annual Convention of the American Association of Equine Practitioners. Lexington (KY): American Association of Equine Practitioners; 2000. p. 150–2.

Wound Care in Horses

Stephanie S. Caston, DVM

KEYWORDS

- Horses • Equine practice • Wounds • Tendons and ligaments
- Healing • Treatment

Wounds are common in equine patients. Due to the horse's nature and the environment in which it lives, wounds frequently involve a significant amount of tissue trauma. Legs caught in fences, panels, wire, or gates are a frequent occurrence, as are lacerations from steel siding, trailer accidents, kicks, and riding accidents. As a result, equine ambulatory practitioners typically see a relatively large number of cases presenting for wound care. Enormous variation exists in treatments, medications, bandages, and bandaging techniques applied to wounds in horses.[1–5] In addition, products marketed to owners for wound care are ubiquitous, numerous, and sometimes dangerous. In some instances, owners may try to treat the wound at home before consulting a veterinarian or they may acquire a horse that has an old wound. This leaves the equine veterinarian treating not only acute wounds but chronic and complicated wounds as well. To further complicate the issue, other factors, including economic constraints, and what is considered an acceptable end result, will often play major roles in the decision-making process.

To develop an intelligent, workable plan for dealing with wounds, an equine practitioner must first have a good working knowledge of anatomy. There is no magic ointment, salve, or injection that makes wound healing easy. The practitioner must be well versed in the wound-healing process and recognize what he or she can and cannot do to assist that process. This will also allow the practitioner to recognize when the wound-healing process is not going according to plan and to ascertain what has happened to complicate the process. This article will review evaluation of a wound, the normal process of wound healing, and general management of full-thickness skin wounds, as well as an approach to managing them.

WOUND ASSESSMENT

The initial assessment of a wound should include careful attention to its anatomical location. Answering a few important questions can help determine what structures the wound affects, and prioritize treatment objectives. First: are structures involved that need more in depth attention? Second: is there involvement of a structure that if

The author has nothing to disclose.

Department of Veterinary Clinical Sciences, College of Veterinary Medicine, Iowa State University, 1600 South 16th Street, Ames, IA 50010, USA

E-mail address: scaston@iastate.edu

Vet Clin Equine 28 (2012) 83–100

doi:10.1016/j.cveq.2012.01.001

0749-0739/12/$ – see front matter © 2012 Elsevier Inc. All rights reserved.

damaged or contaminated could be life threatening or career limiting? Damage to structures such as thoracic or abdominal cavities, large vessels, synovial structures, fractures, flexor tendon, or suspensory ligament damage complicate wound management. Visual examination, careful digital exploration with a gloved hand, palpation and manipulation, ultrasound, and radiographs should all be used as needed to help determine what structures are involved and what is the extent of damage to them.

CATASTROPHIC WOUNDS

Catastrophic wounds should be evaluated in light of the best interests of both the horse and the client; treatment of such wounds can be difficult and expensive. If a wound communicates with the thoracic or abdominal cavity, it should be evaluated for occurrences such as fecal contamination of the abdomen, which might make wound care superfluous. If treatment of a catastrophic wound is desired, or possible, first aid should be applied, if necessary, after evaluation of the structures involved and possibly after consultation with a referral facility. Therapy for shock may be needed; the body cavity should be sealed if possible. Catastrophic wounds are very difficult to manage in the field, and, ideally, should be referred for further care.[6–8] Specific first aid management would best be decided. Complications like pneumothorax and peritonitis are more easily dealt with in a hospital setting.[7–9]

Hemorrhage is generally a cause for alarm for clients of the ambulatory practitioner. If a wound has damaged a large vessel(s) and severe bleeding is occurring, the vessel should be located and ligated or clamped. Ligating a severed vessel will not cause further damage and will stop bleeding; the practitioner should not hesitate to do so. If the source of bleeding cannot be located and bleeding does not cease, it may be necessary to apply a pressure bandage to help control the bleeding and consider anesthesia in the field or at a referral center as appropriate. If they are completely severed, vessels can retract a significant distance from the primary wound, making them difficult to locate. The volume of blood lost and circulatory status should be considered prior to sedation or anesthesia, and doses adjusted, accordingly. Bleeding from smaller vessels is less problematic; most bleeding from smaller vessels can be stopped with pressure from a good bandage. Regardless of the size of the vessel, either ligation or pressure or a combination thereof will almost always stop the bleeding; reassuring the owner that everything is going to be fine presents a separate challenge for the ambulatory practitioner. Under any circumstances, it is rare for a wound to cause bleeding that is fatal.

WOUNDS TO SYNOVIAL STRUCTURES

Wounds communicating with synovial structures can frequently have unfavorable outcomes.[10–14] If the wound is anywhere near a synovial structure, communication of the wound with the synovial structure should be ruled out. Some wounds that do not initially appear to involve synovial structures may actually involve them; the position of the skin and underlying tissues at the time of injury may mislead the ambulatory practitioner, unless further evaluation of the wound is undertaken. For example, a limb that sustains an injury while it is flexed is often then evaluated once the horse is standing with the limb in extension. In such cases, the skin wound may not be directly over the synovial structure. Wounds that may miss synovial structures initially may invade them subsequently; blunt trauma wounds can erode into synovial structures post wounding. Checking for communication of wounds with synovial structures requires familiarity with their anatomy and where to approach them for synoviocentesis and distention of the joint. An excellent field reference is available for joint injection techniques.[15]

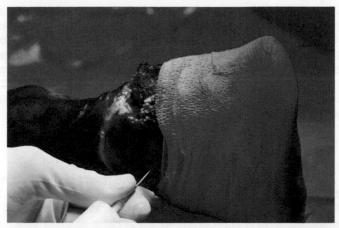

Fig. 1. A needle has been placed in the dorsal pouch of the coffin joint in the left forelimb. The horse is in right lateral recumbency. A solution of saline and procaine penicillin G is being injected, and the opaque, white fluid can be seen readily exiting the wound on the lateral pastern area.

Tips to evaluate whether a synovial structure has been penetrated include the following:

1. Prepare the joint or tendon sheath is routinely as for injection or synoviocentesis at a site remote from the wound, prior to inserting the needle.
2. Save a synovial fluid sample for cytology and culture if fluid is obtained.
3. Distend the synovial structure with a sterile solution, such as saline or lactated Ringer's solution.
4. In most subacute/chronic wounds that have penetrated a synovial structure, the synovium has sealed and it is easy to collect synovial fluid; it is not uncommon in acute cases to not be able to aspirate a sample because the synovial fluid is leaking into the wound. Fluid will normally exit the wound if it communicates with the synovial structure (**Fig. 1**).
5. An idea of the capacity of each synovial structure is useful. Some structures require a larger volume to distend. The veterinarian should avoid administering so much fluid in smaller joints so that they are potentially damaged.
6. Often, leaving the needle in place and disconnecting the syringe after the joint feels pressurized is useful in determining if the joint is intact. The injected solution and synovial fluid will normally come back out of the needle if it the joint capsule is intact.
7. A dilute solution (approximately 1:5) of procaine penicillin G and saline can help aid in visualization of the fluid exiting the wound (see **Fig. 1**).
8. Radiographs are also often helpful in assessing the synovial structures and the surrounding area for fractures, metallic foreign bodies, and air in tissues. A radiographic contrast study may be indicated in some cases to determine if a wound communicates with underlying structures.

Older wounds that communicate with a synovial structure frequently present with severe lameness. However, absence of severe lameness does not ensure the absence of synovial sepsis as an open synovial structure may not allow pressure to build within; intrasynovial pressure is a major source of pain. The possibility of fractures associated with a wound should be suspected if the horse is also acutely severely lame or if there is crepitus or instability on palpation. While most long bone fractures of the limbs are quite obvious due to the degree of swelling, inability to bear weight, and palpation findings, smaller, incomplete, or nondisplaced fractures may not be so obvious. Wounds on the head or face may have depression fractures that are not immediately apparent, especially if there is concurrent swelling. Again, radiographs of any area are rarely contraindicated when evaluating a wound and are frequently quite helpful in determining if fractures are present.

WOUNDS TO TENDONS AND LIGAMENTS

If a wound is on the palmar/plantar surface of a limb and the flexor tendons or suspensory ligament are lacerated or damaged, the wound should be cleaned and a heavy bandage applied. A splint is likely warranted if a tendon or ligament is severed.[16] For optimum outcome, referral to a clinic that can proceed with repair and/or external coaptation is appropriate for these cases as these structures are vital to athletic function and injuries to them can be career ending or even life threatening,[16–18] Selected cases can be managed in the field, although they may require a significant time and money commitment from the horse owner.

Injuries to flexor tendons or the suspensory ligament are in stark contrast to injuries to the extensor tendons that reside on the dorsal aspect of the limb. These tendons are often damaged during a traumatic equine limb wound that involves the dorsal cannon bone area. The extensor tendons can be damaged or even completely severed, and prognosis for return to full function may still be very good in most cases.[16,19] In the early period following disruption of the extensor tendons, a splint or very heavily padded bandage may be necessary to prevent the horse from knuckling over, which may slow healing due to mechanical disruption of the wound.[20,21]

WOUND-HEALING PROCESS

Once the wound has been evaluated and career-ending or life-threatening injuries have been ruled out, treated, or first aid and referral pursued, routine wound care begins. Horses suffering traumatic full-thickness skin wounds heal via a process that is typically divided into 3 phases. These phases—inflammation/debridement, proliferation, and maturation/remodeling—overlap temporally. Any process that prolongs or prevents a phase from proceeding to completion can prevent the next phase from being completed as well. The entire process is a complex occurrence that includes participation of cells, extracellular matrix, and many mediators.[22] This process is described in detail; there are also practical implications for wound management during each stage.

Inflammation

This phase starts at the time of wounding. The magnitude of the inflammatory reaction is directly correlated to the severity of the trauma and amount of tissue damage sustained with the injury.[22] White blood cells—primarily neutrophils—initially migrate to the site of injury to help clean up bacteria and debris, but macrophages will take over as the major inflammatory cell, killing bacteria, and helping in the debridement process, as well.[22] They also recruit other cells and thus initiate the angiogenesis, fibroplasia, and epithelialization of the proliferation phase.

Clinical signs seen by the ambulatory clinician during this period include the classic signs of swelling, heat, redness, and pain (**Fig. 2**). In addition, wounds become larger before getting smaller as tissues swell, retract, are debrided, and even slough

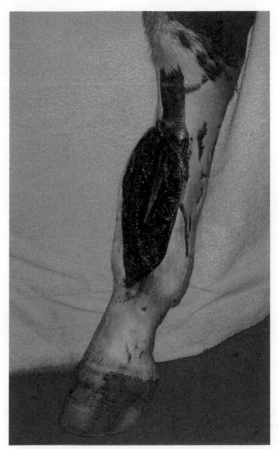

Fig. 2. Signs of inflammation, including swelling, can be appreciated in this wound on the dorsal cannon bone region of the right hind limb. This image was taken during the initial examination of the wound and it is approximately 36 hours since the wound occurred. The cannon bone is exposed in the center of the wound.

tissue.[23–25] In some cases where the injury that caused the wound involved blunt trauma, surrounding tissue that initially appears viable may not be, and skin flaps may not survive.[24] Inflammation that continues for a protracted period either due to ongoing trauma, sepsis, or wound mismanagement will not only prolong the inflammation/debridement phase but can also contribute to exuberant granulation tissue.[22] In addition, factors that prolong debridement such as sequestration of tissues or presence of reactive foreign bodies within the wound can prevent the completion of inflammation and debridement.[25,26]

Proliferation

Ideally, primary closure could be utilized in all wounds to allow for first-intention healing. This is often not possible, so then wounds must heal by second intention using proliferation, maturation, and remodeling. During the proliferative phase of wound healing, granulation tissue starts to fill the wound gap, becoming visible in a wound at about 3–5 days.[22,26] Fibroblasts, endothelial cells, and epithelial cells enter

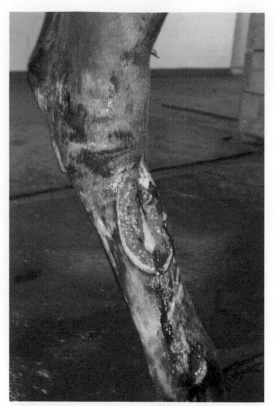

Fig. 3. Wound on the dorsal cannon bone region of a left hindlimb. The wound is approximately 6 days old and granulation tissue can be seen starting to fill the wound as well as a rim of new epithelium around the edge of the granulation tissue. The cannon bone is exposed in the center of the wound.

the wound during this phase, intiating fibroplasia and angiogenesis, along with continued debridement by macrophages. The multitude of new blood vessels along with the fibroblastic stroma gives healthy granulation tissue the classic pink-red "cobblestone" appearance[22] (**Fig. 3**). Not only does granulation tissue provide a surface for epithelial cell migration, but it provides both a physical and a physiologic barrier to infection.[22] If the granulation tissue has defects or is unhealthy, epithelialization can be impaired.[22] Epithelialization can be seen starting to occur around the wound edges at about 4–6 days post injury; its existence at the edges of a wound can give ambulatory practitioners hints as to when the wound occurred in chronic wounds that are being seen for the first time (see **Fig. 3**). During the proliferative period time, wound strength is still relatively poor,[26] and even as new epithelium covers the wound, it is easily traumatized, especially as it becomes thinner near the center of larger wounds.[22,26]

Maturation and Remodeling

The last stage of the normal healing process includes contraction and scar tissue formation. During the period starting about the second week after the wound occurs, contraction usually starts to occur.[23,24] Generally, in horses contraction is advantageous,

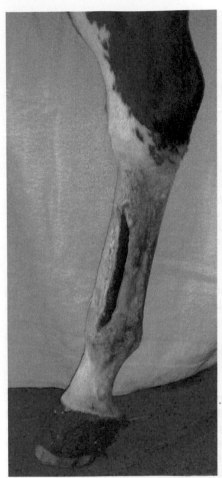 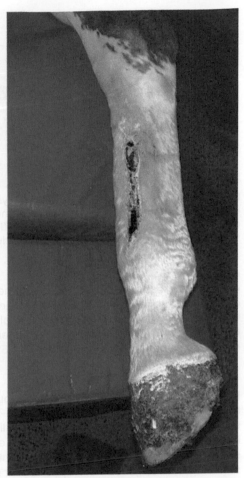

Fig. 4. This is the same case as in **Fig. 2**. The image on the left is at day 42, and the image on the right is at 70 days. The wound has filled in with granulation tissue, epithelialization and contraction are occurring. This horse was treated with bandaging and sequestrum removal.

as it lessens the distance the new epithelium has to cover; as such, it speeds closure of the wound and improves aesthetic appearance and strength[27] (**Fig. 4**). In a few locations, contraction can cause problems with cosmetics or function—notably the eyelid, lips, and ears—as it can distort the tissue, inhibits function, or results in stricture (**Fig. 5**). If the tension in the surrounding skin is too great, then contraction will be inhibited or stop. In addition, contraction will stop in very chronic wounds as the myofibroblast (which are responsible for contraction) numbers drop.[22] More contraction is possible in areas with loose skin than in areas with skin under tension; for example, pectoral wounds can contract considerably, whereas wounds to the distal limbs have a much more limited ability to contract.[22,27] The potential of tissue to contract has important implications in the clinical decision as to whether to try to close wounds by suturing or to simply let the wounds granulate and contract.

If a wound heals by second intention, the eventual end result of granulation tissue is its conversion to scar tissue. This proceeds by collagen synthesis, degradation, and

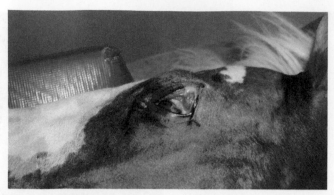

Fig. 5. Healed wound on the left upper eyelid. Loss of tissue and subsequent second-intention healing including contraction of the wound have caused eversion of the upper eyelid and loss of mobility. This horse had difficulty blinking. Recognition of this probability should have prompted a reconstructive procedure to be performed to prevent this end result.

eventually cross-linking and rearrangement. Remodeling of the scar tissue can continue for up to 2 years.[22] Over time, the tissue becomes more organized and less vascular, and the normal ratio of type I collagen to type III collagen (1:4) is restored. It is important for ambulatory practitioners to realize that even when scar tissue reaches full maturity, the wound will be 15%–20% weaker than the original tissue.[22]

TREATMENT OF THE WOUND

Following initial triage of the wound, it should be cleaned. Sedation will frequently be helpful. Treatment with nonsteroidal anti-inflammatory agents to reduce pain and swelling is also appropriate at this time. Clipping the hair around the wound is of use in getting and keeping the wound clean even if the wound will not be closed with sutures. Applying a water-soluble lubricant in the wound or packing the wound with saline moistened gauze can help keep hair out of the wound while clipping. If the area is covered in dried blood or mud/dirt, preliminary cleansing can begin with a hose. The hose should not have a sprayer nozzle attached; the sprayer can force water into tissue planes. The goal is merely to cleanse the surface. After clipping the hair and removal of the bulk of organic debris, the wound can be further cleansed with mild soap, dilute iodine, or dilute chlorhexidine soaps and rinsed with saline or another isotonic fluid. Large volume lavage utilizing isotonic fluids can also dilute contamination and help with the removal of foreign material.

A regional or local anesthetic block can facilitate debridement. Judicious sharp debridement can be used to remove a very thin layer of tissue if foreign material is embedded in the tissues. Skin flaps, especially on the head or below mid-forearm/mid- gaskin, should not be removed during sharp debridement. The viability of skin flaps will become readily apparent over the first few days post injury; any portion of a flap that remains viable can and will be used to aid in the healing process. The paucity of movable skin in some areas makes it such a desirable commodity that skin flaps should be given every possible opportunity to remain. Skin flaps on eyelids should never be removed at initial treatment. It is surprising in some cases, especially on the head and eyes, how much of a skin flap can remain viable. It is very easy to trim skin flaps, but there should not be a rush to do so. If there is any doubt about skin viability, err on the side of caution. Once you remove the skin, you are committed. As

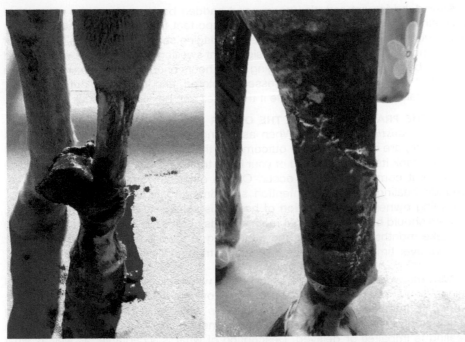

Fig. 6. Degloving injury to a left hindlimb before and after debridement/suturing. The cannon bone and extensor tendon are exposed prior to closure in the image on the left. These structures are covered and the skin flap is held in place in the image on the right.

compared to the upper body, the distal limb has greater skin tension, epithelialization is slower than on the body, and excessive granulation tissue is more likely to occur.[22,28]

Once the wound is cleaned and debrided, an effort should be made to close the wound, or to bring the edges as close together as possible. Suture patterns such as near-far-far-near and vertical mattress patterns—with or without stents—can be used to pull the skin edges together in cases where there is skin missing or there is enough swelling to create significant tension. Many suture patterns have been described for closing specific wounds, and those can be employed as the wound configuration dictates.[29,30] Even if the clinician suspects that a skin flap will later slough or the sutures dehisce due to tension or motion, closure of the wound should be attempted, even if only partially. Even a partial closure can help hold tissues in place, cover underlying structures, and reduce dead space (**Fig. 6**).

If the wound is highly contaminated or a large amount of dead space is present, a drain can be placed and then removed a few days later. A simple Penrose drain exiting the most ventral aspect of the wound or area of dead space is often sufficient.[30] Areas that cannot be closed or that were closed and later dehisce, will heal by second-intention wound healing. It is good practice to prepare owners for that occurrence and to counsel them on what to expect so that they do not perceive it as a failure on your part when dehiscence occurs. High motion areas, deep wounds, and areas that are difficult to bandage, such as those that may occur in the pectoral area or upper hindquarters, may dehisce. Owners should be aware of this possibility. Fortunately, these areas also heal very well as open wounds.[28]

After debridement and closure, a good padded bandage should be placed and maintained. A good bandage is extremely important for reducing the swelling in an acute wound, which can be severe (see Bandaging section) (see **Fig. 2**). In cases of distal limb wounds that already have significant swelling and might otherwise be hard to close because of tension, bandaging for 24 hours prior to wound repair can also be beneficial. The wound can be assessed, explored, and lavaged as outlined earlier, then reevaluated in 24 hours to see if the edges can be apposed under less tension.

WHAT THE PRACTITIONER AND THE OWNER SHOULD EXPECT

1. *Make realistic assessments.* When assessing and treating wounds, practitioners should prepare owners for likely outcomes at the time of the initial exam. The wound will likely look its best at the end of your initial treatment, but owners should be made aware that complications can occur. On the other hand, realistic expectations for wounds healing by second intention sometimes come as a surprise to owners. Informing owners of the duration of healing is something that is often overlooked; owners should be fully aware that most wounds healing by this process (unless small) will take months to heal. Care and bandaging of a wound can become tedious for owners over time, and they may discontinue treatments in frustration.

2. *Monitor wound healing.* The presence of wound fluid and the odor of a wound during bandage changes can disturb some owners and lead them to assume the wound is infected or healing poorly, even in cases where healing is progressing satisfactorily. On the other hand, some owners ignore or fail to recognize when healing is impaired or delayed. Description of what is acceptable, as well as what changes should initiate a call to the veterinarian, should be given to the owner to better their ability to monitor healing and assist in care of the wound. For example, the appearance of a healthy granulating wound versus one that is incomplete because of a sequestrum or foreign body, one that has developed exuberant granulation, or one that exhibits impaired/delayed healing is an example of a complication that might be discussed with clients in practice.

3. *Be prepared for complications.* If bone is exposed, as often happens in lower limb wounds, a sequestrum should be an expected outcome. Good debridement of the wound and the surface of the bone (with a curette or bone rasp) and closure of the skin, if possible, may help reduce the incidence or degree of sequestrum formation, but owners should be aware of a possible additional procedure to remove a sequestrum in the future. Sequestrum formation is usually evident radiographically within 3 weeks[31] and should be suspected if the granulation tissue has a cleft or defect when it has otherwise filled the wound (**Fig. 7**). Most sequestra can also be seen using ultrasound as well. Some horses exhibit lameness during the time the sequestrum is maturing at around 10–14 days; practitioners and owners need to be aware of this possibility. These horses can be up to grade 4/5 lame[32] when this occurs. The lameness is usually transient and can be alleviated with NSAID therapy. Sequestrum removal can often be performed in a standing, sedated horse. If the horse's nature or the location or extent of the wound makes standing removal difficult, short-term anesthesia can facilitate removal. Radiography and/or ultrasound can be helpful in determining if removal is complete.

4. *Consider skin grafting larger wounds.* Wounds that result in the loss of a large area of skin, especially on the limbs, either at the time of initial injury or after sloughing/debridement should be considered candidates for skin grafting. Owners should be advised that some wounds cannot heal, or heal poorly, with contraction and

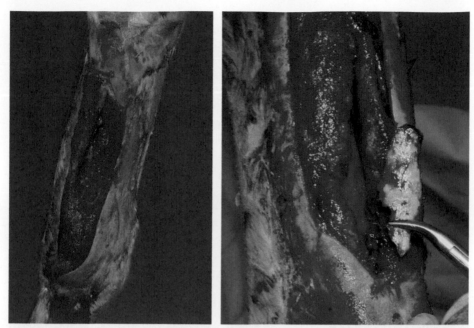

Fig. 7. This is the same case as in **Figs. 2** and **4**. The wound is approximately 3 weeks old, and a cleft can be seen in the granulation tissue in the image on the left. The sequestrum is shown in the image on the right at the time of removal.

epithelialization alone. Grafting can remedy this problem, and decrease healing time for many wounds. There are several techniques for free skin grafting frequently used in horses; the type chosen may depend on equipment available, cost, and expected cosmetic outcome. Pinch or punch skin grafts are relatively inexpensive, graft harvest and implantation can be performed in a standing horse, can be accepted even in less than ideal granulation beds,[33–35] and can be safely performed in the field. Success of each graft is independent of the others, so failure of one or more grafts does not affect the rest[35] (**Fig. 8**). Other grafting techniques, such as sheet grafting or tunnel grafting can cover larger areas and have a more cosmetic outcome but are often relatively expensive and require more specialized instruments than pinch or punch grafts[33–35] and must be performed under general anesthesia, most commonly at referral facilities.[33]

BANDAGING

Even though it can be difficult, and expensive over time, the importance of a good bandage to equine wound care cannot be overstated. While there is some evidence that bandages can promote some degree of exuberant granulation tissue, other evidence suggests that bandaged wounds may heal faster than those that are not bandaged,[36] and a good bandage has many other beneficial effects on wound healing.[28] The qualifier *good* is significant; a poor bandage can, at best, be of little or no benefit to the patient and, at worst, be detrimental. A good bandage can help stop bleeding in an acute wound, prevent further contamination and trauma, restrict movement, provide a moist wound-healing environment, and reduce swelling.[4,21,28]

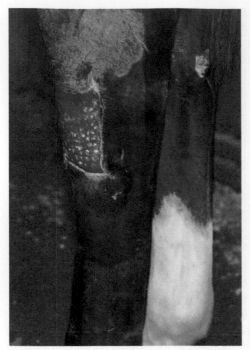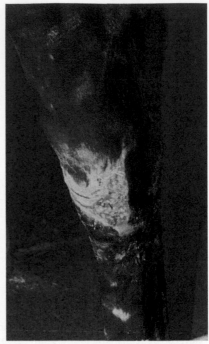

Fig. 8. Wound on the left tarsus that has been treated with pinch skin grafts. In the image on the left, an area where some grafts were lost can be seen in the proximal portion of the granulation bed and successful grafts in the distal and lateral portion of the wound. The image on the right is approximately 4 weeks later, and continued contraction of the wound and epithelialization can be appreciated. Hair is starting to grow from the graft islands as well.

Unfortunately, bandaging is often discontinued early in the process of wound care, is not performed, or is done improperly. This is likely because application and maintenance of a good bandage can be time consuming and require a good deal of work on the part of the veterinarian and owner. Use of an inadequate amount of padding is a very common pitfall. A number of cotton roll products exist, and any can be used to provide this padding. A compressive layer or 2 over the cotton, such as wide brown gauze followed by a self-adherent elastic bandage, will help secure the bandage and provide compression. Sealing the top and bottom of the bandage with an elastic adhesive tape helps keep the bandage in place and helps keep shavings and other debris out of the bandage.

Bandage changes can occur every few days in most cases. Early on, bandage changes may need to be more frequent if bleeding is still occurring or if treatments such as debridement, suturing, or regional limb perfusions are necessary. After the wound is stable, owners can change the bandage every 3–5 days or sooner if it slips down or gets torn, worn through, or very wet. In some instances, owners do not feel comfortable changing the bandage, or the horse requires sedation for bandage changes. In such cases, a heavily padded, very snug bandage fully covered with elastic adhesive tape may last 7–10 days. This seems a long period, but a good bandage should last that long and there should be no worry about leaving a bandage on for that duration if it stays intact—when casts are used to cover a wound, they are often left in place for 14 days or longer. Stall confinement will usually prolong the life of a bandage, but unless the injury requires, it is not essential. While farm setup and management may preclude stall rest in some cases, limiting the activity level of the horse with a limb wound decreases the amount of motion and may be useful in the early phases of wound healing.

When bandaging is discontinued, it may be useful to warn owners that the area being bandaged can become edematous with the cessation of bandaging. Increased exercise, or "weaning" the horse from bandaging by applying a bandage for 12–24 hours, then removing the bandage for 12–24 hours, then bandage for 8–12 hours, then remove, and so on, can help counteract this problem.

TREATMENTS, PRODUCTS, AND CONTINUED MANAGEMENT OF THE WOUND

Unfortunately, there is no "silver bullet" that will speed wound healing significantly. Some treatments, products, and procedures have shown modest benefit, but the degree to which each helps is contingent on the wound properties, location on the body, and stage of healing, and the time and cost of such interventions may not justify the marginal clinical relevance. For the practitioner to search for one product that will heal every wound or heal wounds extremely fast or without complications is futile. Certainly, partial-thickness wounds and wounds that are able to be closed by delayed primary closure will heal quite quickly and often with excellent cosmetic results, but there is no evidence that their healing is helped by various over-the-counter wound products, which only add to the expense of care. Full-thickness wounds that heal by second intention must all go through the same healing process, and while some differences in healing time and quality can be obtained with proper care, no one product or treatment is right for every case, and few have been shown to make a very dramatic difference in healing time.[3,5]

What does seem clear is that wound healing can be impaired or delayed with some practices and with application of some products.[20,21,28] Although desiccation of epithelial cells can result in slowed epithelialization if a moist wound-healing environment is not always maintained, a common misperception among owners is that wounds should "get air to them." Other practices can be more damaging; the author has seen substances such as formalin, pickling lime, silver nitrate, lye, and calcium hydroxide put on wounds. Most are used in an attempt to reduce or prevent excessive granulation tissue but, in fact, such substances delay wound healing and can promote scarring.[28] There are an astounding number of wound treatment products on the market. The ambulatory clinician should carefully scrutinize the ingredients in such products before using any wound treatment; many topical treatments contain agents such as phenols and alcohols or other chemicals that are known irritants, caustics, or drying agents. In addition, some products can damage tissue surrounding the wound or other normal tissue that comes into contact with it.[28]

In some instances, a product applied can be irritating enough to cause self-mutilation and damage to intact skin (**Fig. 9**). If a wound has granulation tissue that is discolored or otherwise unhealthy or that is below the level of the skin, then the application of a caustic treatment should be considered as a cause. Caustic agents are not selective; they are caustic to all of the tissue with which they come in contact. While the intent of these agents is to decrease granulation tissue, they can delay wound healing by destroying epithelial cells. To remedy the urge by some owners to apply products to wounds and avoid potentially caustic or harmful substances, it may be useful to give owners something to apply that will do no harm. In most cases, this is simply generic triple antibiotic ointment.[2,37]

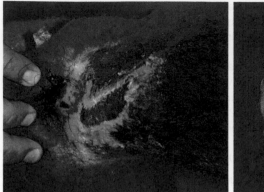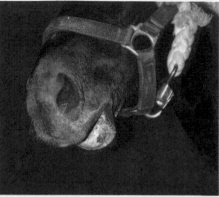

Fig. 9. Thoroughbred weanling that originally sustained a wound to the pectoral area. A commercial wound powder containing caustic hydrated lime was applied to the pectoral wound. This caused self-mutilation, during which contact with the lime caused a wound under the lower lip. That wound—seen in image on the left—eventually contracted and caused deformity of the lip that had to be corrected surgically. (*Images courtesy of* Dr Scott McClure.)

COMPLICATED AND CHRONIC WOUNDS

On occasion, the ambulatory equine practitioner is presented with a chronic, nonhealing wound. These can be difficult cases but should be approached with the wound-healing process in mind. There are many reasons why a wound may not be healing, and a systematic approach can help narrow down the possibilities:

1. Is the granulation bed appropriate and intact? If the granulation tissue bed is not intact, if a cleft is present or if the wound itself is a draining tract, then something is causing continued drainage. Possible causes include a sequestrum, foreign body, motion/trauma, or infection of an underlying structure.
2. If the granulation tissue is intact across the entire bed of the wound—is it appropriate? Bulging of the granulation tissue above the wound surface, or proud flesh, is one example of an inappropriate course of healing. Granulation tissue with an abnormal color or consistency may also be signs that the bed is not healthy.
3. Is something else growing? Sarcoids or squamous cell carcinomas might be suspected if the normal skin edge ends abruptly and a mass begins, rather than a healing epithelial edge being present[38] (**Figs. 10 and 11**).

Proud Flesh

Exuberant granulation tissue, or proud flesh, is one cause for a wound to have delayed or impaired healing. Prevention of this occurrence with good wound management is best, but sometimes it is an inevitable outcome. Small to moderate amounts of excessive granulation tissue can be treated with application of corticosteroid cream and a good bandage, but if there is a large amount of proud flesh, it should be sharply excised.[28] The excess granulation tissue should be trimmed flush with the healing epithelial edge, taking care not to remove or damage healthy surrounding skin or new epithelial tissue. Most horses are amenable to this being performed while standing under sedation. A tourniquet above the area that is to be trimmed can help reduce the amount of bleeding, but because of the composition of

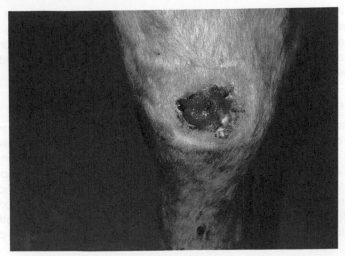

Fig. 10. Sarcoid on the dorsal carpus of a 5-year-old quarterhorse stallion.

granulation tissue, bleeding will still occur. The owner should be prepared for bleeding if they are present for the procedure, as it can appear to be a dramatic amount, especially since horse blood clots slowly. The bleeding will eventually cease with a heavily padded bandage placed over the wound after trimming. In some cases,

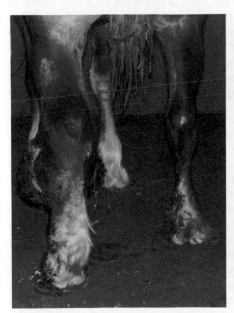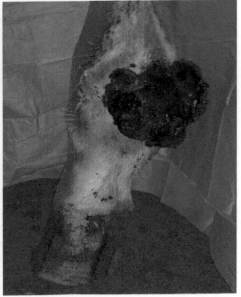

Fig. 11. Two cases with chronic nonhealing wounds. The case on the left has chronic excessive granulation tissue present, while the proliferative tissue in the case on the right is a sarcoid. Both cases underwent treatment for removal of the excess tissue and the underlying wound, but the enlargement of the leg caused by chronic swelling remained in both cases.

repeated trimming of the granulation tissue is necessary.[28] However, if the wound needs repeated trimming of granulation tissue and does not appear to be making progress, causes for delayed healing should be investigated. In those wounds that are simply too large to heal well by second intention alone, skin grafting should be offered as a treatment option.

Summer Sores

Habronemiasis can occur in open wounds and will sometimes have an appearance similar to proud flesh or sarcoids. It can be difficult to tell the difference between these 3 problems and a few other conditions, such as squamous cell carcinoma. Summer sores often contain calcified granules and are can be quite pruritic. Histopathology is recommended for any proliferative nonhealing wound as treatments and expected outcomes may depend on the diagnosis. Debulking the portion that protrudes beyond the skin edge and bandaging is almost always an excellent start to getting any of these conditions under control, and a biopsy can be submitted from the portion that is removed.

Excessive Motion

At times, even if the wound is healing appropriately, a large amount of motion can disrupt the granulation bed and delay healing or result in undue scar tissue.[20,21,28] Areas where this may occur are typically near joints such as the dorsal fetlock or over a bony eminence, such as the point of the hock. Measures to reduce motion including stall confinement, a heavily padded bandage with a splint, or a cast can help limit motion and thus disruption of the healing wound.

Wounds that are chronic and have been left without treatment for a long period of time may have associated limb swelling that could be permanent due to a large amount of scar tissue and disrupted vascular/lymphatic function. Even if the wound is amenable to treatment, if the duration of swelling has been prolonged the owners should be advised of the possibility of a permanent enlargement (see **Fig. 11**). Nevertheless, there are many chronic cases in which treating the wound and bandaging the limb may result in surprising improvement in both the appearance of the wound, as well as in limb swelling.

SUMMARY

Care of equine wounds in the field can be a challenging endeavor. Many times, wound care is complicated by chronicity or by prior inappropriate care in addition to the great degree of tissue trauma that occurred when the horse was wounded. Recognizing involvement of synovial structures, loss of skin, and damage to bone are critical in the initial examination of wounds and will guide future care. Education of clients is also important in that preparing them for possible outcomes during healing may help improve compliance and proper treatment of wound. Owners and trainers often perform much of the daily care and monitoring of equine wounds and thus can greatly assist or impede the progress. Bandaging is important to management of equine wounds—especially on the limbs—and is sometimes overlooked because of its labor-intensive nature and the desire for a spray, ointment, or salve that will heal the wound. The practitioner that improves and utilizes his or her understanding of the wound-healing process in concert with his or her knowledge of local anatomy will be the one who is best equipped to care for wounds in ambulatory practice.

REFERENCES

1. Stashak TS, Farstvedt EF. Update on wound dressings: indications and best use. In: Stashak TS, Theoret C, editors. Equine wound management. 2nd edition. Ames (IA): Wiley-Blackwell; 2008. p. 109–36.
2. Farstvedt EF, Stashak TS. Topical wound treatments and wound care products. In: Stashak TS, Theoret C, editors. Equine wound management. 2nd edition. Ames (IA): Wiley-Blackwell; 2008. p. 137–59.
3. Theoret C. Wound repair: problems in the horse and innovative solutions. In: Stashak TS, Theoret C, editors. Equine wound management. 2nd edition. Ames (AI): Wiley-Blackwell; 2008. p. 47–68.
4. Gomez J. Bandaging and casting techniques for wound management. In: Stashak TS, Theoret C, editors. Equine wound management. 2nd edition. Ames (IA): Wiley-Blackwell; 2008. p. 623–58.
5. Dart AJ, Dowling BA, Smith CL. Topical treatments in equine wound management. Vet Clin North Am Equine Pract 2005;21:77–89.
6. Holcombe SJ. Shock: pathophysiology, diagnosis and treatment. In: Auer JA, Stick JA, editors. Equine surgery. 3rd edition. St Louis: Saunders Elsevier; 2006. p. 1–9.
7. Holcombe SJ. Physiologic response to trauma: evaluating the trauma patient. In: Auer JA, Stick JA, editors. Equine surgery. 3rd edition. St Louis: Saunders Elsevier; 2006. p. 88–96.
8. Hassel DM. Thoracic trauma in horses. Vet Clin North Am Equine Pract 2007;23: 67–80.
9. Hendrickson DA. Management of deep and chronic wounds. In: Auer JA, Stick JA, editors. Equine surgery. 3rd edition. St Louis: Saunders Elsevier; 2006. p. 299–305.
10. Schneider RK. Synovial and osseous infections. In: Auer JA, Stick JA, editors. Equine surgery. 3rd edition. St Louis: Saunders Elsevier; 2006. p. 1121–30.
11. Wereszka MM, White NA 2nd, Furr MO. Factors associated with outcome following treatment of horses with septic tenosynovitis: 51 cases (1986–2003). J Am Vet Med Assoc 2007;230:1195–200.
12. Schneider RK, Bramlage LR, Moore RM, et al. A retrospective study of 192 horses affected with septic arthritis/tenosynovitis. Equine Vet J 1992;24:436–42.
13. Honnas SM, Schumacher J, Cohen ND, Watkins JP, Taylor TS. Septic tenosynovitis in horses: 25 cases (1983–1989). J Am Vet Med Assoc. 1991;199(11):1616–22.
14. Gibson KT, McIlwraith CW, Turner AS, et al. Open joint injuries in horses: 58 cases (1980–1986). J Am Vet Med Assoc 1989;194:398–404.
15. Moyer W, Schumacher J, Schumacher J. Equine joint injection and regional anesthesia. 5th edition. Chadds Ford (PA): Academic Veterinary Solutions; 2011. p. 1–144.
16. Davis CS, Smith RKW. Diagnosis and management of tendon and ligament disorders. In: Auer JA, Stick JA, editors. Equine surgery. 3rd edition. St Louis: Saunders Elsevier; 2006. p. 1086–111.
17. Taylor DS, Pascoe JR, Meagher DM, et al. Digital flexor tendon lacerations in horses: 50 cases (1975–1990). J Am Vet Med Assoc 1995;206:342–6.
18. Foland JW, Trotter GW, Stashak TS, et al. Traumatic injuries involving tendons of the distal limbs in horses: a retrospective study of 55 cases. Equine Vet J 1991;23:422–5.
19. Mespoulhès-Rievère C, Martens A, Bogaert L, et al. Factors affecting outcome of extensor tendon lacerations in the distal limb of horses. A retrospective study of 156 cases (1994–2003). Vet Comp Orthop Traumatol 2008;21:358–64.
20. Stashak TS. Selected factors that negatively impact healingIn: Stashak TS, Theoret Ceditors. Equine wound management. 2nd edition. Ames (IA): Wiley-Blackwell; 2008. p. 71–84.

21. Hendrickson D, Virgin J. Factors that affect equine wound repair. Vet Clin North Am Equine Pract 2005;21:33–44.
22. Theoret C. Physiology of wound healing. In: Stashak TS, Theoret C, editors. Equine wound management. 2nd edition. Ames (IA): Wiley-Blackwell; 2008. p. 5–28.
23. Shumacher J, Brumbaugh GW, Honnas CM, et al. Kinetics of healing grafted and nongrafted wounds on the distal portion of the forelimbs of horses. Am J Vet Res 1992;53:1568–71.
24. Wilmink JA, Stolk PW, Van Weeren PR, et al. Differences in second-intention wound healing between horses and ponies: macroscopic aspects. Equine Vet J 1999;31: 53–60.
25. Schumacher J, Stashak TS. Management of wounds of the distal extremities. In: Stashak TS. Theoret C, editors. Equine wound management. 2nd edition. Ames (IA): Wiley-Blackwell; 2008. p. 375–425.
26. Theoret, CL. The pathophysiology of wound repair. Vet Clin North Am Equine Pract 2005;21:1–13.
27. Wilmink JM, Van Weeren PR. Second-intention repair in the horse and pony and management of exuberant granulation tissue. Vet Clin North Am Equine Pract 2005;21:12–32.
28. Wilmink JM, Van Weeren PR. Treatment of exuberant granulation tissue. Clin Tech Equine Pract 2004;3:141–7.
29. Stashak TS. Selection of suture materials, suture patterns, and drains for wound closure. In: Stashak TS, Theoret C, editors. Equine wound management. 2nd edition. Ames (IA): Wiley-Blackwell; 2008. p. 193–224.
30. Stashak TS. New and innovative approaches to wound closure. In: Stashak TS, Theoret C, editors. Equine wound management. 2nd edition. Ames (IA): Wiley-Blackwell; 2008. p. 225–37.
31. Moens Y, Verschooten F, De Moor A, et al. Bone sequestration as a consequence of limb wounds in the horse. Vet Radiol 1980;21:40–4.
32. American Association of Equine Practitioners (AAEP). Lameness scale: definition and classification of lameness. In: Guide for veterinary service and judging of equestrian events. 4th edition. Lexington (KY): AAEP; 1991. p. 19.
33. Bristol DG. Skin grafts and skin flaps in the horse. Vet Clin North Am Equine Pract 2005;21:125–44.
34. Schumacher J. Skin grafting. In: Auer JA, Stick JA, editors. Equine surgery. 3rd edition. St Louis: Saunders Elsevier; 2006. p. 269–87.
35. Schumacher J, Hanselka DV. Skin grafting of the horse. Vet Clin North Am Equine Pract 1989;5:591–614.
36. Woollen N, DeBowes RM, Liepold HW, et al. A comparison of four types of therapy for the treatment of full-thickness skin wounds of the horse. In: Proceedings of the Annual Convention of the American Association of Equine Practitioners 1987;33:569–76.
37. Stashak TS. Management practices that influence wound infection and healing. In: Stashak TS, Theoret C, editors. Equine wound management. 2nd edition. Ames (IA): Wiley-Blackwell; 2008. p. 85–106.
38. Knottenbelt DCSarcoid transformation at wound sites. In: Stashak TS, Theoret C, editors. Equine wound management. 2nd edition. Ames (IA): Wiley-Blackwell; 2008. p. 585–608.

Lameness and Performance Evaluation in Ambulatory Practice

John S. Mitchell, DVM

> **KEYWORDS**
> - Equine practice • Equine ambulatory lameness practice
> - Horses • Lameness • Performance evaluation

The past two decades have seen a dramatic increase in the emphasis on equine performance. Prior to the 1990s, most people would have associated the phase "equine performance" with racehorses. But today there is pressure on all breeds to perform at a high level. Three-day eventing, show jumping, and dressage are examples of the very competitive nature of the English sport horses. Cutting, reining, rodeo, and team penning are just some of the Western performance horse events. From endurance riding to chariot racing, people are asking horses to perform. Performance evaluation, both before and after purchase, has become an important part of many equine veterinary practices.

Critical to equine performance is the ability to perform free of pain and free of any associated lameness, and this is an important part of ambulatory practice. Ambulatory practitioners are hired by individual owners and/or trainers to provide veterinary care to the horses in their stables, and equine lameness evaluation and treatment represent an important part of that care. As such, the veterinarian can often become (for better or worse) part of a management "team" of owners, trainer, groom, farrier, and possibly other paraprofessionals or lay people who claim expertise in helping improve horses' performance. It is part of the ambulatory practitioner's responsibility—and it is definitely good business—to be proactive in the all the decisions that affect the patient. Coordination of the input and care provided by the entire team can be one of the most challenging aspects of today's equine lameness practice.

COMMUNICATIONS

Equine ambulatory practitioners may be presented with a whole spectrum of situations. The simplest one occurs when an owner is present with the veterinarian to evaluate and provide treatment for the horse on the owner's property; such interactions can be very straight forward and may not involve any "team" effort. The other end of the spectrum is

Equine Associates, 744 Camino Lakes Circle, Boca Raton, FL 33486, USA
E-mail address: johnmitchelldvm@gmail.com

Vet Clin Equine 28 (2012) 101–115
doi:10.1016/j.cveq.2012.01.007
0749-0739/12/$ – see front matter © 2012 Elsevier Inc. All rights reserved.

the horse owned by a group of absentee owners, under the care of an absentee out-of-state trainer, and presented by a groom or an agent.

When there are absentee owners and/or absentee trainers, the need for establishing owner/trainer/veterinarian communications early in the evaluation of the equine patient becomes critical. Often the owner is not aware of lameness concerns with the horse, and sometimes there is a conflict of interest, whereby the trainer may fail to share this information with the owner. Thus, it becomes paramount for both good practice ethics and successful practice outcomes to establish direct owner/veterinarian communication as soon as possible in the lameness evaluation of equine patients with absentee owners. By no means should the trainer be excluded from being involved with or informed of these communications; however, leaving all the owner communications in the hands of the trainer has the potential for unsuccessful outcomes. Under some circumstances, when previous experience with an owner/trainer has revealed good communications and the owner has expressed that the trainer has full authority for all decisions and procedures for their horse, the veterinarian can be comfortable with all communications being handled through the trainer.

The ambulatory practitioner may elect to have a form for his or her practice that spells out these communication responsibilities. It may or may not be combined with a financial responsibility form and, once signed, remains on file for each patient (**Fig. 1**).

Good management principles apply to all horses, regardless of their level of performance, in racing horses, as well as horses that are kept as pleasure and companion animals. Establishing good rapport and communication with all members of a patient's management team helps lead to successful outcomes for the patient and long-term positive relationships with the team members.

LAMENESS AND PERFORMANCE EVALUATIONS—OWNERS AND TRAINERS

Equine lameness and performance evaluation usually begins with a complaint. The owner or trainer contacts the veterinarian with a problem, or the perception of a problem. The *perception* of a lameness problem is an important concept for veterinarians to consider. The owner's/trainer's perception of a lameness problem does not always equate with the horse having a lameness problem. The owner often has certain performance expectations. These expectations can be based on many factors, commonly including the horse's family history of performance or the amount of money invested and/or the expectations promised by the trainer. It seems that a failure of a horse to perform up to expectations is rarely considered to be the fault of the trainer or rider. It may not be considered that the horse is performing up to its abilities; rather, a failure to perform is often ascribed to a physical problem with the horse or an equipment problem. So, for example, when pressured about the horse's performance not meeting expectations, the trainer may defer that pressure to the veterinarian and infer a lameness problem to the owner. Another common scenario is one where the owner, in frustration over the horse's performance, requests that the trainer obtain a lameness evaluation of the horse. While this may be a valid avenue for investigation, the prudent veterinarian must remember that just because the horse is presented for lameness evaluation does not also mean that the horse is lame.

Commonly, owners or trainers will present the attending veterinarian with a diagnosis and not a problem. For example, they may report that, "My horse has a bad knee," or "He needs his hocks injected," or "My horse has sore feet" instead of reporting that, "My horse is limping and not performing well," or "My horse has trouble

AUTHORIZATION FOR EQUINE PROFESSIONAL VETERINARY SERVICES
Generic Veterinary Services
Address
Contact Information

Horse Name_____ Date_____

Horse ID?_____ Age_____ Sex:_____ Color_____ Breed_____

Owner name:_____   Authorized Agent name:_____

Address:_____   Address:_____

_____   _____

_____   _____

Cell Phone:_____   Cell Phone:_____

Other Phone(s):_____   Other Phone(s):_____

Insurance Carrier:_____

Person with horse today-Name:_____Relation:_____

I hereby authorize Generic Veterinary Services (GVS) to examine and treat the horse described above. I understand that such treatment may include diagnostic tests and injections, the administration of vaccines, medications, rectal palpation, ultrasound examinations, diagnostic radiology, and other tests, surgical procedures, anesthetics, or treatments that the veterinarians deem necessary for the health, safety, or well-being of the above described horse while it is under our care and supervision.

Generic Veterinary Services is dedicated to good owner / trainer-agent / veterinarian communications. As designated below the veterinarians and staff will make continued attempts to communicate timely patient information.

As above listed owner of this horse I desire the following communication: (Choose only one)

      ( ) All patient communication is to be handled ONLY by the authorized agent listed above and the responsible trainer /agent / caregiver where the horse is stabled

      ( ) Patient communication should ONLY be shared with the above listed owner(s) and the responsible trainer /agent / caregiver where the horse is stabled

      ( ) The above listed owner should be the primary contact person for patient communication and that sharing of this information with any other owners, authorized agent, and the responsible trainer / agent / caregiver where the horse is stabled is authorized

I acknowledge that ( ) the primary owner listed above, or ( ) authorized agent listed above is fully responsible for payment of any and all professional fees and expenses incurred in connection with the treatment by GVS of the above described horse. Payment is due in full at the time of services.

If I am not the Owner, I affirmatively represent and warrant to the GVS that I am the authorized agent of the owner and that I possess complete power and authority and am fully authorized by the owner to seek medical treatment for the horse described above and to complete this form on the owner's behalf.

This form will be kept on file and apply to this horse until the owner requests changes or a new form.

Dated:_____ Signature GVS Witness:_____

Signature of Owner / Authorized Agent:_____

I hereby authorize Generic Veterinary Services to charge my credit card:
    _____ Balance in full

    Credit Card #:_____ (Visa, MC,AE, Discover)

    Expiration Date:_____ Name on card:_____

    Card Holder Signature:_____ Date:_____

Thank You for allowing us to serve your veterinary needs   GVS Authorization Form:12-1-2011

Fig. 1. Sample form: authorization for professional veterinary Services.

walking out of the stall each morning." When a horse is presented for lameness evaluation with such a diagnosis, the veterinarian must be careful not to focus just on the presenting diagnosis and miss evaluating the whole horse. It is important not to be overly influenced by the presenting problem.

While the presenting "diagnosis" may not, in fact, be relevant to the horse's problem, from a client management standpoint, it is very important to write down the presenting complaint. In the final analysis and consultation, the veterinarian should be sure to address the presenting complaint. Even if the initial "diagnosis" is unfounded, the complaint is real to the owner/trainer. Even if you find significant other findings, you should address their presenting complaint; listening to the client, and attending directly to their concerns, is an important aspect of good client relations. Without such attention, some clients may seek others who will listen to them, despite any expertise that the veterinarian has demonstrated.

The patient's history is very different from the owner's complaint; everything should be taken seriously, and with attention to detail. Listen to the horse's story. In taking a history, it is important to interact with the client. Ask questions and be sure to listen closely to the answers. Owners or trainers usually give the veterinarians good information that may ultimately lead to a diagnosis, even if the initial client "diagnosis" was a red herring.

Establishing good communication with the owner and/or trainer is one of the most important aspects of lameness diagnosis and management. Attending veterinarians should:

1. Discuss the overall diagnostic plan and explain the difference between noninvasive and invasive diagnostic procedures.
2. Discuss the cost estimates and ask about any financial limitations.
3. Set realistic expectations for a definitive diagnosis, improvement, and a reasonable time table for expected results. Owners are never displeased when their horses improve more quickly than anticipated.

LAMENESSS/PERFORMANCE EVALUATION GUIDELINES

When evaluating a horse for lameness and/or performance problems, consider five possible contributing categories:

1. Proper use/genetic potential
2. Problems that may be identified in blood chemistry assays
3. Respiratory/cardiovascular system problems
4. Musculoskeletal/neurologic problems
5. Environmental/management Issues.

Any and all of these categories may affect a horse's ability to perform, and they may also be associated with lameness.

PROPER USE/GENETIC POTENTIAL

In the initial examination, it is important to look at the overall quality and type of horse presented. It may be important to discuss with an owner that the horse is not lame but that it may not have the body type or genetic potential to perform up to the owner's or trainer's expectations. A useful analogy is that you can't buy the best Volkswagen Beetle and compete on the NASCAR circuit. The fact that genetic potential or good breeding does not guarantee performance is sometimes hard for owners, especially new owners, to accept. Royal bloodlines or full sibling pedigrees do not ensure top performing horses in any discipline.

Other factors influencing perceptions of poor performance or lameness include age and experience. A young, green horse may be more difficult to evaluate for lameness or poor performance than an experienced horse. The experienced horse has already established his athletic ability and competitive attitude; however, these traits may be difficult to evaluate in the green horse. The unproven horse may have not developed the mental or physical attributes necessary for the desired performance; furthermore, there is no guarantee that each individual will ever reach these performance expectations. The young/green horse may also be harder to examine due to his fractious nature or lack of understanding with what the veterinarian is trying to communicate in his or her evaluation procedures.

BLOOD CHEMISTRY ASSAYS

Laboratory analysis of a blood sample is occasionally useful in examining the lame horse and can give clues as to performance-related problems. It is important to draw the blood early in the exam, so that evaluations will be on resting horses. In this way, one can obviate concerns that abnormalities were iatrogenic. The author often draws blood samples early in the exam and then decides at the end of the exam the value of submitting the samples for analysis.

Muscle enzyme elevations are diagnostic for exertional rhabdomyolysis (ER). The creatine kinase (CK) enzyme elevates very rapidly (4–6 hours) after an episode of ER and will regress to normal in 3 to 4 days post event. The aspartate aminotransferase (AST) enzyme elevates more slowly and may take 10 to 21 days to return to normal after 1 rhabdomyolysis episode.[1] A common finding in horses that have been affected with ER is a normal CK and elevated AST, indicating a tying-up episode more than 3 days ago but within the past several weeks. Some cases of exertional rhabdomyolysis are subclinical, and the blood analysis can be valuable in identifying this reason for poor performance or obscure lameness. The history obtained on the horse may correlate with the muscle enzyme analysis and help correlate with the poor performance.

The complete blood count (CBC) may have limited use in evaluating poor performance and lameness. Diagnoses of "anemia" should be made reluctantly. Studies have shown little correlation between resting red blood counts and either class of the racing horse or poor performance.[2,3] A suspected low red blood cell (RBC) count should be further evaluated by taking a resting sample and a post exercise sample to determine if the RBCs elevate to normal levels with exercise. The horse routinely stores up to 30% of the RBCs in the spleen, making a diagnosis of true anemia difficult in horses.

An elevated white blood count (WBC) and/or elevated fibrinogen can indicate infection and/or inflammation. A high or very low WBC count should be of concern and should be correlated with a thorough physical exam. Abnormal WBC counts may need to be monitored with repeat samples at several-day intervals.

Some poorly performing horses may have serious infections and normal WBC counts, especially cases of pneumonia and pleuropneumonia. In such cases, plasma fibrinogen is a valuable tool for evaluating subclinical infection and/or inflammation. Fibrinogen is a soluble plasma glycoprotein that is synthesized by the liver. Fibrinogen is converted to fibrin in the coagulation cascade. In the horse, the circulating fibrinogen level may be used as an inflammatory marker. Mild transient variations in laboratory results above or below the laboratory normal may be related to factors such as diet, stress, or recent shipping.

Poor performance may also be an indication of gastric ulcers.[4,5] Horses with gastric ulcers may show poor performance as the first and only clinical sign of gastric ulcers. Gastric ulcers can be evaluated by a gastric endoscopic examination or, less precisely, by "diagnostic treatment." As a diagnostic treatment, a 3- to 5-day treatment with an oral medication such as omeprazole may be used to see if improvement is noted. In the author's experience, most subclinical cases of gastric ulcers show a dramatic improvement when treated. Gastric ulcers may also be a secondary finding in horses with poor performance, secondary to chronic pain, or as a result of regular medication (eg, with frequent doses of nonsteroidal anti-inflammatory drugs). It is also appropriate to discuss diet, supplements, and any medications the horse is receiving. In the author's experience, owners/trainers may have ruled out gastric ulcers in their own mind due to their own treatment efforts, when the horses are in fact very responsive to medical treatment for ulcers.

RESPIRATORY/CARDIOVASCULAR SYSTEM

Poor performance may be related to problems of the cardiovascular or respiratory system. Poor stamina or fading near the end of a race is a common performance problem in racing horses. Blood or mucopurulent discharge from the nares post exercise can indicate a respiratory problem, but many horses show neither of these. Further examination of the respiratory system can demonstrate very significant findings. Coughing or respiratory noise indicates the need for careful evaluation of the respiratory system, including auscultation of the heart and lungs. Other techniques for ambulatory evaluation of the respiratory system include the use of a rebreathing bag, endoscopic examination (resting, post exercise, and dynamic) and ultrasound. The cardiovascular system may be further evaluated by electrocardiography and ultrasound in the ambulatory environment.

LAMENESS

The lameness examination is critical to proper diagnosis and treatment of lame horses, as well as for horses with performance problems. The very best diagnostic equipment is no better than the lameness examination on which the use of this equipment is based. Ambulatory practitioners typically do not have advanced imaging modalities such as magnetic resonance imaging (MRI) or scintigraphy at their disposal. The lack of availability of advanced imaging modalities, or the reluctance of a client to pay for such imaging, should not preclude the ambulatory practitioner from performing a high-quality and detailed lameness examination. A good lameness examination will usually lead to an accurate diagnosis and an effective therapeutic plan. The patient requiring more advanced diagnostic procedures can be referred to the practice's hospital (if it has one) or to a referral center, after a complete lameness workup.

Before delving into a detailed lameness exam or diagnostic procedures, the first aspect of the lameness evaluation should be to assess the entire horse. Owners or trainers should be questioned as to whether the horse has received any anti-inflammatory or pain-relieving medication within the previous 72 hours or any intra-articular injections within the past month; such medications can interfere with the accurate perception of the horse's lameness. While listening to the owner or trainer state the problem and give the history, the environment around the horse should be assessed. How the horse moves out of the stall and to the exam area should be watched. Palpating the horse should be avoided until it has been walked around and its overall condition and attitude assessed. When the history or the physical appearance of the horse indicates a general physical problem, examination, auscultation, and blood sampling for laboratory analysis should be done at this time.

If the history indicates a lameness problem, the horse should first be examined at a walk in a straight line on a firm flat surface. The next step should be trotting in a straight line and, if indicated, lunging the horse. It may be very valuable to lunge horses in circles both ways. Some horses may exhibit lameness only when circled in one direction; for example, it has been noted that some horses exhibit lameness only

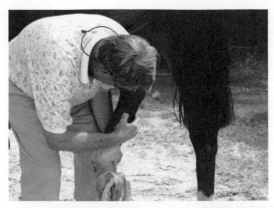

Fig. 2. Palpation of hind suspensory ligament.

when the affected limb is on the outside of a circle. It may be necessary to have the horse ridden or used in a manner that the lameness has been reported to be most apparent. It is best to continue with the in-motion examination until the veterinarian is confident that the lameness is predominantly affecting a certain leg. If the owner/trainer reports the horse is not as lame as normal, be sure to ask again if the horse has received any treatments or medication since the lameness was observed. If the horse has been rested or treated, the lameness may have resolved.

Once lameness has been identified in a particular leg, thorough palpation of the horse should be performed (**Fig. 2**). While some sources of pain may cause some horses to have a classic gait change, there is no particular gait abnormality that is pathognomonic for a particular lameness condition; the same cause of lameness may not have a consistent presentation in all horses. Thus, isolating the source of pain to a specific anatomical location (eg, "I think it's in the shoulder") simply by observing the gait is usually not a very reliable way to achieve a diagnosis.

If the lameness appears to be a left front leg problem, the author will usually start with palpation of the right front leg. Beginning the lameness examination on a limb that may not be the problem for the horse calms the horse and relaxes him to the palpation procedures. Importantly, from palpating a normal limb, how the horse reacts to a normal stimulus can be assessed and compared to the reaction when a suspected sore area is identified. Most horses will noticeably tense or even pull away when the examiner's hands come near the sore area, even before the skin is touched. In the author's experience, this protective reflex, a "menace response," is especially useful in finding muscle injuries and abscesses.

The lameness exam should be done according to the same routine with each patient. By proceeding systematically, the practitioner becomes very confident of what constitutes a normal response and will thus be less likely to miss, or overinterpret, the reaction to palpation or flexion of an area. For example, the response to flexion of a normal fetlock, done before flexing the suspected injured fetlock, can give the practitioner a baseline to assess the response in the affected limb. Similarly, some horses may react to palpation of their suspensory ligament; however, when the other limb palpates the same, it can be recognized that such a response is normal for that horse, although in some cases the horse might have a bilateral soreness.

Next, a thorough hoof tester examination should be performed (**Fig. 3**), followed by observing the horse in motion again as before. This practice will help correlate any

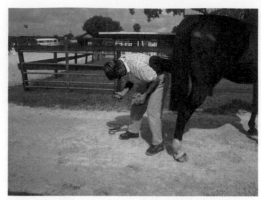

Fig. 3. Hoof testers' examination.

suspicions identified by the hoof testers to the lameness problem, and the hoof tester examination may also exacerbate lameness. For example, certain horses may have exaggerated lameness if trotted off just after hoof tester pressure in a certain area of the hoof or after standing on a small block of wood to put pressure on a certain part of the hoof. Careful comparison to other parts of the foot is necessary to differentiate lameness response from normal response.

After motion, palpation, and hoof testers' examination, the author may next perform a series of flexion tests. The author generally considers that there are 2 types of flexion tests. The most commonly used flexion text involves simply flexing the joint with a reasonable amount of pressure and evaluating the horses' response. Care must be used to attempt to flex only 1 joint at a time (to the extent possible), then compare the response in that joint to the response to flexion of the contra lateral joint. The classic joint for this flexion test is the fetlock joint, but information can be gained by flexing and manipulating all joints, including the spine. The cervical spine can be palpated directly and evaluated indirectly by flexing the neck to each side and flexing the head in a dorsal and ventral plane. Direct palpation of the thoracic and lumbar vertebrae should be performed—direct palpation of vertebrae while shifting the standing horse's weight may elicit pain. These passive flexion tests are usually included as part of the physical examination, which also includes palpation of the legs. If lumbar or pelvic soreness is suspected, it may be valuable to perform a rectal examination, including walking the horse while palpating the pelvic musculoskeletal system.

The second type of flexion test applies moderate pressure to a joint, placing it in a flexed position for a specific time (usually 1–2 minutes, depending on the joint, and the examiner) and then immediately trotting off the horse. The amount of lameness post flexion is compared with the amount of lameness pre-flexion; if lameness is increased, the source of the lameness may be in structures close to the area flexed. While commonly used in lameness evaluation, equine ambulatory practitioners should interpret flexion tests with a degree of caution. A positive response to flexion tests is directly proportional to the length of time that the joint is flexed, the force applied,[6] as well as to the age of the horse (older horses are more likely to have positive flexion tests). Horses are more likely to flex positive when a male examiner flexes the horse than when a female examiner flexes the horse, probably due to increased force exerted by male examiners.[7] Factors such as weight, height, or even joint range of motion do not accurately predict a response to a flexion test.[8] Finally, working horses are less likely to have positive flexion tests than are stabled horses or horses at pasture rest.[9] In short, while flexion tests are commonly used in lameness evaluation, the tests are neither very sensitive nor specific and have significant variation in individual application. Nevertheless, when a horse has a dramatic positive timed flexion test, the flexed area and the surrounding tissues should be further examined for a source of soreness.

If there is still question as to the degree of lameness, the reproducibility of lameness, or conflicting results from the palpation, hoof testers, or flexion tests, the horse should again be observed in motion. It should always be kept in mind that the purpose of the examination is to allow the horse to show a problem, not to make a case for a perceived or suspected lameness. If, after these examinations, the lameness is still difficult to observe or isolate, it is very important to observe the horse performing his intended use. At the standardbred track, this involves watching the horse jog or train on the track; for a dressage or jumping horse, it may involve watching the horse in the ring, performing the maneuvers during which the problem may be seen.

It is not a good practice to force the issue of trying to isolate a lameness on a day that the lameness is very subtle, intermittent, or much milder than reported on previous days. If a lameness is inapparent or seems to be improving, it is preferable to stop for that day and request that an additional examination be performed on a day when the lameness is more obvious. Under such circumstances, it is also entirely reasonable to charge for the professional services rendered for evaluating the horse on both examination days. The ambulatory clinician should explain that the best case scenario is that the condition is resolving and may not require further evaluation. It is important that the practitioner be clear that he or she would like to reexamine the horse on a later date if the lameness reappears.

If the palpation, hoof testers, and or flexion tests isolate a definite area of soreness, proceeding to other diagnostic tests may be indicated, or, in many cases, treatment can be initiated. For example, a suspensory ligament that palpates sore may need ultrasonic examination, a sore flexed joint may require radiographs, or a painful broken bar in a foot may benefit from corrective shoeing. If there is any question about the suspected area being the source of the lameness, the client should be offered the option of diagnostic nerve or joint blocks to localize and confirm the source of the lameness.

TO BLOCK OR NOT TO BLOCK (PICK YOUR BATTLES!)

The success of regional diagnostic anesthesia (blocking a horse) is often based on case selection. In order for an anesthetic block to be successful, the horse must have a significant gait abnormality that is consistent and reproducible. Most "blockable" lameness problems will have either a consistent head nod or pelvic lift. As a rule, any problem should be observed and reproducible at least 3 times during the examination before considering diagnostic anesthesia. In addition, before considering blocking a horse, the veterinarian should make sure that there is time to complete the examination; if a condition is only evident when a horse is ridden, and the only rider is leaving or a rainstorm is pending, then this is not a good time to block.

Diagnostic anesthesia should only be considered after a thorough lameness examination. Not all lameness exams require diagnostic anesthesia to confirm the source of lameness. In addition, thorough palpation may reveal a problem that will not respond to diagnostic anesthesia. Common examples of lameness problems found on examination that would be difficult to localize with diagnostic anesthesia are flexor tendon tears, curbs, and post injection cervical or gluteal muscle abscesses, where, for example, a horse returning to work after a treatment and rest period from pneumonia may have a pelvic lift as a result of soreness from a gluteal antibiotic injection or abscess. The author has been asked to examine several horses for an exaggerated head nod on the track, only to find a sprung shoe that was causing the head nod.

It is important to explain diagnosis of lameness by regional anesthesia to owners and trainers prior to proceeding, in order to help them understand the process. The author has encountered trainers who did not believe in blocking horses; no matter how dramatically a horse improved, they would refuse to see any difference and would not approve additional diagnostic procedures based on the blocks. The author has also had the frustrating experience of initially diagnosing a left front lameness, but when the horse had a dramatic response to blocking the left front foot and switched to being lame in the right front, the owner would not accept this response as diagnostic. Untrained eyes may not be able to see that the horse has switched lame legs; in the untrained eye, after a successful block of one limb, with subsequent lameness in another, the horse is still lame and nothing was learned. If a clinician is not working for a client who has confidence in the clinician and the client will not listen to the clinician's interpretations, proceeding with diagnostic regional anesthesia should be done with caution, and only after a lot of client education.

Fractious horses may be too difficult to inject with local anesthesia without danger: to the horse, to the veterinarian, or to handlers. The author usually does not tranquilize or sedate horses before blocking them; however, some fractious horses that are otherwise impossible to examine become calmer, and may actually show more lameness, after an intravenous dose of 50 to 75 mg of xylazine. It is prudent not to overly restrain a horse during blocking; in the author's experience, excessive twitching or fighting with the horse during the blocking procedure has occasionally resulted in a false improvement in lameness that may be due to a central nervous response and not to the local anesthesia.

When using regional diagnostic anesthesia in horses, it is important to control as many variables between the first observation, blocking, and the second observation. The same gait, equipment, driver/rider, and/or performance should be used for the second observation so that, to the degree possible, the diagnostic block is the only significant variable. For example, standardbreds that are lame when jogged by the groom are often much sounder when jogged by the trainer, who may be carrying a whip; it could be that the horse knows from experience that more is expected by the trainer, and the horse may not appear as lame as a result. Under such circumstances, switching drivers or riders after blocking could result in false-positive blocks.

It may be unwise to evaluate the negative response to a single block repeatedly. Some horses warm out of their lameness, so exercise should be limited between diagnostic blocks once it is established that there has been no improvement. On the other hand, once a horse shows dramatic improvement, exercise should be stopped so as to avoid further damage to the anesthetized area. Very lame horses should only be allowed to take a few sound steps if they show a dramatic improvement after an anesthetic block. Horses can turn a painful incomplete fracture into a complete non–weight-bearing fracture if exercised too much while blocked.

The horse with multiple areas of soreness, especially soreness in several legs, can be a confusing and frustrating one on which to use diagnostic anesthesia. If the practitioner suspects several areas may be contributing to lameness, it may be advisable to skip blocking and progress into other diagnostic procedures and treatments. It is often more productive to treat the obvious problems and then reevaluate later to sort out the remaining lameness with blocking; the time necessary to heal an obvious lameness problem may also allow for resolution of another, less obvious problem.

Conversely, horses with multiple problems may not show one lameness dramatically until another source of soreness is blocked. Diagnostic blocks in these cases can be very valuable in documenting multiple sources of soreness, but the clinician must be diligent in sorting out the primary and secondary sources of the lameness. As stated, it may take several lameness examinations that are spaced days or weeks apart to sort out all the horse's problems.

The cost and the time necessary for a thorough and complete lameness evaluation should be considered and discussed before starting diagnostic anesthesia. The client should be aware that it may take repeated diagnostic blocks to localize the lameness, which will increase the time and cost of the exam. Also, the veterinarian should schedule the blocking session when there is adequate time available; it can be frustrating when it is necessary to block a horse multiple times when one is already behind in his or her schedule.

DIAGNOSTIC ANESTHESIA—GENERAL OBSERVATIONS

Evaluating forelimb lameness with local anesthetic blocks is often easier than evaluating the hindlimb, especially for inexperienced practitioners. The typical forelimb head nod is usually more easily distinguished than are pelvic movements, and a dramatic improvement in gait is often seen when the sore area of the forelimb is successfully anesthetized. Also, generally, in the author's experience, forelimb lameness is more often from a single area of soreness and thus easier to eliminate than hindlimb lameness. In racing thoroughbred and standardbred horses, hindlimb lameness is often from multiple sites of soreness, and only partial improvement may occur when one of the sore areas of the hind limb is blocked.

The "golden rule" for diagnostic anesthesia in the equine limb is, *Start distally and work proximally, up the leg.* This applies to both front and rear limbs. A significant percentage of equine lameness originates in the foot so both the lameness examination and the diagnostic anesthesia should facilitate a thorough examination of this area. If in doubt, the foot should be blocked first. It is very embarrassing to spend a long time conducting a lameness examination and diagnostic anesthesia on a horse and not identify a sore foot, only to have the horse form an abscess at the coronary band a few days later, rupture the abscess, and become sound. It is possible to miss deep abscesses, hematomas, and bruises with palpation, flexion, and hoof testers' exam, but these lamenesses should not escape localizing the lameness in the foot with diagnostic anesthesia.

Beginning local anesthetic blocks distally avoids problems in interpretation that may arise if the initial block is placed more proximally. Anesthetic injected in the middle of the leg may also produce anesthesia in the distal part of the leg and confuse the interpretation of the response to the block if the horse becomes sound. An example would be a resolution of lameness after a horse was initially blocked in the proximal ("high") suspensory ligament area. If the foot and fetlock were not blocked before the proximal suspensory ligament, the veterinarian may be misled as to where the source of the lameness is originating. Many horses with a sore foot will also show secondary soreness to palpation in the proximal suspensory region, presumably from landing abnormally on the sore foot. Blocking the foot first will usually produce a significant improvement in the lameness, and the soreness palpated in the proximal suspensory region can be appropriately diagnosed as a secondary soreness.

DIAGNOSTIC ANESTHESIA—SPECIAL CONSIDERATIONS
General Considerations

1. Preparation of the area of injection is a matter of personal choice. Clipping hair does not appear to be necessary for a clean injection[10,11] and may be objected to in animals that are soon to be presented for race or show.
2. The ideal method of preparation of an area of injection has not been definitively determined. The usual preparation is several surgical scrubs with povidone-iodine or chlorhexidine followed by a clean water/and or isopropyl alcohol rinse. Excessive scrubbing may damage the skin and may result in post-injection blistering of the skin.
3. Aseptic technique should be used for all diagnostic anesthesia. For example, synovial sheaths may be penetrated during perineural anesthesia administration, and aseptic technique may help prevent an infection under such circumstances.
4. The choice of anesthetic, as well as the size of the needle used for injection, is largely based on personal choice. However, research indicates that the use of smaller needles is associated with less contamination from the injection.[11]
5. Several good references are available to help practitioners refresh their techniques, as well as to learn about the pros and cons of specific anesthetic blocks.[1,12–14]
6. The breed and use of the horse may dictate how individual veterinarians may block horses, based on lameness that is typical of those factors.
7. A combination of perineural and intra-articular blocks may be necessary to localize lameness.
8. It is easier to work on a forelimb than a hindlimb. Horses may resent having multiple anesthetic blocks in their hindlimb and become difficult to handle. For certain horses, it may be prudent to try to block larger regions first and observe a response, then to come back on another day to try to block particular areas of concern.
9. Reserve the right to come back on another day to repeat blocks or use different blocks to assess particular areas of concern.
10. Systemic anti-inflammatory medication and/or limb bandaging should be considered to help control limb swelling post anesthetic injection, particularly if multiple blocks, or large volumes of anesthetic, are used.

Perineural Anesthesia

1. The palmar digital (PD) nerve block, arguably the most commonly performed nerve block, is not specific for navicular syndrome and anesthetizes other areas of the foot, including the distal interphalangeal joint.[15,16] Many areas of potential lameness are anesthetized by a PD block.
2. If lameness is thought to be localized to one side of a limb, blocking only the nerve supplying the affected area may be appropriate.
3. There are a number of structures that are potentially blocked with each perineural block; thus, it behooves the practitioner to perform a thorough examination before blocking.
4. Perineural anesthesia may migrate significantly depending on volume, anatomy, and technique. The practitioner should be aware that anesthetic migration may inadvertently anesthetize other areas of the horse's limb and consider this fact in the lameness evaluation.

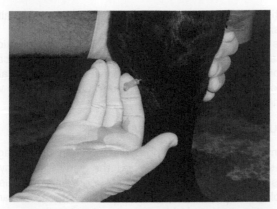

Fig. 4. Joint fluid should be removed from a joint prior to injection, for possible analysis, to ensure entry into the joint space and for ease of injection.

Intra-Articular Anesthesia

1. Removing fluid from a joint prior to injection makes the injection easier and may have therapeutic value. Fluid removed from joints should be examined and collected, if necessary; it can give clues as to the etiology of the lameness problem (**Fig. 4**).
2. The amount of anesthetic used to inject various areas is, to some degree, a matter of personal preference. Larger joints usually require larger volumes of anesthetic.
3. In an effort to avoid problems post joint injection:
   a. Use sterile, noncompounded products
   b. Use sterile technique
   c. Allow fluid to drain back through the needle to help avoid joint contamination
   d. Do not inject unless fluid drains freely, and the injection is without significant resistance
   e. Avoid periarticular injections.
4. Anesthetic placed in the distal interphalangeal joint can anesthetize structures outside of the joint.
5. With time, anesthetic placed in the intercarpal joint can anesthetize the proximal suspensory ligament. Conversely, if one infiltrates the proximal suspensory ligament, it is possible to enter distopalmar pouches of the intercarpal joint and inadvertently anesthetize that joint.
6. There is considerable discussion about anesthesia of the hock, particularly regarding the percentage of horses in which communication occurs between the tarsometatarsal and distal intertarsal joints. Before attempting anesthesia of the hock area, practitioners should be familiar with both the anatomy and the relevant literature.[1,14]
7. In certain situations, some practitioners may choose to mix diagnostic anesthesia and intra-articular treatment medication and administer them at the same time, particularly if a horse is performing in the near future and shows mild lameness and the client wants no further diagnostic workup.
8. Multiple entries into the same joint on the same day are a practice that is eschewed by some but is not necessarily harmful. Waiting for interpretation of diagnostic imaging modalities prior to additional joint entry allows for owner/trainer communication as to the horse's problem prior to injection; however, it may not always be

practical. Multiple injections of the same joint may be especially necessary in a ship-in clinic situation and in some ambulatory situations.
9. In the author's experience, some horses with lameness conditions secondary to sore joints may have a prolonged soundness after mepivacaine injection for several days or weeks. This prolonged positive effect on the pain cascade in the joint can be confusing to owners and trainers. Often the horse will remain sound until hard training is resumed.

LAMENESS VERSUS NEUROLOGIC DISEASE

Differentiating lameness from neurologic disease can be a diagnostic dilemma. Neurologic disease may be subclinical, and the early signs may be very subtle. Neurologic disease may also lead to soreness or coordination issues that present as lameness. Neurologic disease may also present with gait changes that mimic lameness but are not accompanied by soreness to palpation or manipulation.

Listen for neurologic clues in the history. Complaints such as stumbling, knuckling over in rear fetlocks, toe dragging, staggering gait, and attitude changes, usually toward depression, all may indicate a neurologic problem. For example, a history of a horse that is weak, bad gaited, or stumbling a few days after a tiring performance or a long transit, that then improves with rest, may be an indication of neurologic disease.

During the assessment of the horse for lameness, the examiner should always be looking for signs of neurologic disease. An immediate change in a horse's neurologic state after a treatment, especially worsening after corticosteroid treatment, may be suggestive of conditions such as equine protozoal myelitis. Conversely, a positive response to administration of nonsteroidal anti-inflammatory drugs usually rules out neurologic disease; horses that improve dramatically after 3 days of oral phenylbutazone usually have lameness issues and not neurologic disease. The author often uses this "bute test" to attempt to differentiate between lameness, neurologic, and limb interference (cross firing, forging, etc) in standardbreds with difficult subtle gait problems. If the horse is not responsive to 3 g of phenylbutazone per day for 3 days, then the differentials of neurologic disease or limb interference are thoroughly explored.

ENVIRONMENTAL/MANAGEMENT ISSUES

As part of evaluating the lame horse, the veterinarian may also have to help with management issues. Assisting the owner to deal with employees, and especially trainer issues, requires very good communication skills. The reality is that not all grooms, blacksmiths, and trainers are compatible with each horse. Helping the owner match each horse with the proper management is sometimes necessary for the horse to be able to perform at its best. Veterinarians must use great care and diplomacy to maintain good working relationships with the horse's team members. Conditioning, nutrition, and shoeing are very important for maximum performance. Horsemanship skills with tack and equipment vary significantly from stable to stable and influence performance; all of these factors affect the attitude of the horse, and they can occasionally even cause lameness. There is an important saying around performance horses: "Happy horses perform best."

SUMMARY

Lameness and performance evaluation can be one of the most rewarding aspects of equine veterinary practice. There is a misconception that it depends on new sophisticated and expensive diagnostic modalities, when the reality is that knowing where and when to use these modalities form the real art of equine lameness practice.

The most expensive ultrasound machine in the world is not very diagnostic if applied to the wrong limb. The art of lameness practice is vested in knowledge of horsemanship, an understanding of anatomy and function, and inquiring senses to sort out what the horse and his handlers are telling you. The ability to listen to both and figure out a horse's lameness problem will be one of the most valuable services experiences the equine ambulatory clinician can provide for his or her clientele.

REFERENCES

1. Ross M, Dyson SJ, editors. Diagnosis and management of lameness in the horse. 2nd edition. St Louis: Elsevier/Saunders; 2011. p. 818.
2. Van Heerden J, Dauth J, Dreyer MJ, et al. Selected laboratory parameters of thoroughbreds. J S Afr Vet Assoc 1990;61:155–8.
3. Revington M. Haematology of the racing Thoroughbred in Australia, 2: haematological values compared to performance. Equine Vet J 1983;15:145–8.
4. Leahy ER, Burk AO, Greene EA, et al. Nutrition-associated problems facing elite level three-day eventing horses. Equine Vet J 2010;42(Suppl 38):370–4.
5. Tamzali Y, Marguet C, Priymenko N, et al. Prevalence of gastric ulcer syndrome in high-level endurance horses. Equine Vet J 2011;43:141–4.
6. Keg PR, van Weeren PR, Back W, et al. Influence of the force applied and its period of application on the outcome of the flexion test of the distal forelimb of the horse. Vet Rec 1997;141:463–6.
7. Keg PR, van Weeren PR, Schamhardt HC, et al. Variations in the force applied to flexion tests of the distal limb of horses. Vet Rec 1997;141:435–8.
8. Busschers E, van Weeren PR. Use of the flexion test of the distal forelimb in the sound horse: repeatability and effect of age, gender, weight, height and fetlock joint range of motion. J Vet Med A Physiol Pathol Clin Med 2001;48:413–27.
9. Verschooten F, Verbeeck J. Flexion test of the metacarpophalangeal and interphalangeal joints and flexion angle of the metacarpophalangeal joint in sound horses. Equine Vet J 1997;29:50–4.
10. Hague BA, Honnas CM, Simpson RB, et al. Evaluation of skin bacterial flora before and after aseptic preparation of clipped and nonclipped arthrocentesis sites in horses. Vet Surg 1997;26:121–5.
11. Adams SB, Moore GE, Elrashidy M, et al. Effect of needle size and type, reuse of needles, insertion speed, and removal of hair on contamination of joints with tissue debris and hair after arthrocentesis. Vet Surg 2010;39:667–73.
12. Moyer W, Schumacher J, Schumacher J. A guide to equine joint injection and regional anesthesia. Yardley (PA): Vet Learning Systems; 2007.
13. Schumacher J, Schramme MC, Schumacher J, et al. How to perform and interpret diagnostic analgesia of the equine foot. Proceedings of the American Association of Equine Practitioners, Focus Meeting, Focus on the Foot. Raleigh, NC, 2009. Available at: http://www.scribd.com/doc/57341531/How-to-Perform-and-Interpret-Diagnostic-Analgesia-of-the-Equine-Foot. Accessed December 22, 2011.
14. Baxter GM, editor. Adams and Stashak's lameness in horses. 6th edition. Ames (IA): Wiley-Blackwell; 2011.
15. Harper J, Schumacher J, Degraves F, et al. Effects of analgesia of the digital flexor tendon sheath on pain originating in the sole, distal interphalangeal joint or navicular bursa of horses. Equine Vet J 2007;39:535–9.
16. Schumacher J, Steiger R, Schumacher J, et al. Effects of analgesia of the distal interphalangeal joint or palmar digital nerves on lameness caused by solar pain in horses. Vet Surg 2000;29:54–8.

The Equine Practitioner–Farrier Relationship: Building a Partnership

William Moyer, DVM, ACVSMR[a],*,
Stephen E. O'Grady, DVM, MRCVS, APF[b], Harry W. Werner, VMD[c]

KEYWORDS

- Farriers • Horseshoeing • Lameness
- Ambulatory equine practice

Foot problems are thought to be the leading cause of lameness in horses. How a given equine athlete is trimmed and/or shod influences both flight and landing patterns; thus, care of the horse's foot is of great importance. The past few decades have seen a virtual explosion of enhanced diagnostic imaging modalities (digital and computed radiography, ultrasonography, computed tomography [CT], thermography, and magnetic resonance imaging [MRI]), as well as a better understanding of the anatomy and function of the various tissues that make up the equine digit. During this same time span, many more choices for care of the horse's foot have become available; there are myriad medications and therapeutic modalities, a variety of materials used, countless designs of shoes and applications, and differing methods to secure the application to the hoof (nails, glue, screws, boots, etc). By virtue of their training, equipment, and expertise, equine veterinarians have unique ability to more accurately diagnose and understand the plethora of disorders affecting the horse's hoof.

Most, but not all, foot disorders require, or would benefit from, alterations in how the hoof is trimmed. In addition to specific trimming recommendations, management considerations include the optimum schedule for trimming a particular horse and whether shoes and various applications are part of the solution. If shoes or appliances are part of the solution, decisions regarding the design and placement of the shoe or shoes are also necessary. Most equine ambulatory clinicians do not also shoe horses; thus, a close working relationship with the horseshoeing community is not only

---

The editors and authors would like to thank farriers Chuck Esau and Kenneth Crofts for their assistance and suggestions in the preparation of the manuscript.

The authors have nothing to disclose.

[a] Large Animal Clinical Sciences, College of Veterinary Medicine and Biomedical Sciences, Texas A&M University, College Station, TX 77845, USA

[b] Northern Virginia Equine, PO Box 746, Marshall, VA 20116, USA

[c] Werner Equine LLC, 20 Godard Road, North Granby, CT 06060, USA

* Corresponding author.

E-mail address: wmoyer@cvm.tamu.edu

desirable but inevitable and essential. The eventual outcome, in the authors' experience, has been very enjoyable and has been a continuously valuable learning process.

THE VETERINARIAN-FARRIER RELATIONSHIP

Veterinary medicine and horseshoeing are historically "joined at the hip." They are, however, separate professions. While communication challenges do often exist between these 2 distinct subsets of the horse community, the challenges are very manageable. The two professions may share the same goal—keeping the horse's hoof healthy, and the horse moving sound—but they have differing skill sets and educational experiences. Equine practitioners are trained to diagnose and select the best treatment plan; farriers are trained to shape the bearing surface of the foot to best suit the mechanical needs of a given foot. Thus, the partnership of clinician and farrier, when functioning properly, combines to work in the best interest of the horse. Furthermore, clients are very appreciative of such cooperative team efforts.

The relationship between veterinarian and farrier is extremely important not only for the overall health of the foot, but because the treatment of most lameness cases will usually require input from a farrier, who will perform part, or sometimes all of the therapy. Many veterinary colleges and most large equine practices doing a large volume of lameness work have a farrier on staff, or at least have a close association with a certain farrier. The relationship can become more complex for the ambulatory practitioner as many different farriers will be encountered. However, under any circumstances, the total health care of the horse, including the feet, is the responsibility of the veterinarian.

A brief look at the evolution of farrier education may be helpful in helping to appreciate the complexity of the veterinarian-farrier relationship. At one time, the apprenticeship was the accepted standard for learning the farrier trade. It provided a comprehensive learning experience under the tutelage of a skilled experienced farrier. Farriery was taught and applied based on experience, and the structures of the foot, and their proposed functions, served as guidelines for the appropriate farriery. The guiding principles were outlined in horseshoeing textbooks published around the turn of the century.[1-4]

As the population, and their economic means, increased, horses became readily affordable for many individuals, both for recreational and competition purposes. This resulted in an increase in the number of horses, and an increased demand forcare, including hoof care. Thus, horseshoeing schools appeared in 1964. Schools varied between 6-12 weeks in length, and were taught by an individual farrier according to their particular views yet. Even so, most schools recommend working with an experienced farrier when the course was completed.

Still, even as educational efforts began, many farriers were self-taught or had worked for another farrier just long enough to get started in the trade. Suddenly, in addition to these experienced horsemen, there appeared a population of farriers with a diversity of interest, knowledge, skill and experience. Any new farriery methods and shoes/appliances were introduced as a way to improve the health of the foot or address lameness. Unfortunately, many of these developments may have interfered with learning and understanding the basic anatomy, function, and biomechanics of the foot, and thus applying the appropriate farriery with those considerations. As a result, many young farriers may lack knowledge, experience and skill, and may be intimidated when asked to discuss farriery or a lameness case with a veterinarian.

Veterinarians also come from diverse backgrounds, not only in education, but also in levels of experience. Diversity in backgrounds brings diversity in opinions; some based on experience; some on preconception; some from the literature; and some from what has been taught in school. Some more recent graduate veterinarians may not have an extensive equine experience and some may have had little exposure to equine hoof care in veterinary school. This may leave some inexperienced practitioners in the uncomfortable position of making requests of an experienced farrier, even though the veterinarian may not be as fully experienced with some of the concepts of trimming and shoeing, and the physiology and function of the feet. Further complicating communications is the fact that veterinarians and farriers often don't speak the same language when it comes to feet and farriery.

Owners and trainers become confused by their options for hoof care, as they are inundated with a multitude of farriery methods, materials, appliances, products, advertisements, etc. All of them are purported to improve the foot and treat various foot disorders, yet there is generally no mention as to the present conformation of the foot, the preparation of a given foot or how a given product is applied/place on the foot.

Further confusing the situation is the fact that there is often no generally accepted terminology. For example, the term "hoof balance" is open to interpretation, but it is generally agreed that "balance" forms the foundation of a well-trimmed foot prior to shoe placement. In this respect, using guidelines or landmarks such as the hoof-pastern axis, the center of articulation and trimming the palmer/plantar section of the foot to include the frog have been proposed in an attempt to standardize the trimming process.[5–6] The lack of generally accepted standards or terminology should spur credible continuing education opportunities devoted to farriery for both professions; such opportunities are particularly valuable when both professions attend. There is no better way to promote essential knowledge and communication.

Even so, while communication challenges do often exist between these two distinct subsets of the horse community, they are very manageable. Both professions bring important skills to the table. Equine practitioners are trained to examine, diagnose and propose the best treatment plan; farriers are trained to prepare the bearing surface of the foot to best suit the mechanical needs of a given foot. Thus, the partnership of clinician and farrier, when functioning properly, combines to work in the best interest of the horse. Furthermore, clients are very appreciative of such cooperative team efforts.

UNDERSTANDING THE KEY ELEMENTS

An equine ambulatory practitioner is quite likely to experience a wide range of personalities, communication skills, expertise, and experience among the farriers with whom he or she may be asked to work. Useful communication between clinicians, farriers, and owners/trainers depend on many factors, including understanding and appreciating what is involved physically and mentally in caring for the horse's hoof, the varying levels of experience and education of the parties involved, as well as the intended athletic endeavor of the horse.

Veterinary medical education has undergone significant changes in the past few decades. The present traditional 4-year curriculum is literally on "overload" as a result of the "information explosion" and the increasing public demand for greater sophistication from practicing veterinarians. In the 1960s, a diagnostic imaging course was confined to one modality (plain film radiography); now students are educated in the use of digital/computed radiography, ultrasonography, CT, nuclear scintigraphy, and MRI. For every addition to the veterinary curriculum, there has to be a decision as to what comes out, as it is still a 4-year experience. As a result, while today's equine practitioner is more highly trained in clinical science than ever, he or she may be less experienced in more "hands-on" aspects of equine practice, including the basics of hoof care and an understanding of the tools and skills of the farrier. In today's setting, where veterinarians generally do not shoe horses, the practitioner provides the diagnosis and suggested treatment plan; the farrier's role is in the implementation of the treatment plan (assuming it involves trimming and shoeing). How that arrangement is best fostered is of utmost importance for the benefit of all involved.

Continuing education is mandatory to maintain and improve skills. Such efforts are abundant and required for practicing veterinarians. While access to subject matter relating to the equine foot may not have been ideal in the past, it is continuously improving. Often such educational experiences combine veterinarians and farriers, and these can be very valued experiences. Still, the "art and science" of shoeing is for the most part "art and experience" rather than science-based. Thus, some of what is thought to be the "truth" is assumed rather than known. When science confronts belief, belief often prevails; how one questions what another believes to be a fact requires good communications skills.

While veterinary education has certain recognized standards, farrier education is somewhat more difficult to define. In the United States, there are literally no requirements or certification required for an individual to "hang out his or her shingle" as a horse shoer. The United Kingdom, however, insists on a 4-year apprenticeship program and subsequent examination before a farrier can become certified/licensed. Some farriers may grow up in the business in the "father-to-son" mode; others may have attended one of the many, yet varied horseshoeing schools (which also are not regulated as to length or content); some fulfill the equivalent of an apprenticeship by associating themselves with an established farrier; and still others are self-taught. A variety of business models also exist in the farrier profession, from the part-time "weekend" or "cowboy" shoer to an individual working in a sophisticated group setup. Some farriers are only equipped to use manufactured shoes (keg shoes), while others invest in wonderfully equipped trailer rigs and shops. Continuing education for farriers is available but it is not required; however, at least one organization, the newly created American Association of Professional Farriers, is requiring annual CE credits. Farrier short courses designed to serve both farriers and veterinarians are usually very well attended and offer educational opportunities for both entities; unfortunately, they may not be well attended by equine practitioners and, as such, may represent a missed opportunity for continuing education and interaction between farriers and veterinarians.

Shoeing horses is a difficult and, at times, dangerous profession. The likelihood of lasting injury or injuries to farriers is very high. The working conditions vary enormously, as do the abilities of horse handlers to safely manage the process. Farriers do not have, or should not have, the legal and scientific standing to utilize chemical restraint. Thus, their collective ability to remain employed by a given owner is very dependent not only on how they shoe the horse but also on how they are perceived as horse handlers. In addition, farriers face similar challenges as veterinarians when it comes to working with owners and trainers. For example, farriers may be told how to trim and shoe a given horse by the client or trainer (which is something that veterinarians should be aware of before thinking or uttering a criticism of their work).

Most farriers have both an acquired and intuitive knowledge of the form and function of the equine hoof. By virtue of regular contact with individual horses, the farrier (assuming that he or she is regularly employed by a client) has an appreciation of morphologic changes that have occurred that an examining veterinarian would not have. The farrier regularly examines such parameters as the shape and quality of horn or how a given foot impacts the ground. Such information is extremely valuable and should be sought by veterinarians attending to problems of the horse's foot. Thus, farriers can serve as an important source of information about the clinical history of horses being examined by the veterinarian. This may also include very useful information about the horse's behavior, as well as information about a client's personality and his or her ability/willingness to comply with instructions.

Farriers tend to have as many or more work- and social-related associations with horse owners than do practitioners as a direct result of frequent/scheduled visits. As a consequence, many horse owners have a very trusted relationship with their farrier. Farriers are often put into an advisory role regarding their opinion about available equine practitioners. While they are inarguably an important partner in effectively managing a horse's health care, farriers should also be regarded as one of the more important marketing elements/targets in the veterinarian's practice business plan.

THE EQUINE PRACTITIONER'S ROLE IN CARING FOR THE HOOF
Equipment

First and foremost, the attending equine practitioner should always present himself or herself in a professional manner. He or she should be well equipped with both a knowledge base and tools. A basic (minimal) list of equipment need for caring for the horse's hoof includes:

- *A shoeing apron.* Aprons are readily available at farrier supply stores. The authors prefer models that are both nylon and leather as they are light, adjustable, washable, and more comfortable in warm weather than the traditional leather apron. Failing to utilize an apron represents a significant safety risk to the user; aprons protect the examiner's legs from hooves, knives, shoes, and nails. Aprons also help the veterinarian to hold a foot more securely.
- *Hoof knives.* Good hoof knives are critical, and it is very useful to have a variety, including loop knives, which are very convenient for exploring abscesses. It is important that knives are kept sharp (which implies that the practitioner learn how to sharpen the blades) **(Fig. 1)**.
- *Shoeing rasps.* Having more than one rasp is helpful, as they will dull, and they will have a variety of uses. The most frequent uses will be to file nail clinches for precise removal of shoes without damaging the hoof wall and for reduction of hoof wall flares and separations.
- *A steel or wire brush.* A wire brush is the most useful and safe tool to clean and explore the bearing surface of the foot. It is safer than using a hoof knife. There have been, and continue to be, horses whose feet have been injured by someone using a hoof knife as an exploratory instrument. Wire brushes are invaluable, and using them to brush debris from the hoof is often the only means of visualizing bruising and discoloration on the sole, fissures, and wall separations.
- *Hoof testers.* Hoof testers come in a wide variety of length/weight and designs. In the authors' opinion, most hoof testers are too long and difficult to operate unless the user has big hands. Many different styles can be purchased at shoeing supply stores or online. An alternative to purchasing hoof testers is to have a set made by the farrier using a worn-out pair of race track hoof nippers; the heads of the nippers are cut off, and the tool is finished using ½-inch steel rod. When making or modifying hoof testers, it is helpful to flare the ends of the handles to keep them from sliding out of one's grip. The flares also can be used as a hoof pick.
- *Shoe pullers.* Good shoe pullers are essential. There are 2 types: the traditional shoe puller and the single nail (crease) pullers. Single nail pullers allow the veterinarian to remove a single nail—for example, removal of the inside heel nail

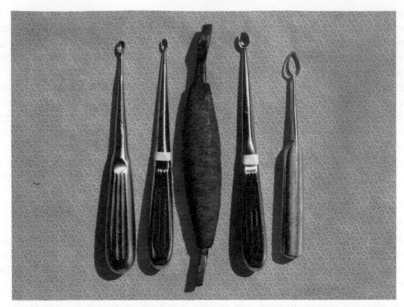

Fig. 1. A selection of good hoof knives is critical for the equine ambulatory practitioner.

(the most difficult nail to place for the farrier without entering or adjoining underlying sensitive tissue) while still keeping the shoe on.

- *Hoof picks.* Hoof picks can be used to clean the hoof but are not always necessary. The authors prefer to clean and explore the frog and clefts with the dull side of the hoof knife and wire brush.
- *Hand-held motorized burrs* (Dremel, for example). These tools have a multitude of uses, and they come with a variety of burrs, small drills, drum sanders, etc. Practitioners not familiar with the use of motorized burrs can safely develop a "feel" for their ability to remove, cut, and sand by practicing on a piece of soft pine wood. Rechargeable varieties of such tools may not be the best choice, as the duration of charge is often less than ideal.
- *No. 2 or No. 3 bone curettes.* Curettes are very useful when exploring hoof wall damage, separations, or opening an abscess and are often safer and easier to use than a hoof knife.
- *Portable radiography equipment.* Radiographs are essential for evaluation of the bony structures inside of the hoof. Radiographic equipment should also include devices to facilitate proper positioning. For example, a means to elevate the foot to center the beam is essential.
- *Digital photography capability.* Perhaps not essential, but digital photography (even if it is a cell phone type) is incredibly useful for the purposes of medical record keeping and follow-up. It is also a useful tool when seeking advice from others about a given problem, for archiving interesting cases, or for educating clients.
- *Ultrasonography.* The hoof is not particularly amenable to ultrasonographic evaluation, but it can be useful in certain settings (eg, evaluation of the navicular bone), assuming one has been trained and is skilled in its use.
- *Hoof angle gauge.* Hoof angle gauges can be occasionally useful for demonstration purposes, but they are not essential.

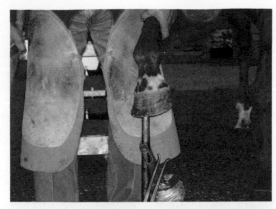

Fig. 2. A portable foot stand can make working on the horse's hoof easier, as well as help minimize wear and tear on the practitioner.

- *Portable foot stand.* Foot stands are not essential, but they are labor saving if one intends on doing regular foot-related work. They clearly can lessen the physical strain on the user (**Fig. 2**).
- A *medical record system* that includes consistent and reliable entries regarding the shape, quality of hoof material, and previous management is very important. This often requires sufficient space for drawings or digital photographs.
- It is very helpful to have ready access to *images of the foot and related anatomy*, or to carry anatomical models, to enhance education of the client. The more the veterinarian is able to effectively educate the people involved in the care of the horse, the greater is the likelihood of client and farrier compliance as well as client retention.

Skills

Veterinarians working on horse's hooves should have the necessary skills to conduct a thorough and proper examination. It has been said that for every case that a veterinarian misses for not knowing, 10 will be missed for not looking. Without the proper skills to adequately evaluate the horse's hoof, proper diagnoses—even obvious diagnoses—can be missed.

Veterinarians must knowing how to properly position themselves under a horse and secure the lower limb in a "farrier's stance" (**Fig. 3**). Proper positioning while holding the hoof is *critical*. While this statement may seem obvious, the number of equine practitioners the authors have observed over the years who fail to hold the limb in proper position is reasonably high. Improper positioning leads to leg fatigue and may result in a less than thorough examination. Additional risks to the clinician from improper positioning include stepped-on feet, injured legs when the horse snatches the leg away, and lower back problems.

Veterinarians should know how to properly and carefully remove a shoes or shoes. Shoe removal is critical to enhance the visual examination of the hoof and/or to take radiographs. The importance of proper shoe removal is 2-fold. First, if the clinches are not properly filed or cut, one can inadvertently tear off hoof wall, making subsequent efforts to shoe or trim the hoof more difficult. Second, a loose shoe is a risk to the horse; when a shoe is not quickly and expertly removed, loosened nails can be redirected into the substance of the hoof, or the partially removed shoe can damage

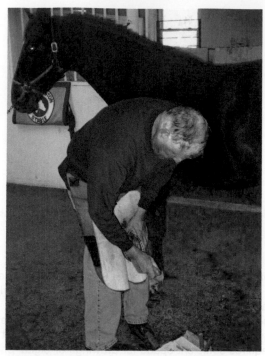

Fig. 3. Proper positioning while examining the horse's foot helps minimize the chance of injury to both the veterinarian and the horse.

the unprotected ground surface of the foot. Once the shoe has been removed, veterinarians should remember that the horse is now barefoot and take measures to protect the hoof until the horse can be shod, such as keeping the horse in an enclosure until re-shod and/or wrapping the feet with protective bandages or boots.

Good skills in taking radiographs are essential for evaluating the horse's foot. Veterinarians should know what is considered to be the standards for creating diagnostic radiographic images of the foot. In most cases, removing the shoe is necessary to obtain diagnostic images. However, in some cases, the owner/trainer may refuse to allow removal of the shoe. In such cases, this should be noted in the record, and especially if a prepurchase examination is performed, since the ability to accurately detect potential lesions is compromised when a shoe is in place.

Skilled ambulatory clinicians know how to use equipment properly, and consistently. For example, hoof testers are one of the few diagnostic tools that one has to detect pain originating in the foot, and in some instances, the device localizes pain to a given region of the foot (**Fig. 4**). Consistent success using this instrument is very user dependent; thus, using it on as many horses as possible is a very useful exercise. Insufficient pressure generated from the testers is likely for some clinicians who lack hand strength or poor positioning under the horse. This may be one reason why an examiner may not get a response with hoof testers, yet still see the horse improve with appropriate local diagnostic anesthesia. Hoof testers are also of use in subjectively determining the quality and strength of hoof tissues.

Veterinarians should know what is generally accepted as "normal shoeing" in their area of practice. Various equine sports often dictate what is considered "normal" (and acceptable). For example, thoroughbred and quarterhorse racehorses are generally shod with aluminum shoes with traction inserts of various shapes and sizes; for these horses, utilizing a flat bar shoe, even though it might be appropriate for a given foot problem, could be a risk to the horse, causing it to slide at speed.

Veterinarians should be familiar with shoeing lexicon. Terms and phrases used by farriers, such as "backing up the toe," or "lowering the heel," may not be immediately familiar to practitioners inexperienced in hoof care. Understanding such terminology is critical for proper communication with farriers. It is so easy to ask or have terms and concepts demonstrated, instead of pretending that one actually knows.

Routine use of diagnostic anesthesia will help veterinarians to be sure the pain and source of lameness is, in fact, the foot. There are many examples of owners/clients spending significant amounts of money on diagnostic imaging only to ultimately find out the problem (pain) is not the foot or vice versa. Still, while local anesthetic blocks are relatively easy to perform, and provide much useful information, they should be applied only after a thorough examination of the foot has been conducted.

Almost equally as important as the technical skills required for examining the foot are communication skills. Developing and improving one's communication skills is key to ensuring that prescriptions for shoeing and trimming are complied with. Communication is part of the "art" of veterinary medicine, and it can be very challenging to an audience that may include the farrier, the owner, the trainer, a stable manager or groom, an insurance adjuster, consultants, or even just a friend who has agreed to be there to hold the horse. In order to avoid communication problems, it is good practice to summarize what has been done and what is expected with regard to aftercare. Veterinarians should also allow for questions as to what is being proposed, and why. Good hoof care is—or at least should be—a team effort.

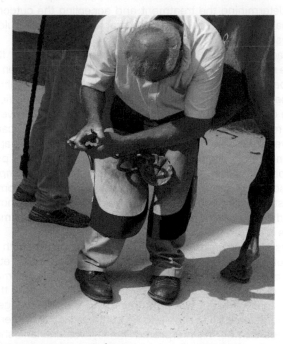

Fig. 4. Hoof testers are essential tools for examining the horse's hoof.

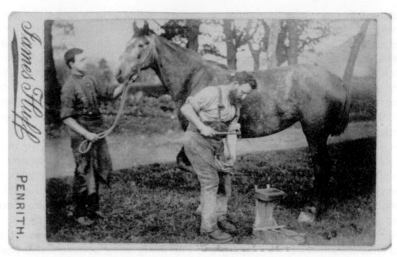

Fig. 5. A good working relationship has been important for good horse care for centuries.

ESTABLISHING AND SUSTAINING WORKING RELATIONSHIPS

Establishing and sustaining a useful and productive relationship with a farrier requires a committed and consistent approach. The most likely way of "starting on the wrong foot" in the veterinarian–farrier relationship is with a demonstration of a lack of respect by either or both parties (clinician and farrier) of the other's knowledge, experience, and expertise. The "I am the Doctor" and therefore know what I am doing routine invariably fails; furthermore, it does not reduce the responsibility placed on the veterinarian for determining the treatment and accepting the outcome. The responsibility to take the lead should rest with the practitioner, who should set the tone as leader of the horse's health care team.

Ambulatory practices tend to have inherent regional boundaries; the same, for the most part, can be said of a farrier's clientele (**Fig. 5**). Therefore, a given busy practitioner is very likely to be dealing directly or indirectly with a significant, although somewhat consistent, number of farriers in their area. The interactions with farriers can vary from very frequently to occasionally, depending on how the work areas overlap.

All successful relationships are based on trust. Ultimately, trust can only be earned over time; however, trust-building can be started with a committed approach from the onset of the veterinarian's interactions with the farriers in his or her practice area. The first impression one provides is important, even though the first impression may not always be in person. An impression could begin with a comment from the client to the shoer, a text message from you regarding shoeing, or perhaps a note you pinned to the stall door, and it is worth the effort for the veterinarians to try to make sure that the first interaction is a good one.

Whenever possible, it is worth the veterinarian's time to visit with a given farrier in person instead of depending on the client/manager/barn help, etc. to accurately provide information. Second-hand information given to the farrier may be inaccurate or may even be perceived as a criticism by the farrier or owner. If the veterinarian is unable to be physically present when trimming and shoeing changes are made, the veterinarian should at least be available to be contacted by the farrier via a cell phone. Even detailed notes can be misinterpreted. Finally, veterinarians should provide the farrier with a business card and a sincere offer of help if the need arises.

DO'S AND DON'TS

For the success of the equine ambulatory practitioner, the importance of building positive, productive and lasting relationships with local farriers cannot be over-stated. As with all worthwhile relationships, the farrier-veterinarian partnership requires on-going attention and nurturing. The following lists of "do's and don'ts" should help the ambulatory practitioner build and maintain a successful veterinarian-farrier relationship:

- Veterinarians should not criticize the way in which a given horse is trimmed or shod in the presence of an owner/caretaker, and especially so if they do not know the relevant history. Veterinarians should also carefully think about and construct comments or statements to avoid them from being construed as derogatory. For example, the veterinarian may believe the toe to be excessively long and comment about the need for trimming. However, the veterinarian may not aware of the fact that the farrier has already made an effort at correcting this problem but had reason to believe that was as much he or she could remove at the time of the last visit. As such, the veterinarian did not see the problem that the farrier was initially confronted with. Furthermore, the excessive toe length may also relate to the fact that the owner does not wish to pay for the ideal frequency of farrier visits and that the problem is therefore not the farrier's fault.
- Veterinarians should be clear in how aggressive they want the farrier to be in correcting the problem. Directions should be communicated directly to the farrier.
- Veterinarians should be aware that they are likely to have long working relationships with local farriers. As such, one consideration is this; what if the shoer who was just criticized is also the best in the area?
- Submural focal infections can occur as the result of a poorly placed shoeing nail. Nails can be poorly placed by the best of farriers, and it can become all too convenient to blame the farrier (even if the veterinarian does not place blame, the client might).

However, it may be useful to think of a "hot" nail in different terms:

1. The nail may have been properly placed, but the shoe moved which moved the nail into or next to sensitive tissue.
2. The individual horse may have very thin walls. In such circumstances (which are all too common), nail placement is always risky.
3. The horse may have been difficult to shoe, and nail placement may have been affected as a result. Veterinarians are certainly aware that if a stomach tube is passed often enough, eventually one or more horses will develop a nose bleed. Sometimes, things happen.

- Veterinarians should be very careful about removing shoes and protecting the unshod foot to avoid hoof wall damage. It can be nearly impossible for a farrier to attach a shoe to a foot from which most of the quarter has broken off. A simple wrap of duct tape or self-adherent wrap is generally insufficient to protect a hoof until such time as the farrier can attend the horse; veterinarians should apply appropriate bandages, or suggest protective boots, to prevent hoof wall damage.
- Veterinarians should make an effort to save the shoes that were removed so as to avoid having the owner to have to pay for an additional set or avoid making the farrier feel unfairly obligated to make new ones for free. Shoes can be taped to stall walls or given to owners or trainers for safe-keeping.

- The phrase "foot balance" is an all too often used description that has no generally accepted definition. The symmetry of the foot is dependent on a variety of factors, including conformation, the limb flight pattern (which influences how the foot strikes the surface), environmental living and working surface environments, athletic working conditions, the presence or absence of lameness, and the frequency and quality of shoeing and trimming. A common example of how "foot balance" can reflect factors other than how the horse is being trimmed is that of a horse with toe-out conformation. Such horses are likely to have a steep medial heel/quarter and a 'flared' lateral toe wall, and the asymmetric "unbalanced" foot may not be the result of the farrier but a result of the horse's conformation, instead. Veterinarians should be very careful about using the term "imbalance" (the opposite of "balance"), as it may lead to the perception that the farrier created it. In fact, in the author's experience, most markedly asymmetric feet are the result of less than ideal conformation, and not the way that the horse is trimmed and/or shod.
- Veterinarians should be liberal in dispensing praise. If the veterinarian is pleased with the way a horse, or group of horses, is trimmed and shod, he or she should let the owner/handler and farrier know! Sincere compliments are often valued more than money. If the owner feels good about how his or her horses are managed, and the farrier knows someone appreciates his or her work, it will also benefit the veterinarian, in both continued work, as well as in potential referrals.
- In prolonged and protracted difficult cases (chronic laminitis being a prime example), veterinarians should let the owner/handler know from the beginning that such cases can be difficult, time consuming, mistake ridden, and expensive ordeals for all involved. Even the best efforts of an involved and accomplished farrier may result in a failure. Owners/handlers should be informed of this at the onset. While communicating with the owners, veterinarians should also elevate the position of the farrier in the process. Under no circumstances should the veterinarian comment on the price for the farrier's services, as that is clearly none of the veterinarian's business.
- If the outcome of a trimming and shoeing procedure results in making the situation worse (ie, more lame) the veterinarian should not place the blame on the farrier. Instead, the blame should be placed on the horse's condition, and the veterinarians should begin to direct plan B.
- If a particular foot problem requires some special shoeing or appliance, the veterinarian should ask the farrier (assuming that the veterinarian does not already know the answer), if this is something that he or she is comfortable with/capable of doing. By doing so, the veterinarian can avoid putting the farrier in a position where the client may perceive that the farrier did not comply with the veterinarian's instructions or was unwilling to help. For both veterinarians and farriers, some cases are clearly better off if they are referred.
- In some cases conflicts may arise, even under the best of circumstances. If a conflict arises on the management of a given problem, the veterinarian should attempt to resolve it in person with the farrier. Differences of opinion and/or experience are normal and often great fun; both veterinarian and farrier can learn from the process. Nevertheless, despite the veterinarian's best intentions, some situations or personalities simply may not work regardless of the effort. In such cases, the horse owner/caretaker should be made aware of such conflicts so as to ensure the health and welfare of the horse.
- Sharing radiographs can be helpful to the experienced farrier in some cases. However, the veterinarian should get permission from the client before sharing

radiographs with any outside party. Interpretation of the radiographs should be perceived as a joint venture rather than the farrier making a diagnosis and developing a treatment strategy.

- Veterinarians should make every effort to honor appointment schedules when dealing with cases requiring the presence of the farrier. Clearly, the veterinarian should treat the farrier with the same courtesy as the veterinarian would hope to be treated.
- Thank the farrier any time he or she helps. The value of kindness and respect is not calculable.
- Veterinarians should subscribe to—and read—readily available farrier publications. This is a great way to understand a variety of issues, techniques, and products that farriers deal with. Being familiar with the materials that farriers read is a great tool for enhancing one's ability to communicate.
- Veterinarians should consider joining internet listservs that are likely to discuss foot related problems, such as the American Association of Equine Practitioners General List and Equine Clinician Network. A more recent addition (2012) is the American Association of Equine Practitioners Podiatry Rounds. Listservs allow for posting questions to colleagues (including) images for consultation or can be simply a location to read and appreciate the thoughts of others regarding the hoof, as well as various other subjects.

SUMMARY

The importance of hoof care in maintaining the health and soundness of a horse cannot be overstated. The aphorism, "No foot, no horse" still holds true. For equine ambulatory practitioners, the time devoted to a thorough understanding of the equine digit and it's care is well worth the investment. The effort devoted to developing good relationships with individuals who will likely be responsible for implementing the changes suggested as a result of that understanding will be rewarded many times over in the course of the equine ambulatory practitioner's career.

ACKNOWLEDGEMENTS

The editors and authors would like to thank farriers Chuck Esau and Kenneth Crofts for their assistance and suggestions in the preparation of this manuscript.

REFERENCES

1. Fisher AT. The Farrier or No Foot, No Horse. London: Richard Bentley & Son; 1893.
2. Lungwitz A. A textbook of Horseshoeing. Philadelphia: J.B. Lippincott Company; 1897.
3. Dollar J. A handbook of horseshoeing. Edinburgh: David Douglas; 1898.
4. Russell W. Scientific Horseshoeing. Cincinnati (OH): Robert Clark Co.; 1908.
5. O'Grady SE, Poupard DE. Proper physiologic horseshoeing. Vet Clin North Am Equine Pract 2003;19(2):333–44.
6. O'Grady SE. Guidelines for trimming the equine foot: A Review. In, Proceedings. Am Assoc of Eq Pract 2009;55:218–25.

The Approach to the Equine Dermatology Case in Practice

Derek C. Knottenbelt, OBE, BVM&S, DVM&S, MRCVS

KEYWORDS
- Equine • Dermatology • Skin • Problem list
- Differential diagnosis • Biopsy • Intradermal skin test

Dermatologic disease in equine practice is always a challenge; there is little that causes more upset in clients than a "bad skin disease" and little that causes so much antipathy between owners and veterinarians when no satisfactory conclusions are produced after prolonged and expensive investigations. Dermatologic examinations are a normal and important part of the physical examination of the horse whether for pre-purchase examination or for clinical reasons. From a clinical perspective, the skin can be affected by primary skin disease; some of these can have systemic or remote implications, where the skin is a secondary component, and often a striking indicator, of an internal disorder. The implications of each of these circumstances are profound and it is the duty of the practice veterinarian to identify and manage the case as a whole.[1]

The skin of the horse is its biggest organ and is by far the most easily examined; it is directly visible and palpable and is easily examined over the entire body. The healthy skin has a lustrous appearance in summer (**Fig. 1**A) and a thick but shiny appearance in winter. There are significant areas on the horse skin that tend to be forgotten, such as the foot; the hoof is simply a modified skin structure and can be a highly informative structure as well as being affected by disease in its own right! In practice, equine skin disease is a common challenge. However, it is unfortunate that owners will almost always have "had a go" at treatment, often using inappropriate/ irrational medications and concoctions that really have little or no chance of successfully treating the problem; cures under such circumstances probably come about despite the treatment, not because of it! This simply serves to confuse the diagnosis—for example, a strong chemical applied to the skin can cause serious deterioration and masking of primary signs, making the clinical investigation much more difficult. The added and common complication of failure to declare the previous "treatments" is another problem for the ambulatory clinician.

The skin is also an effective window on the health or otherwise of many other organs and systems (**Fig. 1**B). The skin can be seriously affected by internal disease, and so it is

The author has nothing to disclose.
Philip Leverhulme Hospital, University of Liverpool, Neston, Wirral, UK CH43 7PT
E-mail address: knotty@liv.ac.uk

Vet Clin Equine 28 (2012) 131–153
doi:10.1016/j.cveq.2012.01.004   **vetequine.theclinics.com**

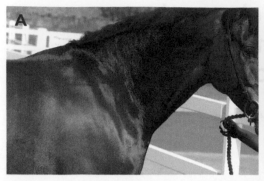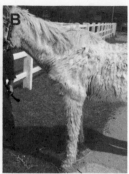

Fig. 1. The normal skin of a horse varies from the highly lustrous short summer coat (*A*) to the longer, denser winter coat. Abnormal coat and obvious lesions are usually very apparent. It is not really the detection of the lesions/abnormalities that is difficult—it is making a diagnosis that is the challenge. In some cases, the signs are pathognomonic or at least suggestive of the diagnosis. (*B*) An old horse with the hypertrichosis (so-called "hirsutism") typical of PPID (equine Cushing disease) is shown. This is in effect the only condition that causes severe acquired hypertrichosis and the dermatologic sign is therefore pathognomonic.

critical to the investigation to consider all the available possibilities and not just the skin itself. For example, an acute onset of an apparent photosensitization affecting the blaze and muzzle could be associated with advanced liver disease or simple ingestion of a primary photosensitizing plant such as St John's Wort (*Hypericum perforatum*) or could indeed simply be a matter of sun exposure (actinic burn). In the former case management of the skin alone would be pointless, while in the latter simply reducing exposure to sunlight by application of sunblock or stabling the horse would be curative. If the problem was being caused by ingestion of a photoactive plant, of course the grazing and management must be investigated and any suspicious plants removed from access. Such a case simply illustrates the importance of an encompassing/holistic approach to the investigation. There should be no assumptions and certainly no speedy conclusions: "Diagnose in haste, repent/regret at leisure!"

Despite the need for a comprehensive approach, intuitive supposition is a common approach to skin diseases. Serious errors can be made by a casual and assumptive approach because of the general clinical similarity of many of the skin conditions. The skin can only respond in a relatively few ways, and many conditions appear broadly similar. It is the nuances and subtleties that make the difference between a satisfying clinical investigation and a disappointing catalogue of failure.

In general, veterinarians will be a called to see chronic skin cases more than those of acute onset; most owners will either have ignored the condition in its early stages (in the hope that it would "go away"), or more usually will have applied some medications (usually ill-advised and inappropriate) in the hope that the condition will be cured quickly and cheaply. This not only makes the investigation and diagnosis more difficult but also often confuses the diagnostic process and treatment and frequently has an additional effect on the prognosis.

INVESTIGATING THE SKIN PROBLEM

The investigation of the dermatology case should always follow a logical and precise structure. Without logic, the process breaks down, and without detail, mistakes are easily made. Logical considerations in the management of skin diseases include the following.

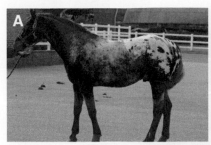 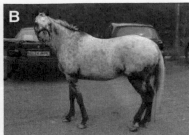

Fig. 2. A 5-year-old appaloosa that was bay with spots until 3 years of age (*A*); by 5 years (*B*), it showed the characteristic and well-recognized fading of the hair color (fading appaloosa syndrome) and thinning of the mane and tail hair (mane and tail dystrophy).

The Signalment of the Horse

The signalment matters in all diagnostic medicine spheres because there are some conditions that are restricted to the specific breed, sex, age, and even color! For example, a nodule in the perineal skin of a gray horse has a very high likelihood of being a melanoma. An old horse presenting with hypertrichosis ("hirsutism") (see **Fig. 1**B) is likely to have pituitary pars intermedia dysfunction (PPID) (equine Cushing disease); this condition is almost unheard of in horses under 12 to 15 years of age. Appaloosa horses suffer from a characteristic mane and tail dystrophy as well as progressive pigmentary changes as they age (**Fig. 2**). Hereditary equine regional dermal asthenia is a well-recognized breed-related disorder in quarterhorses but is occasionally encountered in other breeds. The clinician can sometimes, therefore, at least begin to refine the differential diagnosis from the simple basic description of the animal. The signalment matters! When submitting any diagnostic specimens or clinical information, it is essential that these data are included in every case. It is unfair to the pathologist to simply submit a specimen taken from "a horse!"

Full Long-Term History of the Horse

A full history must always be taken! The history establishes facts about the duration of ownership, management/use, and the previous disease/illness history. The history should establish all the duration of ownership and management details and the disease or accident history of the horse. Each aspect of the normal clinical history has an implication in either supporting later diagnosis or ruling it out! It is also important to make enquiry about animals in contact and whether they have a similar condition. A logical approach is essential; many of the most common conditions can be tentatively diagnosed with clinical and historical information alone. Horses that have been owned for many years will obviously have a more-detailed history than do those that have been recently acquired.

Aspects of contagion may be established from enquiry about peers and in contact animals (**Fig. 3**). Horses that are managed outside may be more likely to be affected by insect bite hypersensitivity than are stabled horses; those that are stabled permanently may be more likely to have management-related disease such as dermatophytosis (see **Fig. 3**).

Some skin diseases occur seasonally, and many become progressively worse. Some skin disease arises as a result of drug eruptions or allergic responses to inhaled or ingested allergens. Concurrent medications can significantly alter the clinical presentation and may mask some of the most diagnostic signs. For example, a horse

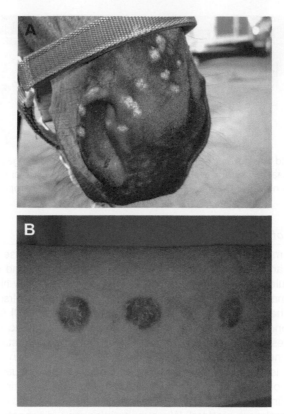

Fig. 3. (*A*) This horse presented with crusting circular lesions on its muzzle, and the owner was also found to have "suspicious" lesions on her arm. (*B*) Equine species of ringworm seldom affect humans, however, and both were infected with *Trichophyton verrucosum* (usually derived from cattle).

that is on long-term steroid therapy for an airway disease problem could easily develop skin infections as a result of immunocompromise, but subtle inflammatory skin disease could be suppressed to the point of nondetection. The clinician needs to be aware of the medications given to the horse and their clinical implications.

The concept of contagion is also an important issue in dermatology, given that the horse has several important ectoparasites. Pruritus is a common frustrating clinical sign. There are quite different diagnostic implications for a single pruritic horse in a group from situations where several or all horses are pruritic. In the former case, an individual disorder is likely, while in the latter, some contagious cause of pruritus such as lice or *Chorioptes* sp mites could be involved.

Detailed History of the "Owner's Complaint"

The clinical signs that the horse exhibits should be explored historically in detail. For example, in a case presented for pruritus it is important to ask if pruritus was the first presenting symptom; it may be the most obvious sign, but there may have been a preexisting clinical condition that the owner failed to recognize as significant. On some occasions, careful questioning will establish that the owner may have developed skin lesions, but it is also possible that this is unrelated. The interpretation of the presenting

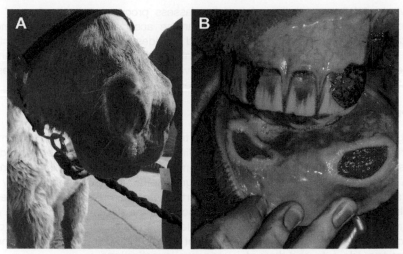

Fig. 4. (*A, B*) This aged gelding was presented because its coat was long and it was losing weight. A diagnosis of PPID was simple to make, but the horse had a serious sinus infection and oral ulcers as part of the syndrome. These concurrent signs altered the outlook significantly and assisted the diagnosis significantly.

signs is a skill that is acquired with experience. Quite often the summary statement made by the owner is a major factor in the investigation, but it can also be misleading. For example, the owner could complain of a localized skin eruption but fail to note that there are concurrent symptoms of weight loss; the converse is also possible (**Fig. 4**). The role of the history is paramount in the investigation and must therefore be taken with care and some understanding; in some cases, the client may be unwilling to divulge some information for fear of criticism or may not understand the detail that is required!

The Physical Examination

A full physical clinical examination is always justified even when the skin signs are limited in severity and extent, and even when they seem trivial. The examination need not necessarily be exhaustive, but the full range of body systems should always be considered because there are skin diseases that occur secondarily to other, sometimes more serious, diseases and there are also skin diseases that have secondary systemic implications. It is remarkable how often a fully physical clinical examination is not carried out, and how easy it can be to miss significant features such as icterus, hemorrhages, or polydipsia/polyuria as a result. Concurrent lameness problems could have a significant diagnostic implication in some skin diseases; similarly, neurologic signs or weight loss detected in a horse with putative photosensitization could be very significant.

Detailed Dermatologic Examination

The focused dermatologic examination provides a detailed description of the types, location(s), and extent of the various recognizable morphologic lesions. It is important to recognize the various options for lesion description and to make a proper diagrammatic map of the distribution and numbers of the detectable signs. This may seem tedious for a busy practitioner but it can be a reputation saver. In the event that treatment is successful, a record can be kept and evidence-based publications can even be made! In the event of failure or the need to follow/assess progression in the face of client skepticism or criticism, the true picture can be accurately followed. Mapping the detectable signs serves several purposes and provides an accurate starting point from which changes in the distribution and extent, progression or improvement, and responses to treatment can be assessed objectively. Photographic records are professionally satisfying and a very effective way of assessing the progress of a case.

THE PROBLEM LIST

Having completed the clinical examination, the clinician should construct a problem list. This is simply a list of any detectable clinical abnormality, whether derived from the history or the physical/dermatologic examinations. The problem list must include all the detected skin signs and any other signs. Some signs may seem initially to be irrelevant or trivial, but some could be important. For example, small mouth vesicles and blisters can be a significant feature of some of the autoimmune disorders of the skin. In some cases, several individual problems can be tied together to add to their diagnostic value. The process of refinement of the diagnosis is developed through eliminations/rule-outs and through supportive investigations.

THE DIFFERENTIAL DIAGNOSIS

From the problem list, it should be possible to formulate a differential diagnostic list in order of likelihood. Nothing should be excluded, no matter how rare or unlikely. There is a strong tendency in clinical practice to jump to conclusions or to bypass this stage completely, and to move directly to a set of diagnostic tests. Both of these approaches should be resisted strongly, no matter how tempting. The process of diagnosis gives job satisfaction and enhances professional reputation. Time spent in clinical thought is never wasted and costs nothing!

Some possibilities can be set aside at an early stage for epidemiologic, geographical, and historical reasons. For example, a linking series of ulcerated nodules in a horse in the United Kingdom or the United States would not (not normally at least) be due to epizootic lymphangitis! Sarcoids, or ulcerative lymphangitis due to *Corynebacterium* infection, would be far more likely. The conditions that are encountered in southern Africa may be very different from those in North America. The significance of local knowledge should not be overlooked.

Establishing a definitive diagnosis is the primary objective of the clinician in practice. Once that is done, the prognosis and the sensible treatment options can be derived from evidence-based publications or from consultation with expert colleagues. Many clinicians have a tendency to use intuitive supposition as the mainstay of their diagnosis. While this often works well for experienced clinicians, it is still an unwise method of diagnosis because many different conditions present with common clinical signs! For example, tail pruritus could be a result of parasitic infestation, allergic, atopic or neurologic disease, or even be physical in origin (**Fig. 5**). A nodular lesion on the inguinal region of an old gray horse may well be a melanoma, but it could also be a sarcoid, lymphoma, or even a collagenolytic granuloma. The outlook and treatment options for the various possibilities are very different; a mistake might, at best, be a waste of both time and resources, but at worst it could convert a treatable case into a disaster through mistreatment or undue delay.

For the most part, equine skin disease can be usefully divided into infectious and noninfectious disease. The former involve virus, bacteria, fungi, protozoa, and internal and external parasitic conditions. The latter include congenital/developmental conditions, allergic or immune-mediated disease, traumatic injuries, and neoplastic

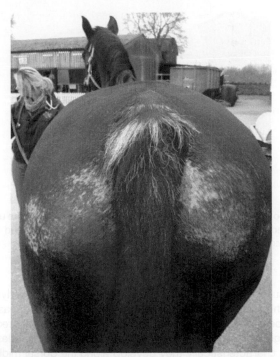

Fig. 5. This mare was presented with severe perineal pruritus that had resulted in marked hair damage (not alopecia!). It was assumed to be insect bite hypersensitivity but failed to respond to all the normal "treatments." It was in fact the result of a severe *O equi* infestation.

disease. Additionally, equine skin conditions can be due to endocrinologic, nutritional, or neurologic problems; others are secondary to vascular disease or from iatrogenic damage to the skin. Often the main concern for clients is the prognosis; once the prognosis is established, the rest follows! Most conditions that have an acceptable prognosis have management or therapeutic measures that will either resolve the condition or at least allow it to be managed.

The clinician should explore the differential diagnoses for the relevant disease category to ensure than every diagnostic possibility is considered, no matter how rare any one might be. The objective is to consider them all and eliminate them on grounds of likelihood and clinical and supportive examinations. The maxim that when one hears hooves, one should think "horses" is apt, but one should always remember that there are also donkeys and zebras and they do occur under particular circumstances!

Noninfectious skin diseases are very common in horses.

1. Genetic or developmental skin disorders are seldom recognized because each of the recognized disorders is rare. Cutaneous agenesis and *epidermolysis bullosa* are very rare—the latter has a genetic origin and is more often encountered in the Belgian breed. The large majority of congenital or developmental conditions are manifest early in life—possibly within the first few days—but some are much later. Hereditary equine regional dermal asthenia/cutaneous asthenia/fragile skin disease may only be detected when the horse is harnessed in some way or is injured at some later age. In this condition, the skin lacks adequate strength in its connection to the subcutaneous tissues, and so traumatic injury or excessive

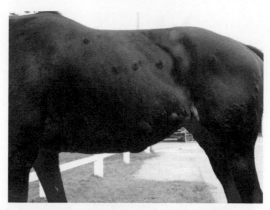

Fig. 6. This 4-year-old thoroughbred colt in training suffered from severe urticaria every time he ate cereal-based feeds. Treatment with drugs was not possible and dietary avoidance strategies were successful in allowing the colt to race (and win).

movement results in vascular disruption and necrosis of the overlying skin. Wounds fail to heal, or heal very slowly. Scarring is extensive; no sooner has one area healed than another becomes affected. Dermoid cysts are commonly recognized in adult horses; although they are a congenital deformity of the hair follicles and glands in a localized area, characteristically they develop along the dorsal midline. Probably the most common congenital skin condition is the nasal atheroma, a dermal inclusion cyst that is usually only of incidental cosmetic significance.

2. Allergic and immunologic diseases of the skin are important in horses. The most common "allergic disease" in horses is surely urticaria, but despite the high prevalence in the horse, there remains considerable controversy over its etiopathogenesis. For example, some specialists believe that it is due to vasoactive amines in the diet, and that by simply reducing the feeds responsible, the condition will resolve. Others believe that there is a genuine underlying hypersensitivity to inhaled, ingested, or contacted allergens (**Fig. 6**).

The diagnosis of the allergic and immune-mediated diseases (whether autogenous or not) is often problematic due to poor pathologic and clinical descriptions in the literature, and possibly unjustifiable extrapolation from other species. For example, terms such as lupus erythematosus may be inappropriately used to describe a particular dermatologic condition, but while the signs may be somewhat similar, no lupus cells have been identified in the horse; the name equine SLE-like syndrome is therefore probably better justified. The range of immune diseases does, however, include all the recognized hypersensitivity options including atopy (a congenital IgE-related hypersensitivity to environmental allergens either ingested or inhaled—seldom via contact!). Insect hypersensitivity (mainly to *Culicoides* spp midges) is probably by far the commonest cause of seasonal pruritus; fortunately, the seasonality and specific circumstances within that seasonality/management make the diagnosis relatively straightforward. Things may not be some simple, however; recent research has confirmed that in many cases the same signs can be due to similar antigens derived from other insect bites (Sloet, 2005). Furthermore, it is sometimes difficult to separate a hypersensitivity response to a few bites from severe clinical response to a swarm challenge. Autoimmune conditions of the pemphigus group appear regularly in equine practice. The early signs can easily be missed or misdiagnosed. For example,

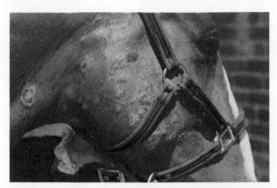

Fig. 7. This 14-year-old hunter-type gelding developed circular crusting lesions over the whole body, and histologic confirmation of pemphigus foliaceus was made by biopsy. The condition had been treated as ringworm for about 12 months.

the focal early lesions of *Pemphigus foliaceus* can easily be mistaken for dermatophytosis (**Fig. 7**). Treatment for the latter will not resolve the problem, of course; even after many months, some cases still have not been diagnosed properly. Whether an early diagnosis improves the prognosis for these cases is a matter for discussion, but under any circumstance, wasted treatments and resources are disappointing. Unless the clinical signs demand immediate intervention, it is far better to delay treatment until a diagnosis can be made.

Immunocompromising disease, ranging from the congenital immunodeficiency conditions (fell pony and SCID syndromes) to the old-age cortisol-related compromise of equine Cushing disease, results in rapid development of skin infections. An individual presented with an unlikely or unexplained infection should be investigated for possible underlying immune compromise. It is also important to remember that some viral infections, deficiency diseases, and chronic debilities also impair the natural skin defense system, and a whole range of cutaneous clinical signs can develop in such cases.

3. Traumatic skin injuries are extremely common in practice; the management of wounds is a significant dermatologic issue. Failure to understand the structure of skin and its response to injury means that wound management is inevitably compromised.
4. Chemical and toxicity problems in skin disease can arise from internal ingestion (either primarily affecting the skin or secondarily as a result of internal organ damage). While major toxicities, such as arsenic, have largely disappeared, there are others, such as selenium, that have become more prevalent. Selenium toxicity results in significant dermatologic signs including severe laminitis (it's a dermatologic problem!) and hair loss (including the mane and tail). It is an unfortunate fact that many owners will apply all manner of concoctions to the skin of a horse that they would not dream of applying them to themselves (**Fig. 8**); these include engine oil, battery acid, thermal heat, chemical blisters, and so on. Furthermore, in many cases, owners (and sometimes veterinarians, too) may be inclined to panic and use overly strong medications. These can be equally dangerous. An accurate history then is sometimes hard to get— confessions are not a standard approach with most horse owners.
5. Nutritional deficiencies are rare in horses, but some, such as zinc, are important causes of generalized skin disease. Although there are reports of vitamin A deficiency, it is hard to visualize how that situation could arise in normal stable circumstances or in any situation where the horse has access to food that is green

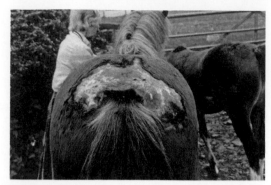

Fig. 8. This extensive chemical burn was caused by the use of strong iodine solution in an attempt to resolve a persistent dermatophilosis infection. Reaching a diagnosis was very difficult since it had a long history.

in color. Severe nutritional deprivation may lower immune status (this applies especially it seems to selenium deficiencies), and so secondary skin infections may develop in such cases. The major part of the signalment relates then to the secondary problem, but failure to consider the underlying disorder will inevitably delay or prevent resolution.

6. Neoplastic diseases of the skin are relatively common but for the most part involve a limited number of easily recognized tumor types such as the sarcoid (**Fig. 9**), squamous cell carcinoma, mast cell tumor, melanoma, and lymphoma. Beyond this, there is a wide range of rarer skin cancers of various types. Equine dermatology suffers badly from the lack of significant numbers of cases in the latter group—most literature reports are for single or few cases, and so it difficult to devise treatment protocols for these. Nevertheless, neoplastic disease is very

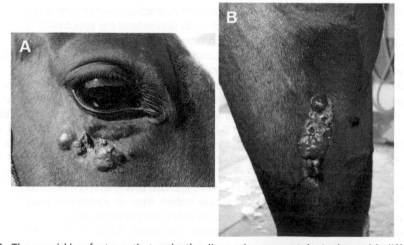

Fig. 9. The sarcoid has features that make the diagnosis more certain. Lesions with different clinical appearances (*A*) and recurrences at sites of surgery (*B*) are typical of the disease. Biopsy is, of course, the definitive differentiation method but is not without hazard.

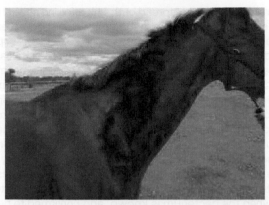

Fig. 10. Localized sweating syndromes are relatively common and are usually associated with autonomic nervous system damage. In this case, there was a cervical vertebral fracture of C7.

important, even though limitations in treatment are bound to be encountered in the horse, as in other species. An additional conundrum arises from non-neoplastic nodules, which can be very difficult to differentiate clinically.

7. There are even some neurologic and endocrinologic conditions of the skin; localized sweating and focal alopecia associated with altered blood flow or local pruritus from a trapped cervical nerve are good examples (**Fig. 10**). Skin disease related to the abnormal behavior of the neuroendocrine system such as PPID (equine Cushing disease; **Fig. 1**B) is also well recognized.

8. Iatrogenic skin damage is common. It is an unfortunate fact that many owners will have caused skin disease through inappropriate use of chemicals on the skin (soap powders, strong antiseptics, overly strong medications, etc) (see **Fig. 8**). Establishing the history in this respect is often highly problematic. It sometimes helps to ask, "What is this that has been put on the skin?" rather than "Has anything been applied to the skin?"

9. Despite all the diagnostic skills that can be brought to bear, there are still some cases that cannot be diagnosed; these can be categorized as "idiopathic." Usually idiopathic cases are managed conservatively, and only broad conclusions can be drawn from the results of treatment and management alterations. There are, in fact, few such disorders, and failure to reach a diagnosis may simply mean that something has been left out of the investigation process. Diagnostic tests may help in some cases at least to understand the nature of the pathologic responses and inform the treatment options.

INFECTIOUS DISEASE

Skin infections should be considered in each of the following categories:

1. *Viral disease:* There are many viral conditions of the skin of the horse, and some are potentially very significant epidemiologically. For example, coital exanthema is a venereal transmitted skin disease caused by equine herpes virus 3. A mare that is infected after service indicates that the stallion had the infection or is likely to have acquired the infection from the mare. In either case, there may be important issues relating to management, even though the disease itself has limited clinical implications in the individual horse. A yearling presenting with viral papillomatosis (grass warts) may

simply be the first of a more widespread outbreak affecting several peers on the same pasture. Close examination of others in the group may show either the early signs or evidence of healed lesions that may not have been noticed. The implications for future years may need to be discussed with the owner of the studs because once the virus is present in the pasture sequential crops of foals may become infected.

2. *Bacterial disease:* Bacterial diseases of the skin are common. Some are well recognized. The reality is that the natural flora of the skin comprises a wide range of bacterial species (as well as some fungi, too!). This complex relationship normally affords protection against pathogens, and most bacterial infections require particular types of circumstance to develop. Therefore, most bacterial infections of the skin are probably best thought of as secondary events. However, since they are often significant, specific targeted treatment is usually used. A problem with treatment of bacterial skin infections is that systemic antibacterial therapy (even when the bacterium is known, and confirmed to be sensitive, it often fails to reach an MIC in the skin itself). Even large doses administered frequently often appear to have little effect. Topical applications rely on skin penetration and that can be very problematic. Commonly skin antiseptics such as chlorhexidine or povidone-iodine are also used as broad-spectrum therapy, but they too often fail to penetrate effectively into the hair follicles.

Common skin infections include dermatophilosis (*Dermatophilus congolensis*), staphylococcal folliculitis/farunculosis, and streptococcal dermatitis. In most cases, there is a dominant species, but in some, a complex infection is involved. Some very serious conditions can arise when the life of the horse is threatened. Most of the severe bacterial skin infections are, fortunately, rare. Diseases such as streptothricosis or glanders have been largely eradicated from much of the Western World, but methicillin-resistant *Staphylococcus aureus* and other staphylococcal infections can become generalized, and in some circumstances, septicemia or bacteremia can develop. Bacterial skin disease is common, but it is also commonly overlooked or belittled. It is very important in terms of treatment and prognosis to know what species of bacterium is present. A good example of the complexity of bacterial infection of the skin occurs in the pastern dermatitis syndrome, where subtle differences in the onset, appearance, progression, and pain levels can be very helpful in diagnosis. Recognition for example that the infection is a superficial dermatophilosis as opposed to a deep staphylococcal folliculitis will inform the most logical and effective treatment.

3. *Fungal disease:* Fungal skin infection is a common and challenging diagnosis in equine practice. Dermatophytes are a regular problem in large yards where they occur recurrently year after year, and especially where cattle and rodent contact is close. Poor stable hygiene is a common feature in extensive outbreaks of fungal disease. Stables that have had previous cases of ringworm will usually get them again. These spores are highly resistant to environmental factors, and the diseases tend to be highly contagious. However, for fungal infections to become established, the skin needs to be damaged; as such, lesions tend to be seen first (at least) around areas of skin trauma such as girth, sides, face, and other tack contact areas (**Fig. 11**). In some cases, fly bites can transmit the infection from site to site and from horse to horse; in such cases, the pattern of the bite/lesion can be helpful diagnostically. Most of the dermatophytes are zoonotic but it seems that equine species of both *Trichophyton* and *Microsporum* are less liable to human transmission than other species.

4. Protozoal disease: It is a rare cause of skin infection but it should not be entirely forgotten—*Besnoitia* sp does cause some skin lesions in donkeys in some parts of the world!

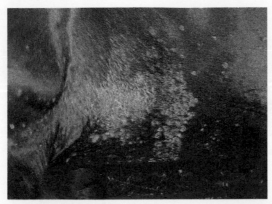

Fig. 11. *T equinum* var *equinum* infection resulting from the use of a contaminated girth. Several horses in the yard were similarly affected. It is important to know the species of ringworm involved because this provided information on the origin and therefore informs the control measures that need to be used.

5. *Parasitic diseases* are a common cause of pruritus and dermal skin lesions.
   a. Ectoparasites are important in horses and are potentially contagious between horses via direct and close contacts. In the author's experience, up to 80% to 85% of pruritic horses will have a parasitic origin (although that does not necessarily mean that parasites cause 80% of pruritus cases in horses, of course). Finding ectoparasites on some horses can be difficult because there is no pathognomonic itch, neither for a particular parasite, nor for the number of those parasites. Some horses will itch severely with a few mites or lice, but others will be almost (or completely) symptom free when they are severely affected. The concept of a symptom-free "carrier" horses is particularly important in *Chorioptes equi* infestations; in such cases, epidemiologic questions need to be asked about management, and in contact horses, it may be wise to examine other animals as well in some circumstances.

   Control of parasitic infestations (whether internal or external) is important. The efficiency of treatment and prevention will depend on the veterinarian knowing the species involved and the life cycle of the insect or worm. The life cycle can be used to identify weak spots—spots in the parasitic life cycle where access and control can be more effective than others.

   C equi causes pruritus and mild to severe scaling in many cases, but some horses have heavy infestations without any apparent signs. There may be some hypersensitivity component in those horses that are intensely pruritic when only a very few mites are present. Lice of both the scale-feeding and blood-sucking varieties occur in horses; both cause pruritus and a moth-eaten skin appearance. The sucking louse (*Haematopinus asini*) can cause significant anemia, further emphasizing the value of a full clinical examination in all dermatologic cases.

   Some ectoparasites cause signs that are not immediately ascribable to parasitic organisms. Relatively common in some parts of the United States, *Habronema musca* is becoming more prevalent in the United Kingdom (although it is still, by any token, rare). It can simply present as a flat ulcerated wound that fails to heal (characteristically on the face below the medial canthus of the eye). The parasite is transmitted by

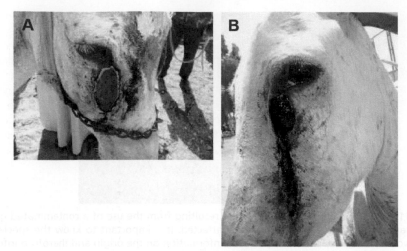

Fig. 12. (*A, B*) Typical cases of habronemiasis. This is seasonal condition, the severity of which is usually dependent on an individual's susceptibility. Many cases are affected year after year and usually the signs are worse each succeeding season. The condition can also affect wounds.

Muscid flies and so is strongly seasonal, hence its name "summer sores." Interestingly, there appears to be a strong recurrence rate in individual animals, implying some sort of genetic susceptibility and no effective immunity lasting from year to year. Some animals are resolutely resistant! (**Fig. 12**).

Seasonality is an important issue in ectoparasitic skin disease (for example, trombiculidiasis only occurs in autumn months). Careful questioning may establish this and therefore narrow the diagnostic options significantly. There are also geographical aspects that should be considered; for example, *Trombicula autumnalis* is restricted to chalky soiled areas, and so is an unlikely diagnosis is springtime on clay soils. There are many "casual"/opportunistic ectoparasites that affect horses, including the poultry mite (*Dermanyssus galinae*) and the forage mites. Even low numbers of these blood-sucking mites can cause serious skin disease accompanied by moderate to severe pruritus, but the circumstances are usually obvious.

   b. Endoparasites

   It is easy to ignore internal parasites as a cause of skin disease, but over recent years several causes of onchocercosis (microfilairiasis/*O cervicalis*) have been diagnosed in the United Kingdom, and the condition is not uncommon in some parts of the United States. The signs are usually fairly dramatic; the characteristic feature is the development of a florid necrotizing focal dermal lesion following the use of ivermectin anthelminitic. *Oxyuris equi* is an occasional cause of tail and perianal rubbing (see **Fig. 5**); the primary disease is probably incidental but the effects can be considerable, and the condition needs to be considered in the differential diagnosis of perineal/tail base rubbing/pruritus).

COLLECTION OF DIAGNOSTIC SPECIMENS

The skin can only respond in a defined number of ways for a wide range of etiologies. Thus, it is common practice to collect samples for the laboratory support of diagnoses and diagnostic rule-outs. Diagnostic aids, including specimens of hair, brushings, scrapings, and biopsies, are frequently taken in equine dermatologic investigations. Samples are usually readily obtained with a minimum of trouble. In some cases, a definitive diagnosis can be established, while in others, the chronic nature of the condition and/or the complications caused by secondary trauma or infection make samples difficult to interpret. Pathologically useful information is usually restricted to early, carefully selected lesions, and a good outcome is heavily dependent on the correct sampling methods of lesions that are truly representative of the primary (underlying) disorder.

There are a limited number of simple basic tests, but their simplicity should not be taken to indicate that they are of limited value. Of course, each test should be considered carefully; by judicious case selection, it should be possible in most instances to establish at least the basic pathology, and in many cases a definitive diagnosis can be made. For example, if samples are correctly taken, it should be possible to confirm a diagnosis of pemphigus foliaceus. Washing and scrubbing of the biopsy site will result in the loss of the pathognomonic acanthocytes, which are to be found in the superficial crust and scale. Under such circumstances, it is unfair to expect pathologists to "make the diagnosis," especially if the full clinical information is not provided.

Skin Scraping

Skin scraping is primarily designed to identify burrowing skin mites, which are in any case uncommon in horses. The commonest mite in the United Kingdom is *Chorioptes equi*, which is a surface feeding mite and so groomings are usually better. Scrapings can also be useful in dermatophytosis (ringworm) diagnosis but plucking hair is probably better and easier.

Using a No. 22 scalpel blade, selected areas are shaved directly into sterile containers. The areas can be slightly moistened with mineral oil and applied to a slide directly. Either type of sample should be covered with enough mineral oil to allow the placement of a cover-slip and the sample is examined under $\times 10$ and $\times 20$ objectives. *Demodex* spp will only be found if scrapings are deep and taken with gentle squeezing of the skin during the procedure. *Demodex* is a commensal in the eyelids and muzzle regions of some horses—it is extremely rare to find any at all, and pathologic states are almost unheard of.

For ringworm examination, the sample may be examined directly, but it may be better to digest the keratin with warm 10% KOH before examination. Most ringworm cases in the Europe and United States are caused by equine dermatophytes including *Trichophyton* spp. Dermatophytes from other species are also found with some regularity. The *Trichhophyton* sp has endothrix spores and does not fluoresce under ultraviolet light. Identification of the species involved is important since it informs the veterinarian what control measures are required. For example, if a bovine or rodent species is involved, the source of the infection must be sought and controlled. Equine species are probably less zoonotic.

Skin Groomings

Using a small dustpan or Petri dish and a stiff brush, the hair is groomed into the dish or onto a black tile and carefully observed for moving mites and lice. This is a simple and effective aid for identifying harvest/forage and poultry mites; lice (**Fig. 13**) (both *Damalinia* and *Haematopinus*) can be readily identified. A dissecting/stereo microscope is very useful, as are a magnifying glass and a black tile. This technique also collects scale and crust and some hairs; a lot of information is available from a simple, cheap test.

Groomings can also be used to help diagnose some superficial skin conditions, such as infestation with *Habronema* spp parasites. The same basic process can be

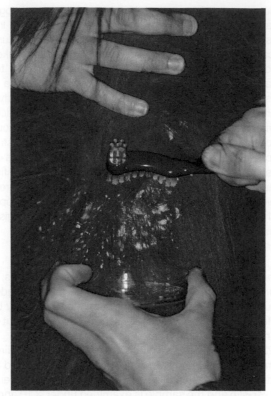

Fig. 13. This case illustrates the skin brushing technique for harvesting parasites from the surface of the skin. The advantage is that it harvests from a large area. A denture toothbrush is a very cheap and effective method. It is possible to examine the groomings with a magnifying glass alone and get enough diagnostic information. It also "harvests" crust and scale for examination.

used to harvest *Habronema* larvae and *Thelazia lacrimalis* from the conjunctival sac **(Fig. 14)**.

Hair Plucking

Where dermatophyte infections or dermatophilosis is suspected, there is usually some scaling or crusting and hair loss. Hairs should be plucked using a pair of hemostats from the fresh margins of young lesions. After plucking the hairs (which are placed in an unsealed, nonairtight sterile bottle/universal), the area can be slightly cleaned with spirit. At least 4 or 5 samples are then taken from the margin and placed in sterile bottles **(Fig. 15)**.

Acetate Tape Preparations (Sellotape)

This technique is used primarily to identify *Oxyuris* eggs on the perianal region. Four-centimeter lengths of clear adhesive tape are stuck onto the skin around the anus and perineum. The tape is then removed and stuck onto a glass slide, onto which a drop of mineral oil has been applied (this helps to disperse the bubbles and artefacts, which can be confusing). It can then easily be examined under low power for the characteristic oval-triangular operculate eggs (90 μm $\times$ 30 μm) **(Fig. 16)**.

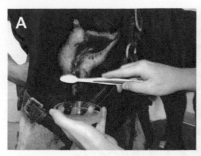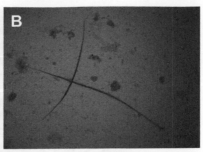

Fig. 14. Skin brushings can also be used to harvest bacteria, fungi, cells, and parasites from open wounds. A soft toothbrush and a Petri dish of saline (*A*) were used to harvest *Habronema* larvae from this Poitou donkey. The larvae were obvious on gross and microscopic examination (*B*).

Skin Biopsy

The value of biopsy cannot be overstated. Many conditions can be definitively diagnosed by skin biopsy. Unfortunately, some very different conditions can produce similar histopathologic effects; other conditions produce very nonspecific pathologic findings. A good example of that is in urticaria; biopsy is frequently very disappointing even in severe cases because the edema fluid drains out during fixation. This may make it difficult or impossible for the pathologist to provide a definitive diagnosis. While it is unreasonable to expect the pathologist to be able to help in every case, often the pathologist can eliminate significant differentials and thereby narrow the diagnostic possibilities. It is very helpful to the pathologist to provide as much information as possible (including sending in a copy of the full history and clinical findings). The clinician and the pathologist are in the same team, and providing as much information as possible helps make it more likely that a definitive diagnosis can be reached.

Skin biopsy samples are taken for the following reasons:

1. To establish a specific diagnosis
2. To eliminate defined clinical conditions (rule-out)

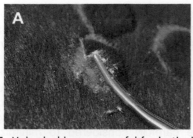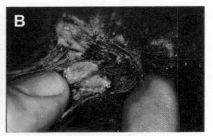

Fig. 15. Hair pluckings are useful for both direct microscopic examination and culture for some bacterial and fungal disorders. They can also provide information on the stage of hair growth, although trichogram use is not widely reported in horses. (*A*) Typical dermatophytosis lesion (*Microsporum equi*). (*B*) Typical dermatophilosis lesion (rain scald) on the back of a horse. In the former case, ectothrix spores and fungal mycelia was seen on direct microscopy and culture was positive. In the latter, the plucking was simply used to make a smear, which showed the typical "rail-track" organisms when stained with Wright-Giemsa (Diff-Quik).

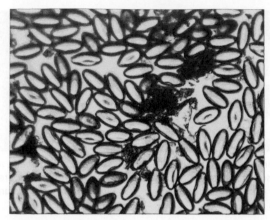

Fig. 16. The typical operculate eggs of *O equi* harvested on an adhesive strip preparation from a horse with perianal pruritus.

3. To monitor the course of disease
4. To confirm the completeness of surgical excision of tumors.

A single biopsy will seldom answer all of these questions. It is useful therefore to obtain multiple samples from defined types of lesions (the pathologist should be told the site and the nature of the lesions as far as possible). In pruritic disorders, the pathology can be profoundly altered by self-inflicted damage, and the lesions may also become secondarily infected, which affects the diagnostic value of the biopsies.

- Biopsies of papules or pustules are prime examples of suitable lesions for biopsy.
- Most neoplastic lesions provide definitive biopsies but can be complicated by concurrent infection or granulation tissue.
- Immune-mediated and autoimmune disorders can be difficult to biopsy effectively. They may also require specialized immunohistochemistry.
- Ulcers and crusts often provide less definitive information.
- Chronic lesions, superficial inflammatory changes, and lichenified crusted dermatoses gain little from biopsy.

Note: Skin biopsy is not usually helpful when the skin changes are very chronic or when there has been self trauma or iatrogenic interference. For this reason, the site of biopsy is not scrubbed or washed at all, and if possible, local anesthetic should not be used immediately adjacent to the site.

The area selected for biopsy should not usually be shaved or scrubbed prior to biopsy. Most biopsy samples are small, and there is a greater danger from misdiagnosis if the skin is scrubbed before biopsy. The patient may require sedation and local anesthesia; it is vital that the site is not infiltrated with local anesthetic agents. Placement of local anesthetic should be carefully considered to minimize the inflammatory effects that they create in the skin. Often biopsy can be performed with regional nerve blocks or even without any local analgesia in a sedated and twitched horse. If local infiltration is used, it is useful to leave the needle in situ so that a small amount can be used and the biopsy site can be accurately located after a few minutes. A scalpel blade or a biopsy punch should always be used; scissors cause severe crushing artefacts. Squeezing with rat tooth forceps is also potentially harmful

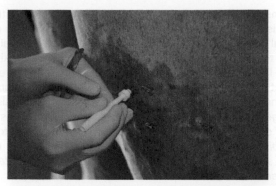

Fig. 17. A punch biopsy being taken from a wide area of changed skin. Note that the needles used for injecting the tiny bleb of local anesthetic are left in situ so that the exact site can be biopsied.

to the subsequent histologic examination. The specimen must be treated very carefully so that maximal information can be obtained.

Punch Biopsy

Sterile disposable skin punches (4-, 6-, 8-mm diameter) are available. Unfortunately, while the smallest punches create the least damage, they are also frequently the least useful! Very small specimens may not be diagnostic and may undergo significant distortion, making both the collection and the handling problematical. The site also may dictate the size of the biopsy; coronary band biopsy and eyelid or limb skin should be protected by the use of a small biopsy. but this also carries risks of failure to get enough tissue to establish the pathology.

The collection process is simple (**Fig. 17**). Here are some tips to increase the diagnostic value of the procedure:

- A 25-gauge needle can be used to remove the biopsy from the underlying fat; it should not be grasped with rat tooth or plain forceps.
- It is sometimes useful to obtain a normal biopsy sample from adjacent area if an interface between normal and abnormal tissue is not obtained.
- The wounds from punch biopsies heal very rapidly and there is no need to suture them.

Excisional/Wedge Biopsy

Careful selection of the biopsy site is important. Regional or local anesthetic is wise to use in almost all circumstances. Depending on the nature of the pathology and the differential diagnoses, it might be acceptable to prepare the biopsy site aseptically, but in general this is not desirable.

Wedge biopsies can be used for larger lesions. A full-thickness scalpel incision (NOT scissors!) through abnormal tissues and normal skin including the interface is made; the so-called cake slice method can be used, but the cake slice needs to be the opposite way round so that a small amount of normal skin is taken with a greater area of pathology! An elliptical incision is made to include all tissues down to panniculus muscle. The site can be cleaned and sutured after the biopsy sample is taken if necessary. Excisional biopsies are useful for vesicles and pustules, especially if the skin can be excised without breaking the lesions open.

In some circumstances, abnormal and normal skin is required, either in one sample (usually to establish the margins of a lesion) or a second biopsy is collected from an adjacent "normal" site. All pathologists will know what normal skin looks like; therefore, unless there are compelling reasons for taking normal skin, there is usually no need for that. It is far better to ensure that a truly representative sample is taken, and that sufficient pathologic skin is collected to maximize the return, in order to give the pathologist the best chance of achieving an accurate diagnosis.

Note. It is suggested that surgical wedge and excisional biopsies are laid down on a small square of card for about 1 minute to allow them to adhere to it before placing in the fixative. This helps to prevent curling and distortion of the biopsy in fixative. Larger pieces of skin should be pinned to card in their natural state. Commercially available specimen meshes are helpful.

It is wise to consult with the pathologist if there is any doubt as to what the best specimen and fixative are for particular circumstances.

Recommendations When Taking Biopsy Samples

- Do not overstretch samples during or after biopsy.
- Use a scalpel, NOT scissors.
- Use a needle to remove the sample, NOT forceps (if possible).
- Samples should be reduced to less than 1 cm in size allow good fixer penetration.
- Multiple sections are useful from large specimens.
- Large samples should be cut in serial section and placed in consecutively numbered containers.
- Attempts to wash the sites after the biopsy has been taken often simply carry infection into the site. They are best left alone to heal.
- Generally, samples for histologic examination are fixed in 10% formol-saline. Where special requirements are required, pathologists can usually supply the correct fixatives.
- For electron microscopy (eg, poxvirus, etc), place 1-mm cubes in glutaraldehyde.
- Place bacteriology specimens in transport medium or in ice for transport to the lab.
- Complete large specimens can be sent in formalin saline, but it may help fixation if the mass is partially incised/sliced.
- Small specimens less than 4 mm are barely adequate. Crushing and distortion artefacts are common.

Fine Needle Aspiration

Fine needle aspirates can be useful in some cases, but generally are less useful than in other species. This probably reflects the poor state of knowledge about many skin masses—in other species, a definitive diagnosis can usually be achieved because much more interpretive experience is available. Simply aspirating the contents of a fluid-filled skin mass may confirm the presence of pus in an abscess. Blood and serum/plasma may indicate a hematoma. A milky white fluid is characteristic of the dermal inclusion cysts known as an atheroma, a developmental cystic lesion that occurs predominantly in the nasal region Aspiration from a melanoma is instantly pathognomonic, but while the cells are typical of the condition, they seldom provide enough pathologic information for an accurate prognosis since the relationship between the cells and blood supply is not clear. Fine needle aspirates are possibly the most misused diagnostic test of all in dermatology. Some tips for improving the diagnostic return are:

- Use a small needle (23 gauge) and a small syringe (2–5 mL only). The concept that a "big needle and a big syringe will get better samples" is absolutely not the case!
- Sample from the edge of the lesion NOT the center—the center may be necrotic and have overt inflammation; those areas are not going to provide the best diagnostic cells!
- Prepare the slides beforehand so there is no delay in making the slide preparation; the slides should be premarked on the frosted part in PENCIL with the name and case details.
- Make the preparation as quickly as possible—do not try to repeat the harvesting process with the same needle since cells will have dried within it, and a short time between harvesting and smear preparation maximizes the cell quality.
- Do not fix the slides unless asked to do so by the pathologist. Air dry them quickly and seal them into a slide carrier.
- The veterinarian should not try to interpret slides by himself or herself. They are difficult and it is easy to misinterpret cell morphology. A skilled cytologist will get the most out of a well-prepared sample submitted carefully with the correct back-up information.

Intradermal Allergy Testing

Over many years there has been an increased interest in the use of intradermal testing for allergic conditions in small animals and humans. Opinions are strongly divided as to the value of these tests in equine diagnosis. Intradermal tests are usually performed by injecting small (threshold) doses of allergens into the skin on a pre-prepared area of the neck. To perform the test, the patient must be under no concurrent drug medication, and the material must be injected intradermally, at defined sites on a previously prepared (clipped and washed) area of the skin of the lateral neck. The responses are measured at 12, 24, and 48 hours post injection. The responses are compared to a saline-negative control and a histamine-positive control site (**Fig. 18**).

A discussion in the 2011 World Veterinary Dermatology Conference showed that the overall opinion was that while intradermal testing can help in some cases, the results are hard to interpret and that the panel of available allergens was possibly not

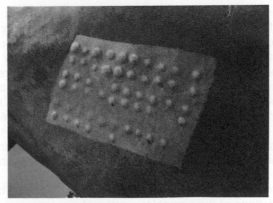

Fig. 18. An intradermal allergy test showing the test area after 2 hours. Note that there are many positive tests (noticeable lumps at the site). The test uses a comparison with a histamine-positive control and a water-negative control (usually at the upper left corner of the test area).

the most appropriate for horses. Furthermore, there was no correlation between the histologic responses and the physical responses to the test even in animals known to be hypersensitive. An alternative patch testing procedure is used in some centers and the reports are possibly better.

IgE Testing of Blood

IgE blood testing carries similar problems to the skin tests. There is little repeatability on the tests; the same patient may present different results from day to day. Again, the tests are limited to around 125 to 150 rather arbitrary "substances and mixtures of substances." The tests are simple to perform, simply requiring a standard blood sample. The blood sample is then subjected to specific IgE ELISA to detect abnormal elevations of particular IgE proteins. The test has little or no value; at present, it lacks specificity, sensitivity, repeatability, and reliability. Hopefully, further development will lead to a more useful test.

TREATMENT

The treatment of skin disease is outside the remit of this report. However, since there has, of late, been a greater respect for dermatology as a specialist subject, treatment options have improved dramatically. There is far less guesswork involved in the investigatory process than previously, and as result treatment is becoming less available and in many countries there is a heavy reliance on drugs that are approved for small animals and humans rather than for horses. This applies in particular to ectoparasiticidal drugs. The equine skin is tolerant of damage and will usually recover reasonably well if the inciting cause is removed. In some cases, however, this is easier to say than do; secondary changes and iatrogenic interference can confuse the appropriate treatment markedly, and in some conditions the cause cannot be treated. Secondary skin disease, such as hepatic-failure derivation photosensitization, simply points the clinician in the direction of the (usually) more important underlying disease. Secondary changes resulting from iatrogenic or self-trauma interference may force the clinician to address the secondary effects first, and then to restart the diagnostic process when the clinical syndrome is clearer.

SUMMARY

A logical and thorough clinical investigation should provide the best basis for the diagnosis of skin diseases. Where no diagnosis can be reached despite a full range of investigations, the clinician can justifiably attempt symptomatic treatment, but it is always better to focus treatment on a specific condition based on properly accumulated and tested clinical evidence. Unfortunately, in equine dermatology there are few text descriptions of the majority of the conditions encountered in practice. While a few diseases are well recognized, there is still little consensus on the best treatments for many of them. Individual veterinarians will have treatments that they rely on, but frequently the same treatment applied by another person inexplicably fails to work in the same way. In dermatology cases, there is no substitute for experience. Referencing to quality textbooks and to colleagues who might have encountered the condition before is often advisable.

Unusual presentations are frequently encountered in horses. For example, there are many manifestations of the pemphigus group of diseases, and not all will have a clear diagnostic pathway. It is important to remember that the skin is one of the biggest organs in the body and yet little is known of its function and pathology! While there are many significant primary dermatologic conditions, there are also important systemic diseases that have more or less pathognomonic secondary dermatologic signs; this makes the proper clinical examination even more imperative.

One of the biggest problems with equine dermatology is the dearth of scientific reports. Many experienced clinicians have much useful information, but this may never reach the rest of the profession. Also there are few useful reference textbooks dedicated to the equine species. Equine dermatology most likely suffers the most of all disciplines in this respect. As a result, every clinician is expected to reinvent the wheel! There is a need for publications and discussions about the problem cases; even the commonest skin diseases are poorly understood.

To make the most use of the supporting specialties of microbiology and pathology, it is important to involve the relevant specialists in the diagnostic process. This means that these specialists must have as much information as they can get; it helps enormously if a photograph can be taken of the disease. Without such information, pathologists and microbiologists may make gratuitous statements about treatment options. For example, a biopsy from an upper eyelid lesion might be easily diagnosed as a sarcoid, and any statement concerning wide surgical excision might be both misleading and nonsensical but would be totally avoidable had the specialist been provided more information.

The approach to the dermatologic case requires a logical and exhaustive clinical investigation involving a thorough history and a detailed clinical examination. Diagnostic tests should be carefully selected to rule-out or confirm a suspected diagnosis. Frequent reexaminations are often required because it is sometimes difficult to establish the primary condition: this is often due to extensive self-inflicted trauma or iatrogenic interference by the owner. By proceeding in a systematic and stepwise manner, equine ambulatory clinicians can frequently bring dermatologic problems to a successful resolution.

REFERENCE

1. Sloet von Oldruitenborgh-Oosterbaan MM. Equine allergic skin disease. Adv Equine Dermatol 2005;5:349–59.

Ophthalmology in Equine Ambulatory Practice

Ann E. Dwyer, DVM[a,b,*]

KEYWORDS

- Ophthalmology • Equine • Horse • Ambulatory • Cornea
- Uveitis

The equine eye can be examined with simple portable equipment and many pathologic conditions can be diagnosed with stall-side tests. Inexpensive digital cameras are effective for imaging the periorbit and anterior segment. Ambulatory practitioners can institute many effective treatments, including installation of subpalpebral lavage tubes for delivery of topical treatments for corneal disease, and standing ocular surgery using regional anesthesia and sedation. Prompt diagnosis and appropriate treatment of ocular problems can be sight saving and is an invaluable service to patients and clients.

KNOWLEDGE AND EDUCATION

Between 5% and 10% of horses are reported to have important ophthalmic lesions that affect vision or function.[1] Experience and study are required to discern the difference between the normal eye, the eye that has a variant that is clinically insignificant, and the eye that has a serious problem. Several illustrated textbooks[2–4] are available as training resources.

Owners must be taught that a veterinarian should see horse eye problems and that applying medication without an examination, or neglect of a painful eye, can cause serious complications, including vision loss. Client seminars, newsletters, and social media posts are good ways to teach horse owners the basics of equine eye conditions.

EQUIPPING THE AMBULATORY VEHICLE

Essential tools for field eye examination include a direct ophthalmoscope (Welch Allyn, Skaneateles, NY, USA), a bright light source (Finnoff transilluminator, or bright penlight), a 14 to 20 D magnifying lens, and a digital camera. Some practitioners may

The author has nothing to disclose.
[a] Genesee Valley Equine Clinic, PLLC, 925 Chili Scottsville Road, Scottsville, NY 14546, USA
[b] Flaum Eye Institute, University of Rochester Medical Center, 601 Elmwood Avenue, Rochester, NY 14642, USA
* Genesee Valley Equine Clinic, PLLC, 925 Chili Scottsville Road, Scottsville, NY 14546.
E-mail address: adwyer@rochester.rr.com

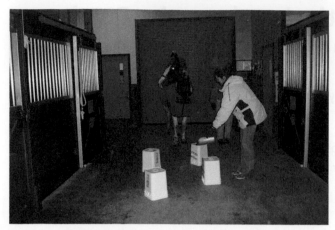

Fig. 1. Maze testing is easily performed in a barn aisle and provides general confirmation of unilateral vision.

invest in a battery-powered handheld slit lamp (SL-15; Kowa Co, Nagoya, Japan) and a tonometer (Tonovet; Icare Vet, Helsinki, Finland, or Tono-pen Avia; Reichert, Depew, NY, USA). In addition to standard sedatives, antibiotics, local anesthetics, and systemic anti-inflammatory medications, the ambulatory vehicle should be stocked with several items for eye examination, including topical ophthalmic anesthetic, tropicamide solution, Schirmer tear test, and fluorescein and Rose Bengal dye strips. Commercial subpalpebral lavage kits (Mila International, Erlanger, KY, USA) are needed for management of serious corneal disease. A variety of topical ocular topical antibiotic, antifungal, anti-inflammatory, mydriatic, and hyperosmotic ointments and solutions will be required for therapy.[5] This author dispenses many ophthalmic medications in small plastic "write-on bags" (Associated Bag Company, Milwaukee, WI, USA) with the treatment schedule written on the bag. Medication schedules for complicated cases are charted on spreadsheets printed off the vehicle laptop computer.

VISION TESTING

Stables are good stages for simple maze tests that allow nonquantitative assessment of vision in horses with a history of poor performance or signs indicative of vision loss. A barn aisle is cleared of hazards, and exit doors and stalls are closed. The unsedated horse is positioned at one end of the hall, and a towel is wrapped over the halter to blindfold 1 eye. About 6 overturned buckets are arranged to create a simple obstacle course along a 20-foot section of the aisle way. The horse is turned loose. A person stands at the other end of the aisle, shaking a tub of grain to encourage the horse to walk in that direction (**Fig. 1**). The clinician observes how the horse picks its way through the maze to reach the grain tub, noting whether the horse avoids the obstacles. The test is repeated with the other eye blindfolded. Horses that have reduced vision may run into obstacles when the affected eye is uncovered. Horses that are unilaterally blind may refuse to move when the visual eye is covered.

EXAMINATION INDICATIONS

Ophthalmic examination should be part of the routine examination of a neonate as well as the workup of older ill foals, as perinatal problems are frequently

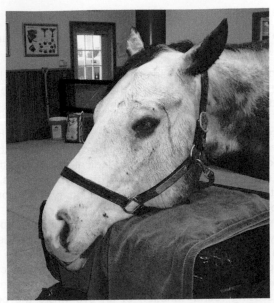

Fig. 2. Stacked bales provide a handy head support for working on the eyes of a sedated horse.

accompanied by ocular disease.[6] Ocular examination is an important part of prepurchase exams[5,7] as well as annual wellness visits for adult and geriatric horses.[8] Owners schedule eye exams when they notice altered appearance or perceive a behavior or performance change. Urgent ocular examination is indicated for eyes that are painful or traumatized.

Making an "Exam Room" in the Field; Optimizing Patient Restraint and Position

A barn aisle or stall is the typical stage for field ophthalmic examination. Prior to examination, these areas can be turned into "exam rooms" by closing doors or windows to darken the area and reduce wind disturbance. Ophthalmic equipment, diagnostic supplies, and medication can be placed nearby on a pair of portable tables (Champagne Pet Products, Southampton, MA, USA; www.champagnetables. com).

While simple ophthalmic examinations can be conducted on awake horses, sedation is indicated for painful eyes. Restraint of these cases is facilitated with passive head support. Oil drums, recycling totes, or stacked bales can be used to create home-made "head tables" (**Fig. 2**). Stabilization of the head facilitates examination, image acquisition, diagnostic tests, subpalpebral lavage (SPL) placement, and standing surgeries.[5]

During the examination, the handler is directed to stand on the opposite side of the horse so that the veterinarian can inspect the eye of interest closely and is coached to steady the head in any position requested. Exposure of the dorsal sclera and limbus is increased when the poll of the horse is twisted away from the examiner. Short people may need to stand on a stool to examine tall horses, while miniature horses and ponies are most easily examined while sitting down. The handler and examiner will "switch sides" when the second eye is inspected.

REFLEX TESTING

Five reflexes are tested on each globe using a bright light and simple tactile stimulation.

1. *Menace response:* The horse should blink or withdraw the head if a hand is waved toward the eye or a cotton ball tossed at the globe. A pathologic lack of a menace response could indicate a lesion in the retina, in the visual cortex or in cranial nerve (CN) II or VII.
2. *Dazzle response:* The horse should partly close the lid or retract the globe if a bright light is suddenly directed into the eye. This response is a subcortical reflex. A pathologic lack of a dazzle response could indicate a lesion in the retina or in the rostral colliculus or the supraoptic nuclei of the hypothalamus. It could also be related to functional inability to close the lid secondary to a lesion in CN II or VII or the orbiculus oculi muscle.
3. *Pupillary light response:* A bright light directed toward the temporal fundus should cause pupillary constriction in that eye. The papillary light response evaluates intact function of the retina, CN II, midbrain and CN III. An observer who is watching the opposite eye should also note simultaneous slight constriction in that eye (consensual light response). The consensual light response is particularly valuable in assessing retinal function of an eye where the posterior segment cannot be visualized.
4. *Blink reflex:* Touching of the periocular skin should cause eyelid closure. Facial nerve paralysis associated with damage to CN II or CN VII causes lack of a blink reflex.
5. *Corneal reflex:* Tactile stimulation of the cornea should also cause eyelid closure. Deficits in CN V or CN VII will affect the corneal reflex, as will any condition that prevents eyelid closure.

SEDATION, TOPICAL, AND REGIONAL ANESTHESIA

Sedation and/or regional anesthesia is needed for inspection and treatment of fractious patients and horses with painful eyes. Intravenous administration of xylazine provides effective sedation for simple exams, photography, and sampling procedures. Completion of standing surgeries usually requires detomidine. Butorphanol tartrate may be added for complex standing procedures, but this drug may induce troublesome head tremors.

Proparacaine or tetracaine solutions that come in dropper bottles are commonly used to induce topical ocular surface anesthesia. Application of the solutions involves drawing a dose of 0.3 to 0.5 mL into a small syringe using a 23- or 25-gauge needle. The needle shaft is broken off and the agent is dripped or sprayed onto the ocular surface through the needle hub. It is also acceptable to spray 2% lidocaine onto the cornea for topical anesthesia.

Periocular regional nerve blocks are required if blepharospasm or severe pain prevent full examination or appropriate therapy. A 5/8-inch 23- or 25-gauge needle is inserted into the target skin area. A small syringe containing the anesthetic is then attached to the needle hub for injection. Motor block of the orbicularis oculi muscle and subsequent paralysis of the upper eyelid are accomplished by injecting 1.5 to 2.0 mL of mepivacaine or lidocaine over the auriculopalpebral nerve in 1 of 3 sites: (1) where the nerve can be felt beneath the skin traversing over zygomatic arch, (2) just lateral to the highest point of the zygomatic arch, or (3) at the caudal border of the ramus of the mandible just below the ear. Sensory block of the medial two-thirds of the upper lid involves injection of 0.5 to 1.0 mL of local anesthetic over the frontal (supraorbital) nerve as it emerges from the supraorbital foramen. The foramen can be palpated medially at the superior orbital rim where the supraorbital process of the frontal bone begins to widen. Other regions can be desensitized by infiltrating the skin over the corresponding margin of the orbital rim.

SKULL, PERIORBIT, AND ADNEXA INSPECTION

Both eyes should be observed from the front, side, and rear to judge symmetry and direction of gaze. Depressions or alterations in the skull or sinus contour and periorbital masses are noted as the horse's head is examined. The medical record should detail observable signs of inflammation like epiphora or blepharospasm as well as altered globe size, dynamics, or position.

Eyelids are checked for swelling and traumatic margin defects. Masses, abnormal meibomian gland appearance, or aberrant cilia position is noted. Eyelash orientation is assessed as unilateral downward orientation of the cilia may signal subtle pain or inflammation. The nictitans and bulbar and tarsal conjunctiva are examined for masses or inflammation. Visualization of periocular masses is aided if a cotton swab is used to lift the area of interest away from its resting position.

GLOBE EXAMINATION

Globe inspection begins with examination of the anterior segment with a bright light and proceeds from the outer to inner aspects of the eye. Several references describe operation of ophthalmic diagnostic equipment and the examination process.[9,10]

The appearance of the tear film is evaluated; normally the ocular surface is uniformly shiny. The cornea should be checked for transparency. Any regions of edema, scarring, pigmentation, or vessel infiltration are noted. Masses, obvious facets, ulcers, or areas of roughening are significant findings. The practitioner should estimate the depth of abnormalities of the cornea using observation with a bright light or slit lamp combined with application of fluorescein dye to the corneal surface. The limbus is evaluated for edema and vascularization. The trabecular meshwork is inspected to assess robustness of the drainage angle.

The anterior chamber normally contains only clear aqueous humor. Transillumination will reveal flare, fibrin, hypopyon, hyphema, or other abnormalities. *The size and shape of the pupil is sometimes overlooked by novice practitioners but are critical to evaluate.* Miosis, mydriasis, anisocoria, synechiae, or granula iridica that are cystic or atrophied should be noted as well as any color change of the iris.

Most ambulatory practitioners use a direct ophthalmoscope to assess the posterior segment. Inspection is facilitated by dilation of the pupils, which is induced about 15 minutes after 0.3 to 0.5 mL of tropicamide (Mydriacil) is sprayed or dripped on to the surface of the cornea (**Fig. 3**).

The lens should be transparent and suspended in a vertical plane behind the iris. Any cataract or lens luxation should be described. The vitreous is normally transparent and has a gel-like consistency in young horses. The vitreous of aging eyes is often an oily liquid containing visible filaments and clumps of cellular debris ("floaters"). Inflamed eyes may show vitritis, which may obscure fundic detail and produce an abnormal orange tint to the optic nerve head. Fundic examination includes assessment of the optic disc, the tapetum, and the nontapetum with a direct ophthalmoscope. Scars, pallor, pigment, and vessel abnormalities of the papillary and peripapillary region may indicate focal or regional dysfunction of photoreceptors with associated visual deficits.

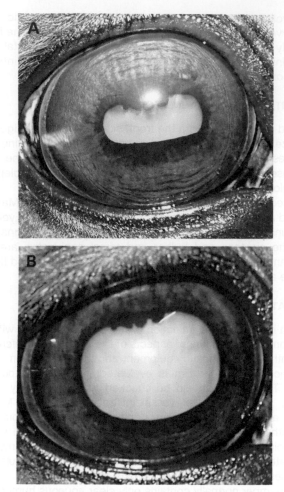

Fig. 3. (*A*) This horse has a cataract. (*B*) Visualization of the lens is aided by dilation of the pupil.

The medical record should list findings at each anatomic level and state if the pupils were dilated. Any abnormal regions noted in one eye are compared to the fellow eye. Descriptions of lesions on the cornea or iris can cite the "clock hour" of the lesion (using the limbus as the reference clock face) and describe the location of the problem using adjectives that relate position to the visual axis, limbus, or orbit (eg, "axial," "paralimbal," "peripheral," "dorsal," "ventral," "nasal," "temporal") (**Fig. 4**). The color, shape, and depth of any abnormality should be described. Size of masses or ulcers can be measured using the ruler on a Schirmer tear test strip. Cataracts should be classified according to their anatomic location within the lens ("capsular," "cortical," "perinuclear" "anterior," "posterior," and so forth), their shape ("punctate," "floriform," "elliptic," "web-like," and so forth), extent ("diffuse," "multifocal," "occupying X% of the lens structure," and so forth), and stage of progression ("immature," "mature," "hypermature").[11] Fundic abnormalities may be described by citing the "clock hour" that relates the lesion to the elliptical optic

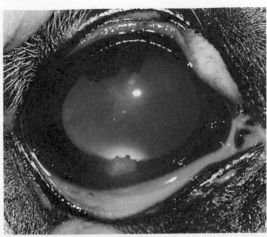

Fig. 4. This lesion on the cornea can be described as a 4 mm diameter, stellate ventral paralimbal opacity that is located at 6:00 o'clock.

nerve head and descriptive adjectives detailing the lesion(s) as a percentage of a disc diameter away from or adjacent to the disc margin.

DIGITAL PHOTOGRAPHY

Imaging of the periorbit, lids, and anterior segment is valuable to record abnormalities and follow injuries, infections, or neoplasias. Many inexpensive compact digital cameras produce excellent images. Superior results can be obtained with careful staging of the patient and the camera.[12]

Imaging is best done in a dark stall or aisle. The glossy cornea will reflect light like a fish eye lens, so the horse must be positioned so that there are no ambient light sources behind the photographer. The camera should be set to the "macro" (flower icon) setting to focus on close objects and placed in "Program" automatic mode (P icon). Novice photographers often hold the camera too close to the eye of the horse, with a resultant blurry image. Most cameras function best if the camera lens is positioned between 5 to 27 inches from the eye (**Fig. 5**). The autofocus system of the camera engages when the shutter button is pressed half way down. If the camera is aimed properly, brackets framing the eye will appear on the viewfinder. The image should be taken as soon as the target region is focused.

The horse's head and the camera must be very still for crisp images. Sedation and/or nerve blocks will facilitate globe exposure if the horse is fractious or has blepharospasm. Obliquely angled images may be supplement standard lateral-to-medial images aimed at the axis. Lens abnormalities are best demonstrated with the pupils dilated.

Once images are stored, the camera is a powerful client education tool. The positioning arrows and "digital zoom" feature are used to center and magnify lesions on the viewing screen. Owners may not appreciate an ocular lesion looking at the horse but can readily see the problem magnified on the camera. Images may also be downloaded to a computer, cropped, and emailed to clients. Electronic transmission of digital images will allow clients to follow progress of cases. Digital photography also facilitates communication with specialists for referral.

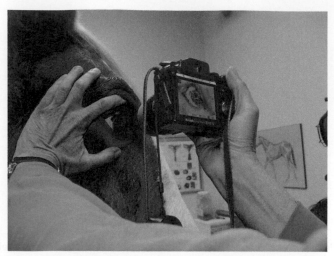

Fig. 5. Digital cameras function best if the lens is positioned 5 to 27 inches from the eye.

ULTRASOUND, RADIOGRAPHY, AND ADVANCED IMAGING

Ultrasound examination of the periorbit and adnexa is indicated for horses that present with a suspected orbital fracture or chronic eyelid swelling, as imaging may detect fractures, foreign bodies, abscesses, or lacrimal gland inflammation.[13] Imaging of the globe and retrobulbar region is useful for horses with exophthalmos, lens luxation, retinal detachment, or vitreal densities.

Ultrasound is performed with mandible head support. Convex or microconvex probes of 7.5- to 10-MHz frequencies commonly used for orthopedic imaging produce serviceable ophthalmic images. Ultrasound of the eyelid or orbital rim is performed by placing the probe on adjacent skin lubricated with transmission gel. Imaging of the globe and retrobulbar space is done by placing the probe on a lubricated closed eyelid, directing the beam through the anterior and posterior segments of the globe. References are available that detail specifics of technique and interpretation.[10,14]

There are fewer indications for radiography in equine ophthalmology, but radiography can be helpful in assessing trauma, sinus disease, globe deviation, and periocular neoplasms. Interpretation is aided if radiodense markers like skin staples or BB pellets are taped to a landmark on the skin.[5,14]

Horses that present with exophthalmos, traumatic or nontraumatic asymmetry of the periorbital region, or globe neoplasia may benefit from referral for computed tomography scanning or magnetic resonance imaging. These modalities image the periorbital sinuses, retrobulbar space, and brain as well as the globe. The prognostic information obtained is valuable in decisions on surgery or other interventions.[14]

OPHTHALMIC TESTS

Ambulatory clinicians should be prepared to perform the tests listed in **Table 1**. Descriptions of test specifics are widely available.[2–4]

Ambulatory clinicians should consider becoming skilled in obtaining cytology samples from serious corneal ulcer cases.[5,10] Corneal cytology specimens stained

Table 1
Descriptions of tests

Test	Materials Needed	Indication
Schirmer tear test	• Schirmer tear test strips • Watch	• Unexplained ocular pain • Dull appearance of cornea
Fluorescein stain of corneal surface	• Fluorescein stain strips • Cobalt blue light	• Test for loss of corneal epithelium, exposure of stroma or Descemet's membrane • Test for aqueous leaking through cornea, or tear film break up time
Rose Bengal stain of corneal surface	• Rose Bengal stain strips • 3-mL syringe, saline	• Suspicion of inadequate tear film • Suspicion of fungal organisms
Corneal culture and sensitivity	• Thioglycollate broth tubes and sterile scalpel blades OR • Calcium alginate culture swabs OR • Blood agar plate and sterile scalpel blades	• Suspicion that a corneal defect harbors bacterial or fungal infection • Therapeutic sensitivity information
Corneal cytology	• Sterile scalpel blades (blunt end used for sample collection) • Plastic slotted box for slide transport • Diff-Quik stain reagent set • Gram stain reagent set • Microscope with ×100 lens	• Sampling of ocular surface in subacute or chronic corneal ulcers • Sampling of abnormal appearing sectors of the cornea thought to harbor foreign bodies, infection, or inflammation

with Diff-Quik and gram stain can be interpreted in the clinic laboratory, using these questions as a guide (**Fig. 6**).

1. Is an inflammatory infiltrate (neutrophils, occasionally eosinophils) present?
2. Are infectious elements (fungal hyphae, bacteria) present? If there are bacteria, are they intracellular or extracellular, rods or cocci, gram negative or gram positive?
3. Is any kind of foreign body (vegetative material, mineralized crystals, other object) present?

These questions are important because a rational choice of ulcer therapy depends on assessing the degree of suppurative reaction and determining the nature of infectious agents or foreign bodies that are present.

Clinicians with a special interest in ophthalmology measure intraocular pressure (IOP) on many patients. Two instruments are available: the applanation tonometer (Tono-pen Avia) and the rebound tonometer (Tonovet). Both instruments may be used in ambulatory practice. The Tonovet rebound tonometer is this author's preferred instrument because it operates well in cold temperatures, does not require topical anesthesia, and has demonstrated reliable sequential readings of IOP on normal and diseased eyes under field conditions. IOP readings are been most consistent with the Tonovet if the horse is lightly sedated with xylazine, an auriculopalpebral block is administered, and the head is positioned with the mandible slightly above the point of the shoulder.

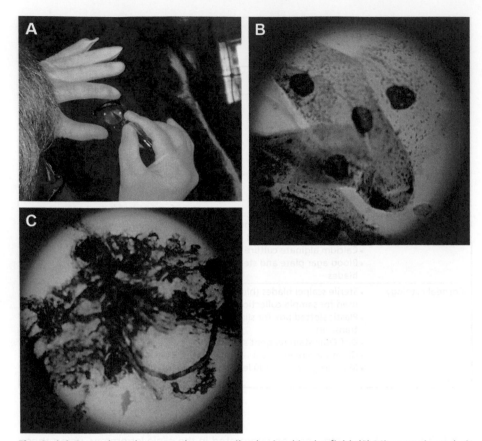

Fig. 6. (*A*) Corneal cytology samples are easily obtained in the field. (*B*) Microscopic analysis of this sample confirms intracellular infection with rod-shaped bacteria (Diff-Quik stain, ×100 magnification). (*C*) Microscopic analysis of this sample confirms fungal keratitis (Diff-Quik stain, ×100 magnification).

MANAGING THE HORSE PRESENTED FOR AN ACUTELY PAINFUL EYE

A common emergency in equine ambulatory practice is the horse with a painful, partially closed eye. Such cases should be seen on a same day basis and both eyes should be examined thoroughly. Of particular importance is notation of pupil size, as miosis signals intraocular or surface inflammation, while a midrange pupil suggests an extraocular inflammation.

The most common cause of a partly closed eye is a corneal ulcer. Corneal epithelial disruption is readily demonstrated by fluorescein stain retention. Fluorescein-positive lesions range from simple abrasions where just a small section of epithelium is missing, to ulcers that extend midway into the stroma, to very deep defects. Fluorescein applied to near full-thickness defects will not adhere to Descemet's membrane; such lesions show a dark, nonstaining center surrounded by green stain adherent to adjacent stroma.

Simple abrasions on the corneal surface treated promptly usually heal quickly with 5 to 7 days of topical therapy (apply a broad-spectrum antibiotic 4 times per day and

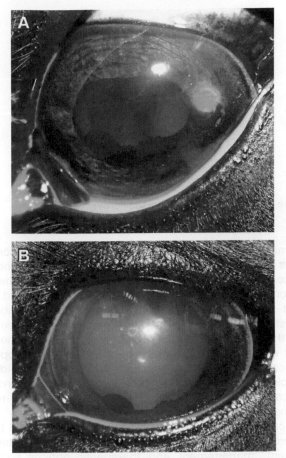

Fig. 7. (*A*) Fluorescein stain at 2:00 o'clock outlines a shallow corneal ulcer examined on the day of injury. (*B*) Three days later: topical antibiotic, atropine, and serum therapy resulted in rapid pupil dilation and epithelialization of the defect.

atropine to effect). Discomfort is readily managed with oral phenylbutazone or flunixin meglamine.

Shallow ulcers can usually be treated with topical ointments. Rapid improvement occurs if appropriate therapy has been chosen. The pupil should dilate within 24 hours, and blepharospasm, tearing, and sensitivity to handling should improve within 2 to 3 days. Lesions should epithelialize in 5 to 7 days (**Fig. 7**). If prompt improvement is not noted, cytologic sampling should be done and therapy changed.

Complicated ulcers that are chronic or involve a significant amount of corneal stroma cause severe pain and are difficult to manage. They may take weeks to heal and may be infected with bacteria or fungi. Host neutrophilic cytokine activity may cause stromal melting, and very deep ulcers risk ocular rupture or iris prolapse (**Fig. 8**). Owner education is critical as treatment is labor intense and expensive, and case progress must be monitored frequently. If the clinician or the owner lacks the resources to manage the case aggressively, referral should be offered *early* for optimum outcome.

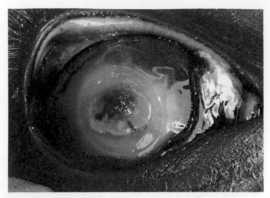

Fig. 8. Iris prolapse has occurred in this infected corneal ulcer.

If the case is managed on the farm, the clinician should collect corneal culture and cytology samples and obtain digital images of the eye. The lesion should be debrided using sterile cotton-tipped swabs and flushed with sterile saline. Therapy will include topical application of a mydriatic (atropine) to dilate the pupil and treat secondary uveitis, frequent application of appropriate anti-infectives (antibacterials and/or antifungals) to sterilize the corneal surface, as well as frequent application of anticollagenase therapy (equine serum, EDTA, or acetylcysteine solutions) to block detrimental host cytokine activity. Choice of anti-infectives is dependent on what organisms have colonized the lesion. Decisions are aided by same-day interpretation of cytology samples, combined with historical efficacy of various antibacterial and/or antifungal medications in the practice region. All cases should receive systemic NSAIDs; some may require concurrent oral gastroprotectants.

Complicated cases and fractious horses must be treated with topical solutions administered through a commercial SPL tube (**Fig. 9**). A detailed description of SPL placement, management and therapeutic options has recently been published.[5]

Ulcers that have eroded into the middle or deep aspects of the stroma take weeks to epithelialize so progress is difficult to gauge. Initial monitoring must be done at 1- to 3-day intervals. Positive responses include rapid dilation of the pupil, clearing of corneal edema, and reduced blepharospasm, tearing, and discharge. Negative signs include persistent miosis, decreased corneal transparency, melting, and increased blepharospasm. Ulcers worsening in the face of treatment merit referral or additional diagnostics, altered therapy, and increased treatment frequency. Some serious ulcers require surgery for resolution.[3,15]

A second common cause of a closed, painful eye is equine recurrent uveitis (ERU) (**Fig. 10**A). In ERU, the cornea will show no fluorescein dye uptake but may demonstrate an even pattern of edema most pronounced around the limbus. Often a brush border fringe of deep vessels is apparent at the corneoscleral interface. The anterior chamber may contain flare, hypopyon, or hyphema. The pupil is miotic and the iris may have a muddy color. The fundus image may appear hazy and orange tinted. Horses with chronic disease may have synechiae, cataracts, lens luxation, or retinal lesions. Ancillary diagnostics may include blood testing for spirochete infection, particularly leptospiral serology.

ERU is a serious, chronic condition with a guarded long-term visual prognosis.[16,17] Candid counseling is important to prepare owners for future recurrences, inflammatory

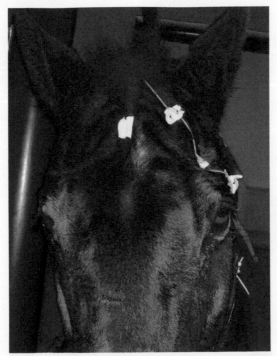

Fig. 9. Subpalpebral lavage tube inserted through the upper lid to facilitate treatment of a complicated corneal ulcer.

sequelae, complications, and possible vision loss. Treatment of acute cases includes topical atropine to control pain, reduce iris vessel "leakiness," and dilate the pupil. Topical corticosteroids (dexamethasone or prednisolone acetate) are applied 3 to 4 times per day to mediate the ocular immune response. Systemic NSAIDs (flunixin meglumine or phenylbutazone) are administered to reduce pain and inflammation. Systemic corticosteroids are used in select cases.

Surgical implantation of a sustained-release suprachoroidal cyclosporine device is a referral option for long-term management of ERU cases. The cyclosporine implant surgery must be performed when the eye does not demonstrate active inflammation. The device is associated with an improved prognosis for many horses.[18]

An important differential diagnosis for the painful eye that is negative for corneal fluorescein stain uptake is a stromal abscess (see **Fig. 10**B). Features that differentiate stromal abscesses from ERU are the presence of a focal round tan or yellow infiltrate in one sector of the cornea, with associated vascularization and/or edema that is *asymmetric*.[15] Stromal abscesses are serious problems that require intense medical therapy with topical mydriatics, antibacterial and antifungal medication, and NSAIDs. Surgical intervention is often necessary for resolution. The use of topical corticosteroids is *strictly contraindicated*, so a stromal abscess must be ruled out before treatment is initiated for ERU.

Less common causes for the horse that presents with a painful or closed eye include immune mediated keratitis, eosinophilic keratitis, corneal foreign body, parasitic keratitis, calcific band keratopathy, endothelial dystrophy, corneal neoplasia,

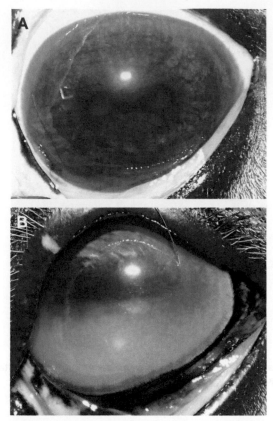

Fig. 10. (*A*) Uveitis. Note the miotic pupil, symmetrical, circumlimbal corneal edema, and lack of focal opacity. (*B*) Stromal abscess. Note the focal yellow infiltrate at the 5:00 o'clock position and the asymmetric corneal edema.

trichiasis, dry eye syndrome, blepharedema, blepharitis, and chemical burns.[2,3,15] Ambulatory clinicians should be familiar with diagnostic characteristics and treatment options for all these conditions.

MANAGING THE HORSE PRESENTED FOR A GLOBE THAT "LOOKS DIFFERENT"

Calls requesting evaluation of a horse that acts comfortable but has one eye that "looks odd" are common. Triage of the issue at hand can be simplified with a few questions:

1. *Is the horse on any ocular medication?* Mydriatics that dilate the pupil allow the observer to see reflection of light off the tapetum. A bluish appearance of a dilated eye may be a normal artifact.
2. *What color is the area that looks odd?* Red may indicate vascular changes on the cornea or hyphema. Red may also accompany corneal surface neoplasia or keratitis. Neoplasias on the nictitans or other conjunctival surfaces will also present as odd red regions. White on the globe surface may indicate corneal fibrosis, calcium or lipid deposition, corneal striae, or immune-mediated keratopathy. White inside the eye may indicate fibrin in the anterior chamber or a dense cataract. A

robin's egg blue color usually means corneal edema accompanying glaucoma, bullous keratopathy, or endothelial dysfunction. A yellow color on the ocular surface suggests a cellular infiltrate. Yellow inside the eye may mean a hypermature cataract or anterior lens luxation. An abnormal brown or black area may be caused by focal pigmentation of the cornea, synechiae of the iris, cystic enlargement of the granula iridica, or intraocular or adnexal neoplasia.

3. *Is the whole eye affected or just part?* Partial color change implies a focal problem where the affected sector has dysplasia, scarring, neoplasia, dystrophy, or local inflammation. Complete color change implies a problem affecting the entire anterior segment or globe such as glaucoma, extensive neoplasia, or intraocular inflammation.

4. *Is one eye a different size than the other?* If one eye appears much larger than the other the clinician should screen for glaucoma or an orbital or periorbital mass that has displaced the globe. One eye that is smaller than the other may be found to be phthisical and blind.

The list of differentials that create an altered appearance of one eye is long, ranging from harmless clinical variants (enlarged granula iridica) to chronic serious ocular problems (glaucoma, lens luxation) to life-threatening conditions (orbital or sinus neoplasia). Common causes of altered appearance in an eye that is the same size as the fellow eye include corneal scarring (focal white leukomas or areas of brown pigmentation), immune-mediated keratitis (cornea shows multiple white dots, blotches, or focal islands in the anterior stroma or epithelium), and cataract. Less common conditions include corneal or conjunctival neoplasia, dysplasia or dystrophy of the cornea, and endothelial dysfunction. Common causes of one eye appearing smaller than normal are phthisis bulbi and posterior lens luxation. Causes of one eye appearing larger than the other include glaucoma and retrobulbar or sinus masses.

Treatment options will vary with cause. Some cases (cystic granula iridica) require no treatment. Others (phthisis bulbi, corneal leukoma) have no therapy that will restore a normal appearance. Surgical intervention is indicated for others (neoplasia of the nictitans). Some cases of altered ocular appearance signify conditions that require lifelong monitoring and medical therapy (glaucoma, immune-mediated keratitis).

MANAGING THE HORSE PRESENTED FOR ADNEXAL OR ORBITAL TRAUMA

Torn eyelids are a common emergency in equine practice. Many stable objects, particularly the "J"-shaped handles of water buckets, can catch the thin margin of the eyelid if a horse rubs its face. Due to the size of the animal, extensive damage may occur if the horse pulls backward.

Fortunately, the blood supply to the eyelids is excellent and a cosmetic, functional repair can usually be achieved in the field with prompt attention and careful technique[19] **(Fig. 11)**. Key elements include:

1. Use of a bale table to support and steady the horse's head. Use of a strap on head light on the surgeon.

2. Heavy intravenous sedation (detomidine or xylazine). Thorough infiltration of local anesthetic into the damaged skin, coupled with an auriculopalpebral motor block and a frontal sensory block of the upper lid.

3. Minimal debridement of the torn tissue margins.

4. Careful apposition of the subconjunctival tissues, with 4-0 or 5-0 absorbable suture. Use no more sutures than necessary, and bury the knots to avoid corneal irritation.

5. Careful apposition of the skin, using 4-0 suture in a simple interrupted pattern. Closure of the tarsal margin with a figure-of-eight pattern.

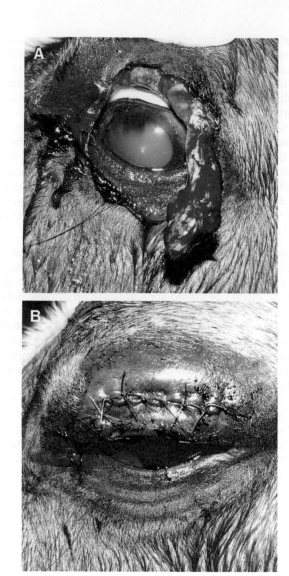

Fig. 11. (*A*) Acute torn upper eyelid. (*B*) Same lid after 2-layer repair.

6. Systemic and topical antibiotics and systemic NSAIDs for 3 to 7 days.

Most eyelid lacerations are simple linear or Y-shaped tears, but some involve multiplanar margin separation with extensive disruption of the palpebral conjunctiva. Other horses have chronic eyelid injuries that were never properly repaired and suffer resultant complications from trichiasis, entropion, ectropion, or lagophthalmos. Some of these cases benefit from referral.[19]

Blunt trauma to the skull, globe, and/or orbit often follows kick injuries or struggles within a horse trailer or starting gate. Orbital rim and sinus fractures are common and may sometimes alter globe position or impede extraocular muscle movement. Worrisome signs include strabismus, miosis, hyphema, corneal edema, or obvious

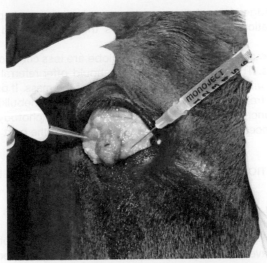

Fig. 12. Excision of the nictitans is indicated if a mass is present on the leading edge.

skull fracture. Negative prognostic signs include hyphema that fills more than 50% of the anterior chamber, lens luxation, detached retina, or rupture of the globe. Treatment principles include topical pupil dilation with atropine and systemic NSAIDs to relieve pain and treat secondary uveitis. Topical steroids are indicated if the corneal epithelium is intact. Owners of horses should be counseled that some horses develop a dense cataract in the months following the insult due to phacoclastic uveitis.

MANAGING THE HORSE PRESENTED FOR ADNEXAL OR GLOBE MASSES

Periocular and ocular masses represent about 10% of all equine neoplasias.[20] The most common neoplasias of the periocular region are squamous cell carcinoma, sarcoid, melanoma, and lymphosarcoma. Horses at risk for squamous cell carcinoma include paints, appaloosas, haflingers, Belgian draft horses, and any horse that lacks pigment along the tarsal margin of the eyelid.

Small periocular masses (<0.5-cm diameter) may be treated in the field with excision and/or local cryotherapy or immunotherapy. Surgical options for larger lesions are constrained by the need to preserve eyelid margin function; removal of enough tissue to provide a generous tumor free margin on all sides is generally impossible. Most horses that present for periocular masses greater than 0.5 cm will benefit from specialist evaluation. Optimal surgical therapy may include excision or surgical debulking accompanied by eyelid reconstruction. Adjunctive therapy such as cryotherapy, hyperthermia, brachytherapy, or photodynamic therapy is indicated to try to prevent recurrence.[17] Histopathology should be performed on periocular masses as optimal therapy selection depends on the type of mass present, and nonneoplastic conditions such as habronemiasis and fungal granulomas can mimic tumors. Prognosis will depend on the tissue of origin, the extent of infiltration, and existence of metastasis in other parts of the body.

Masses on the nictitans are usually first seen on the leading edge of the third eyelid (**Fig. 12**). Standing excision of the nictitans can be performed in the field[21] and has not been shown to have deleterious effects.[22] Excision is recommended for masses that are on the leading edge of the nictitans and surrounded by normal appearing mucosa. Referral or enucleation is advised for masses that have spread onto the bulbar conjunctiva.

Masses on the ocular surface or inside the globe are less common than periocular or nictitans masses. The ambulatory clinician should offer referral for these cases. Advanced imaging will be used to define the extent of the mass. If preservation of the globe is possible, treatment involves surgical excision or debulking of the mass, combined with adjunctive therapy such as brachytherapy or photodynamic therapy.[19] If the mass is advanced or inoperable, enucleation may be the best option to prevent tumor spread.

OCULAR EXAMINATION OF THE HORSE WITH BEHAVIOR CHANGE OR POOR PERFORMANCE

Clinicians are often asked to perform eye examinations on horses that exhibit poor performance or behavior change. In this author's experience, a minority of these horses have clinical ocular findings that are associated with the observed behavior while the majority have normal eyes. In either case, a thorough inspection of both eyes should be performed as previously described. Ancillary tests may include Schirmer tear testing to evaluate quantitative tear production and tonometry to check intraocular pressure. Maze testing is valuable to determine how the horse navigates when only one eye is receiving light and may educate the owner about the horse's general visual status.

OCULAR SURGERY

Specialists perform most procedures that involve deep dissection, suturing, or grafting of the cornea with biomembranes, conjunctiva, or donor corneal tissue. Other referral surgeries include eyelid reconstruction, laser ablation of granula iridica cysts, cyclosporine implants for ERU, phacoemulsification of cataracts, cyclophotocoagulation surgery for glaucoma, and cosmetic prosthetic orbital implant surgery.[3,4]

Ambulatory equine practitioners can perform a number of simpler surgical procedures including removal of small eyelid masses, repair of periocular traumas, neonatal entropion correction, minor eyelid revision, chalazion curettage, nictitans removal, and installation of subpalpebral lavage systems.

Enucleation is indicated for neoplastic globes or eyes that suffer chronic pain secondary to intractable uveitis, infection, globe rupture, or glaucoma and is offered by many equine practitioners. Equine practitioners often perform the surgery under general anesthesia[4], but in the past decade, practical techniques for enucleation of the standing horse have been published.[23,24] Standing enucleation must be done in stocks under heavy sedation, using mandibular head support and regional local anesthesia combined with a retrobulbar block of the orbital cone tissues (**Fig. 13**), The procedure has a low incidence of complications, and this author has found it to be a good option for horses at risk for general anesthesia (large draft horses, very old horses, and so forth).

BLINDNESS

Despite recent advances in equine ophthalmology, vision loss is still a common endpoint for many horses that sustain serious ocular trauma, infection, neoplasia, or uveitis. Horses that are blind in one eye function well due to the panoramic monocular visual field of the fellow eye, and are usually ridden and handled with little trouble.

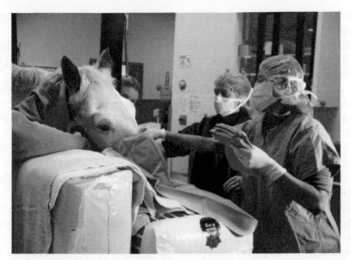

Fig. 13. Horse being prepared for standing enucleation.

Most equestrian competitions and racing jurisdictions allow participation of half-blind horses.

Bilateral blindness is a common endpoint of chronic uveitis, especially in the appaloosa breed.[17, 25] Some owners opt to euthanize horses that are blind for safety or economic reasons. Other horse owners choose to maintain blind horses as pets, and a few blind horses are ridden. Horses with quiet temperaments may adapt well to blindness. Clients who own horses at risk for losing vision should be directed to online resources (www.blindhorses.org) or printed materials[25] that describe management and training of blind horses.

SUMMARY

Equine practitioners examine patient eyes on a daily basis. Indications range from inspection of normal anatomy to treatment of traumatized eyes to workups of sight threatening inflammatory or neoplastic ocular conditions. Assessment of equine eyes requires practitioners to take time to create a good "exam room" in the field and administer appropriate restraint, sedation and/or regional anesthesia to facilitate thorough examination. Accurate diagnosis and treatment of equine eye problems requires skill in ocular surface staining and cytology, and basic proficiency in standing surgery. Expertise in digital photography optimizes client education and case management. As some equine eye problems benefit from intense medical treatment or advanced surgical care, practitioners should be familiar with the options offered at specialty centers, and recognize cases that would benefit from referral. Finally, blindness is not uncommon in horses. Practitioners can counsel clients that own blind horses on the best options for managing sight loss.

REFERENCES

1. Hurn SD, Turner AG. Ophthalmic examination findings of Thoroughbred racehorses in Australia. Vet Ophthalmol 2006;9:95–100.
2. Barnett, KC, Crispen SM, Lavach JD, et al. Color atlas and text of equine ophthalmology. 2nd edition. London: Mosby-Wolfe; 2004.

3. Brooks D. Ophthalmology for the equine practitioner. 2nd edition. Jackson (WY): Teton New Media; 2009.

4. Gilger BG, editor. Equine ophthalmology. 2nd edition. St Louis: Elsevier Saunders; 2010.

5. Dwyer AE. Practical general field ophthalmology. In: Gilger BG, editor. Equine ophthalmology. 2nd edition. St Louis: Elsevier Saunders; 2010. p. 52–92.

6. Labelle AL, Hamor RE, Townsend WM, et al. Ophthalmic lesions in neonatal foals evaluated for nonophthalmic disease at referral hospitals. JAVMA 2011;4:486–92.

7. Karpinski LG. The prepurchase examination. Vet Clin North Am Equine Pract 2004; 20:459–66.

8. Cutler T. Ophthalmic findings in geriatric horses. Vet Clin North Am Equine Pract 2002;18:545–74.

9. Carastro SM. Equine ocular anatomy and ophthalmic examination. Vet Clin North Am Equine Pract 2004;20:285–99.

10. Gilger BC, Stoppini R. Equine ocular examination: routine and advanced diagnostic techniques. In: Gilger, BG, editor. Equine ophthalmology. 2nd edition. St Louis: Elsevier Saunders; 2010. p. 1–51.

11. Matthews AG. The lens and cataracts. Vet Clin North Am 2004;20:393–415.

12. Dwyer AE. How to take digital photographs of equine eyes in practice. Proceedings of the 56th Annual Convention of the American Association of Equine Practitioners, 2010, p. 228–37.

13. Reimer JM, Latimer CS. Ultrasound findings in horses with severe eyelid swelling and recognition of acute dactryoadenitis: 10 cases (2004-2010). Vet Ophthalmol 2011; 2:86 –92.

14. Ramirez S, Tucker RL. Ophthalmic imaging. Vet Clin North Am Equine Pract 2004; 20:441–57.

15. Clode AB, Matthews AG. Diseases and surgery of the cornea. In: Gilger BG, editor. Equine ophthalmology. 2nd edition. St Louis: Elsevier Saunders; 2010. p. 317–49.

16. Gilger BGDeeg C. Equine recurrent uveitis. In: Gilger BG, editor. Equine ophthalmology. 2nd edition. St Louis: Elsevier Saunders; 2010. p. 181–266.

17. Dwyer AE, Crockett RS, Kalsow CM. Association of leptospiral seroreactivity and breed with uveitis and blindness in horses: 372 cases (1986-1993). JAVMA 1995;10: 1327–31.

18. Gilger BG, Wilkie DA, Clode AB, et al. Long-term outcome after implantation of a suprachoroidal cyclosporine drug delivery device in horses with recurrent uveitis. Vet Ophthalmol 2010;5:294–300.

19. Giuliano E. Equine ocular adnexal and nasolacrimal disease. In: Gilger BG, editor. Equine ophthalmology. 2nd edition. St Louis: Elsevier Saunders; 2010. p. 133–80.

20. Sundberg JP, Burnstein T, Page EH, et al. Neoplasms of equidae. JAVMA 1977;170: 150–2.

21. Harper J. How to surgically remove the third eyelid in the standing horse. Proceedings of the 56th Annual Convention of the American Association of Equine Practitioners, 2009. p. 380–5.

22. LaBelle A, Metzler AG, Wilkie DA. Nictitating membrane resection in the horse: a comparison of long-term outcomes using local vs. general anaesthesia. Equine Vet J 2011;43:42–5.

23. Pollock PJ, Russell T, Hughes TK, et al. Transpalpebral eye enucleations in 40 standing horses. Vet Surg 2008;37:306–9.

24. Hewes CA, Keoghan GC, Gutierrez-Nibero S. Standing enucleation in the horse, a report of 5 cases. Can Vet J 2007;48:512–4.

25. Dwyer AE. Practical managemont of blind horses. In: Gilger BG, editor. Equine ophthalmology. 2nd edition. St Louis: Elsevier Saunders; 2010. p. 470–81.

Reproduction in Ambulatory Practice

Ron Friedman, MS, DVM

KEYWORDS

- Equine • Ambulatory • Practice • Reproduction

Equine reproduction in an ambulatory practice setting is far more common than are in-house clinic facilities. Although ambulatory settings sometimes require adaptation and ingenuity, most procedures for a successful breeding season are readily adaptable to the ambulatory practice. This article will describe practice procedures that are feasible for most ambulatory settings.

PROCEDURES: MARES

Transrectal Exam

Successful broodmare management requires serial examinations of the mare before and shortly after ovulation. These procedures ensure that the stallion is used efficiently and the mare is bred in a timely manner. As a general rule, the goals of breeding management, ambulatory or otherwise, should be to:

- Utilize the stallion and mare as economically and efficiently as possible
- Achieve pregnancy in as few breedings, as close to ovulation, as possible
- Ensure that the mare's uterus maintains a suitable, contaminant-free environment ready for the maintenance of pregnancy.

The fundamental diagnostic procedure in mare reproduction is the transrectal uterine and ovarian palpation examination. Long a mainstay in equine reproduction, the transrectal exam remains diagnostically useful, adding information unavailable via other methods. Other basic reproductive procedures that require transrectal palpation as a prerequisite are:

- Uterine culture
- Uterine cytology
- Uterine biopsy
- Artificial insemination (AI)
- Uterine treatments: infusion and lavage.

The author has nothing to disclose.
The Oregon Equine Reproduction Center / Friedman Veterinary Service, PO Box 695, Lake Oswego, OR 97034, USA
E-mail address: rfdvm97034@yahoo.com

Vet Clin Equine 28 (2012) 175–187
doi:10.1016/j.cveq.2012.02.002
0749-0739/12/$ – see front matter © 2012 Elsevier Inc. All rights reserved.

vetequine.theclinics.com

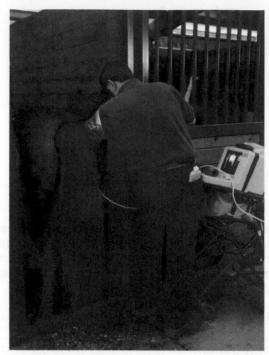

Fig. 1. Using a stall wall as protective barrier.

While ambulatory equine reproductive practice requires minimal equipment, an ultrasound unit with 5-MHz probe is almost indispensible. These machines have been around for many years, and a used, relatively inexpensive machine is not difficult to find. Even so, for a veterinarian only called upon to breed a few mares annually, the investment in an ultrasound machine may not be economically feasible. And while mares without complication can be successfully managed without ultrasound, it is indispensible for management of twins (previously the largest cause of abortion in mares), as well as some other common problems, such as management of excessive uterine edema or delayed uterine clearance and detection of biofilm.

Due to the nature of mare reproductive procedures, safety is critical for the veterinarian, handler, and horse. The veterinarian should always consider the possibility of serious injury and take precautions to minimize this risk. Gynecologic procedures should rarely be conducted without some form of barrier, restraint, or sedation; it is unsafe to palpate a mare with the examiner in the corner of a stall. Most mares need to be restrained, or possibly sedated, prior to any reproductive procedure. While standing stocks are a helpful tool, they are often unavailable to the ambulatory practitioner. If mare behavior or handler inexperience necessitates, the lip twitch and lip chain and/or sedation can minimize risk of injury and facilitate the reproductive exam or procedure in an efficient and safe manner.

The doorway of a stall can provide a means to decrease the risk of injury to the veterinarian. Reproductive procedures can be performed with the mare's hind legs standing at the stall doorway while the stall door or wall is used as a protective barrier (**Figs. 1** and **2**). Although not eliminating the risk of injury, these simple precautions can minimize risk and provide an obstacle to the sudden kick from a mare.

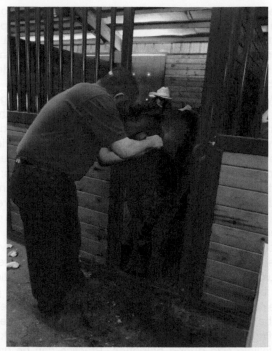

Fig. 2. Using the stall door as a barrier decreases the risk to the veterinarian.

Adequate lubrication not only facilitates the transrectal exam but is a safety consideration for the mare. Carboxymethyl-cellulose and mineral oil are the most commonly used lubricants and help decrease rectal straining; although straining is not necessarily a prerequisite for a rectal tear, it can contribute to this potentially catastrophic injury. Sedation with xylazine or detomondine at recommended dosages may help improve mare handling and safety but may not relieve rectal straining.

In addition to the mare's safety, excessive rectal straining can be a significant impediment to any procedure requiring transrectal palpation. The addition of a local anesthetic such as xylocaine HCl to the lubricant or applied to the rectal mucosa may reduce rectal straining. Intravenous N-butylscopolaminium bromide (Buscopan; Boehringer Ingelheim GmbH, Ingelheim, Germany) at recommended doses will eliminate rectal straining around the arm for a short time and allow for a thorough examination or any procedure requiring transrectal manipulation of the uterus or ovaries. Mares being palpated for the first time commonly strain and resist palpation. Some mares never acclimate to the procedure and will continue to strain during subsequent exams. Even experienced mares who are normally unperturbed by palpation will strain if the procedure exceeds a few minutes. In these instances, not only will N-butylscopolaminium bromide decrease the risk of rectal trauma but it will also facilitate the speed, efficiency, and accuracy of the exam findings.

The procedure for and the findings of transrectal reproductive palpation have been described.[1,2] The diagnostic goal of rectal palpation of the mare is to evaluate the size and tone of the uterus, ovaries and follicles, and cervix. An enlarged uterus, either from pregnancy of approximately 60 days or from a diseased state such as pyometra, is readily palpated. Differentiation, possibly difficult by palpation alone, can be accomplished if the fetus is balloted. Ovarian size ranging from the peanut sized ovary of anestrous to the abnormally enlarged ovaries formed by a follicular-ovarian hematoma or granulosa cell tumor can also be palpated. Differentiation of varying causes of ovarian size changes is difficult without ultrasound, and definitive diagnosis is achieved by serum hormonal parameters.

Reproductive cyclic changes will affect uterine tone. These changes range from the relaxed tone with edematous endometrial folds during estrus to the increased tone and tubularity found in diestrus and early pregnancy. With careful digital palpation of the uterus, endometrial folds of estrus can be detected as small "ridges," as can the tight tubularity found in early pregnancy and, to a lesser extent, diestrus. The hormonal effects on cervical tone are similar to those of the uterus: relaxation during estrus, increased tone, tightening, and tubularity during diestrus, and more so during pregnancy. Palpation of the normal pregnant mare's cervix will reveal a very tight "cigar"-like cervix, while the estrus cervix will flatten upon pressure or may be difficult to differentiate from the uterine body due its flaccid tone.

Even with the routine use of ultrasound for mare reproduction, ovarian palpation of follicular characteristics remains diagnostically valuable in detecting impending ovulation. As estrus progresses toward ovulation, the dominant follicle(s) will enlarge, soften, and often be painful to the mare when palpated. These physical follicular characteristics are not readily detected by ultrasound. With practice, determination of follicular size can be very precise with palpation. Knowing the dimensions of parts of your fingers (eg, fingertip width, distance from fingertip to knuckle, etc) facilitates determination of follicle size during palpation. Practice can be gained not only by palpating mares but also by touching objects all around. Accuracy is improved by estimating the size of objects by using your fingers and estimating dimensions of objects. Repetition will lead to increased ability to estimate the size of an object by feel alone.

Pregnancy diagnosis is readily accomplished both by ultrasound and by transrectal exams. Diagnostic findings of these exams are described elsewhere.[3,4] Management of early twin pregnancy is only feasible with the use of ultrasound; the detection, separation, and elimination of early embryos, although readily accomplished in an ambulatory setting, all require visualization of the early embryonic vesicles. With as many as 20% to 35% of mares double ovulating, the need to address this issue is not uncommon.

Elimination of one twin is most easily accomplished between days 12 to 15 of gestation, before cessation of the vesicle mobility phase on day 16. During the mobility phase, the embryonic vesicle will move throughout the uterus as one mechanism of maternal recognition of pregnancy. During this time the embryos will often be found adjacent to each other and can be manually separated by gently pressing the ultrasound probe between vesicles. Elimination of one twin can be accomplished with as little as 0.5-cm distance between vesicles, although a 1-cm separation is preferred. Once separated, pinching the vesicle between thumb and index finger or by pressing the vesicle against the pelvis with the ultrasound probe is possible and has been previously described.[5] The author's preferred method is a rapid "flick" of the vesicle with the ultrasound probe, and in the author's hand, the procedure is significantly less time consuming and requires much less manipulation of the uterus. Although several reports in the past indicated that treatment with exogenous progesterone or flunixin (a prostaglandin synthesis inhibitor) had no effect on the viability of pregnancies following twin reduction,[5,6] this therapy appears to be commonplace.[7] More recent reports indicate that treatment with flunixin and exogenous progesterone at the time of twin reduction resulted in delivery of more live foals than in untreated mares.[7] The author prefers to start these treatments 24 hours before, and continue for 3 days after, twin reduction.

Preparation of Mare for Intrauterine and Intravaginal Procedures

Prior to any vulvar or vaginal surgery or intrauterine procedure (AI, intrauterine treatment, uterine culture, cytology, biopsy, and vaginal speculum exam), the mare's tail must be secured out of the way. Even without a handler holding the tail, this is easily accomplished by wrapping and tying the tail with a reusable neoprene tail wrap, gauze roll, or self-adhering cohesive bandage or with a rectal exam sleeve. When using a reusable neoprene tail wrap, the base of the tail is incorporated into the wrap and the end of the tail is folded on itself distal to the last coccygeal bone, making a loop of tail. One end of a long piece of string is placed inside the loop of tail, wrapped around the tail 2 or 3 times and tied off at the halter or around the mare's neck with a quick release knot or held by the mare handler (**Fig. 3**A–C). When using gauze or flexible self-adhering cohesive bandage roll, the tail is wrapped from the base of the tail distally, knotted, and then tied off as just described. Incorporating small strands of the tail hair will keep the gauze wrap from slipping (**Fig. 3**D–F). When using a plastic rectal sleeve, the tail is folded and placed within the sleeve and taped tightly with porous tape at the base of the tail. A piece of string is pushed through the loop of tail and secured with a quick release loop. The other end of the string is secured as described (**Fig. 3**G–I). Once the mare is adequately restrained, the tail positioned out of the way and the mare is properly cleaned, and intravaginal or intrauterine procedures are readily accomplished in an ambulatory setting.

Endometritis: Diagnostic Procedures

The major cause of mare infertility is endometritis. In the past it was thought that endometritis was primarily due to bacterial infection. Current research, however, indicates that a more likely etiology for endometritis arises from a delay or failure in the uterine clearance of sperm and inflammatory byproducts normally found in the post-breeding mare, as well as bacteria.[8,9]

Endometrial culture and cytology are common and widely used to determine the presence of endometrial infection and inflammation respectively, either as a diagnosis for infertility or as a prerequisite of the stallion owner prior to live cover or semen shipment. Recent studies suggest that swabbing the endometrium may be insufficient to detect certain bacteria and that culture of uterine fluids or uterine biopsy samples are more sensitive.[8,9] Retrieval of uterine fluids is accomplished via lavage and does pose some challenges to the ambulatory practitioner, as discussed later.

While a uterine biopsy is not as commonly performed as a bacterial culture, it is a valuable technique to determine the degree of uterine fibrosis and endometritis and to determine the ability of the uterus to maintain a pregnancy to term. It should be considered for breeding soundness exams, in mares bred for 3 or more cycles without a resultant pregnancy (repeat breeders), mares with early embryonic death, and prior to any genitourinary surgical correction for infertility. If the biopsy predicts that the uterus is incapable of maintaining pregnancy to term, the need for the proposed surgery would be negated.

Diagnostic procedures, techniques, and interpretation have been widely reviewed and discussed. They are valuable in assessing mare fertility, and most are readily performed in an ambulatory setting.[10]

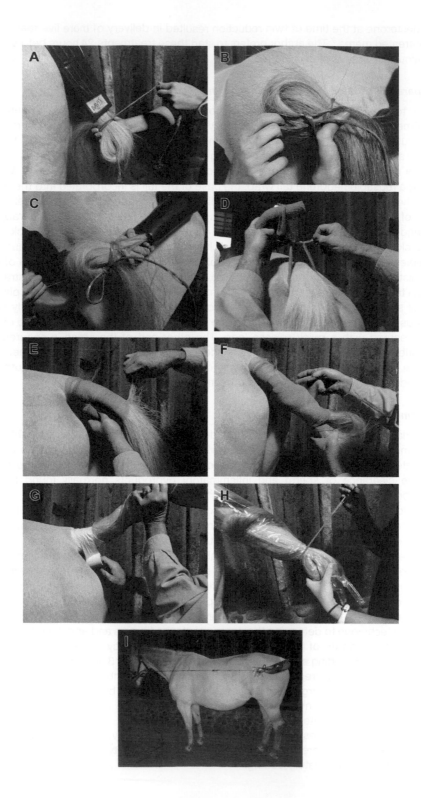

Endometritis: Therapeutic Considerations

Common reproductive therapies in the mare include antibiotic infusion into the uterine lumen, systemic antibiotics, systemic steroids to lessen the post breeding inflammatory response, as well as endometrial irrigation (lavage) and ecbolics to augment uterine clearance.

Techniques for intrauterine infusion are identical to those for AI, but uterine lavage requires adaptation or the help of an assistant for the veterinarian. For example, inflatable balloon-tip equine uterine flush catheters (Equine uterine lavage catheter; Animal Reproduction Systems, Chino, CA, USA) help seat the catheter within the uterus but can be cumbersome to inflate with one hand while the other is holding the catheter in place. As uterine irrigation usually involves the use of several liters of sterile saline or lactated Ringer's solution in single-liter containers, similar challenges are encountered when sequentially changing containers.

Recent findings suggest that coliforms and yeast produce a host immunosuppression secretion called biofilm. Biofilm is effectively treated with mucolytics such as N-acetylcysteine. Indications and protocols are reported and all are readily performed in ambulatory practice.[8,11]

Cervical Speculum Exam

Visual examination of the cervix is a valuable aid in assessing the mare's reproductive status.[12] In addition to visual inspection, if the speculum is pressed against the cervix and rotated (from 10:00 o'clock to 2:00 o'clock position) before withdrawal, a sample of cervical mucus may be obtained on the end of the speculum for examination. Mares in diestrus or pregnant will have pale, tight cervices raised above the vaginal floor with a tacky, sticky mucus film. In contrast, the estrus mare will have a relaxed, hyperemic cervix, possibly down on the vaginal floor with varying amounts of stringy fluid instead of normal cervical mucus. On occasion, cervical mucus, if produced in sufficient quantities and not having been "flushed" by urination, may be detected just inside the exterior vulva prior to introduction of the speculum. This mucus may also be found upon withdrawal of an instrument or a finger during any intrauterine procedure. Fluid cervical mucus can be detected in mid to late estrus and shortly after ovulation; its presence is a reliable indicator of estrus and if observed during a pregnancy exam suggests the mare is either not pregnant or is in the process of aborting the fetus.

Artificial Insemination (AI)

The convenience and opportunity afforded mare owners to breed to a worldwide roster of stallions, without having to transport their mares, along with the high success

---

Fig. 3. Preparing the mare for intrauterine and intravaginal procedures. (*A*) Fold the tail on itself, put the string through the fold, and wrap around tail twice. (*B*) Make a quick release loop through the string as it passes through the fold of the tail. (*C*) Tighten loop: the quick release knot can be easily opened by pulling on the loose end of the string. (*D*) Tie a half hitch at the top of the tail. (*E*) While wrapping roll over tail, incorporating a few tags of tail hair will secure wrap in place. (*F*) Fold the tail on itself and incorporate into wrap, forming a loop for securing tail. (*G*) To apply plastic sleeve as a tail wrap, place sleeve over folded tail, and secure to base of tail with adhesive tape. (*H*) As in *A–C*, wrap string around tail and through fold in tail. (*I*) Tail can be secured around neck of mare, tied to halter in quick release knot, or held by mare handler.

rates of chilled shipped semen and, to a lesser extent, frozen semen, have made AI commonplace in ambulatory practice. Equipment and supplies required are minimal: shoulder length sleeve, sterile lube, syringe, and AI pipette. Achieving positive results with AI can pose several challenges to the ambulatory clinician, because determination of the stage of cycle and accurate prediction of ovulation are essential for success. Several farm visits are often required until the stage of cycle is determined. Reproductive cycle manipulation is highly utilized and may include prostaglandin injections or 10 days of progestins followed by prostaglandin. Hormonal manipulation of the mare's reproductive cycle will decrease the number of farm visits and mare exams required, significantly increasing efficiency and economy, and will also synchronize insemination dates with the shipping companies' days of operation.[13]

The mare is examined daily or every other day during estrus until ovulation can be reliably predicted. Ideally, when using shipped semen, semen is ordered for insemination 1 day pre-ovulation. Ovulation induction agents are commonly used to shorten the interval between insemination and ovulation. When using frozen semen and as ovulation nears, the mare is examined multiple times daily or examined and inseminated using the timed protocol discussed later.

Because thawed frozen semen has a shorter life span compared to chilled semen, it requires insemination much closer to ovulation than with shipped semen or live cover, ideally within a few hours. Precise prediction of ovulation is difficult; 2 basic breeding protocols have gained popularity for AI by frozen semen.[14]

The first breeding protocol for AI by frozen semen requires examination every 6 to 8 hours as the gravid follicle matures, with insemination at the time ovulation is detected. As the life span of the ova is, at most, 12 hours, this examination protocol ensures that sperm are introduced to the ova no more than 8 hours after ovulation and in practice often less than 6 hours after ovulation.

The second frozen semen protocol is timed around the administration of ovulation induction agents and uses 2 breeding doses of frozen semen. In this scenario, the mare is examined once daily until a 35-mm follicle is detected. At that time, the mare is administered an ovulation induction agent (human chorionic gonadotropin or gonadotropin releasing hormone). AI is then performed at 24 hours and 40 hours after administration of the ovulation induction agent.

Both protocols for AI with frozen semen have their drawbacks in ambulatory practice: the first protocol requires numerous trips to the mare, and the second protocol requires 2 breeding doses of frozen semen. An additional challenge to using frozen semen in an ambulatory setting is that specialized AI "guns" may be recommended by various semen producers. These "guns" hold 0.25- to 0.5-mL straws and typically require the use of multiple straws of frozen semen, using 1 straw at a time. Their use may also require additional assistance, which is not always available in ambulatory practice. Additional equipment is required for thawing frozen semen. Although recommended, an electric hot water bath is not required since an accurate thermometer and a thermal insulated mug, a large sink, or any insulated container can be adequate for thawing frozen semen.

Two AI techniques are commonly used in the mare: traditional AI and deep horn artificial insemination (DHAI). Traditional AI technique deposits the semen into the uterine body. DHAI deposits semen at the apex of the uterine horn, ipsilateral to the gravid follicle, close to the oviductal papillae. The technique is described elsewhere.[15] DHAI has been recommended for use with semen containing the lower numbers of sperm per breeding dose that are often found with frozen semen. Some advocate the use of endoscopy to facilitate DHAI, but utilization of this technology often requires additional assistance not always available in an in ambulatory setting. DHAI can be mastered transrectally using commercially available AI pipettes manufactured for the technique (Universal Insemination Pipette and Gun; 55- and 65-cm lengths, Minitube of America, Verona, WI, USA). Both techniques, when applied in appropriate circumstances, provide similar pregnancy rates.

Another challenge to AI in an ambulatory setting is assessing the viability of the semen used. Insemination does not always result in a pregnancy and not all causes of nonpregnancy originate from actual infertility. Some arise from errors in semen handling and processing. Ideally, semen should be examined prior to insemination, or shortly afterward, to eliminate such potential causes of infertility. Although precise correlations between percent motility and pregnancy may be difficult to quantify, finding less than 30% motile sperm in a shipped semen sample is a cause for concern. The semen collection, processing, and handling procedures should undergo further scrutiny if low semen motility is noted. While mares can be bred with semen that has not been assessed for viability, it is impossible to adequately assess all potential common causes of infertility without such examination.

Motility assessment is the most commonly used method of semen viability and requires that sperm be handled as close to physiologic temperatures (37°C) as possible. Slide warmers and microscopes are essential for this. An inexpensive alternative to a slide warmer is a disposable styrofoam chick incubator with a light bulb to heat slides and coverslips. This is followed by rapid observation of sperm under a microscope. Care must be taken that semen and supplies are maintained close to 37°C. Although the problem is not insurmountable, evaluation of semen motility can be difficult for the ambulatory practitioner when working with the low numbers of semen and the small volume of frozen semen.

Embryo Transfer

Embryo transfer is not easily adaptable to ambulatory practice. Flushing embryos from donor mares requires transport of equipment and supplies, including, but not limited to, sterile intrauterine catheters, specialized tubing with fittings, embryo filters, embryo locating dishes, dissection microscopes, and other equipment, as well as several liters of heated embryo flush and holding solutions. Additional personnel are needed for the flushing procedure and restraining the mare. Keeping the mare adequately restrained and immobile without stocks for the duration of the procedure will be problematic, as many mares become mildly agitated or anxious when their uterus is distended with flush solution. Thus, clients who are interested in embryo transfer should be referred to facilities equipped for the process.

Foaling and Post-Foaling

Foaling management of mares in the ambulatory practice has some distinct limitations inherent to the rapid progression of the mare from stage 1 to stage 2 of labor. These limitations are directly proportional to the distance the practitioner must travel to the patient. As the time to render assistance to mare and foal increases, so does the likelihood of complications. Fortunately, mares rarely require obstetric assistance since more than 95% of foaling mares are able to successfully deliver a foal to term without intervention.

When dystocias are encountered, they are a true emergency and ambulatory practitioners should be prepared to respond in 30 minutes or less to maximize the possibility of preserving the life and health of the mare and foal. Longer response times can result in lower survival rates for the foal and/or mare.

Before vaginal intervention, the mare's tail should be wrapped and the hind quarters and vulva thoroughly cleaned. Correction of dystocia is facilitated with copious amounts of clean water-soluble lubricant. This is most effectively introduced with a sterile or sanitized nasogastric tube and pumped around the foal as much as possible. A word of caution is given about using polyethylene polymer powder (PEP) lubricant in the foaling mare (J-Lube; Jorgensen Laboratories, Loveland, CO, USA): although PEP obstetric lubricant has been used for many years to successfully manage equine dystocia, this powdered lubricant can cause acute fatal peritonitis if exposed to the peritoneal cavity.[16] Thus, it should be used with care and restricted to mares not considered for surgical intervention.

To deliver a foal during dystocia, it is essential to ascertain if the foal is alive, along with its presentation (cranial, caudal, transverse), position (dorsal, ventral), and posture (reflected head, carpal flexion, etc).

Repulsion and correction of fetal presentation, position, and posture can be physically demanding and difficult due to mare contractions, the weight of the intestines, constriction of the pelvic canal, and fetal malformation. Systemic anesthetics will not only decrease the mare's contraction and straining but also act as fetal cardiodepressants. They should be used with caution if the foal is alive, and foal resuscitation equipment should be readily available. If the mare is sedated, lifting the hind end higher than the thorax relieves much of the weight from the abdominal contents and is a significant benefit. This can be accomplished with ropes and tractors with hydraulic lifts or with the use of pulleys and overhead beams. With enough help, the mare can be pulled onto an inclined sheet of thick plywood. Reducing mare straining and contractions can be achieved with a caudal epidural injection of lidocaine or xylazine. It can also be achieved with the systemic administration of tocolytic clenbutarol or, preferably, an intravenous injection of N-butylscopolaminium bromide.

If referral to a surgical facility is an option, speed is critical to optimize foal survival and to limit obstetric injury in the mare. If surgical referral is not an option and the dystocia uncorrectable, fetotomy should be considered. Specific methods for dystocia management and fetotomy are described.[17]

Post-Partum Care: Retained Placenta

One of the more common post-foaling complications is retained placenta. If the fetal membranes are retained for more than 3 hours, treatment should be instituted. Oxytocin, nonsteroidal anti-inflammatory agents, and systemic antibiotics are frequently the first line of therapy. Gentle traction should be approached with caution as placental microvilli can be torn off, leading to metritis and sepsis. If fetal membranes are not intact or other complications of parturition diminish uterine involution or cause endometrial infection, uterine lavage is indicated. Regardless of the cause, if lochia appears purulent (other than the normal "brick red" color) or involution is not progressing normally, uterine lavage with dilute povidine solution (100 mL per gallon water) followed by oxytocin injections will help stimulate uterine clearance and involution.

A valuable but often overlooked therapy to relieve retained intact fetal membranes is the Burns technique. A clean and disinfected nasogastric tube is placed into chorioallantoic space and tied off with string. Fluid (the author uses 5 L of clean water with 100 mL of povidine-iodine solution) is slowly pumped into the lumen, resulting in the distention and detachment of microvilli from the chorioallantois and the endometrium and release of the placenta.[18] Extensive in-depth descriptions of the management of both retained placenta and postparturient complications have been given.[19]

PROCEDURES: STALLION

For the most part, stallion reproduction in ambulatory or referral settings revolves around 2 fundamental procedures: semen collection and semen transport. Reproductive procedures on stallions are inherently more complicated than those on the mare simply because they commonly require the presence of a mare and accompanying personnel. Occasionally, when working with the highly trained and experienced stallion that has been trained for collection on a phantom mare without an estrus mare being present, additional assistance is not necessary.

Semen Collection

Stallion semen collection in ambulatory practice, although not a difficult procedure, does pose some hurdles not encountered when working on mares. In most cases, a receptive mare is essential, which rarely poses a problem if the estrus mare used is the mare to be bred. If the semen is to be shipped, having an estrus mare that coincides with the time semen is requested can be problematic and, without preparation, unreliable.

Semen collection can be accomplished on a mare displaying estrus or on a "phantom mare" breeding mount if available. Either method requires additional assistance because handlers are needed for both the mare and the stallion, as well as a person handling the artificial vagina (AV). In contrast to reproductive procedures carried out on mares, experienced horse handlers are critical in semen collection because sedatives and tranquilizers for the stallion are not a viable option. Without experienced personnel, collecting semen from stallions can be a dangerous procedure, and ambulatory practitioners who do not have access to trained personnel and proper equipment would be best served to refer to facilities that specialize in this procedure.

Because of the very nature of the procedure, collecting a sexually stimulated stallion in close proximity to, or on the back of a mare, who may or may not be compliant, can rapidly lead to some unexpected and unpleasant situations extremely quickly. Semen collection and the equipment required, as well as the methods to produce an estrus mare, have been widely described.[20]

Packaging and Shipping Semen

Once collected, processing and packaging semen requires assessing motility, determining sperm concentration and total numbers, and diluting semen with semen extender. Although not difficult procedures, they require the transportation of additional equipment and supplies.

Processing semen for chilled shipment is often a simple matter of mixing semen extender and gel-free semen. However, attention to detail is a prerequisite for success. Preheating supplies (syringes, AV, semen extender) that come into contact with semen to 37°C prevents cold shock. This may be difficult to achieve in some ambulatory situations. Microscopy is also needed to ensure that sperm in the semen are alive and motile. Selection of the optimum semen extender may be problematic in some stallions. Fortunately, the majority of stallion semen is compatible with nearly all commercial semen extenders. Details of handling and processing semen for shipment are described elsewhere.[21]

Containers for shipping semen vary widely in style and expense. Fortunately, most popular models available today are adequate for the majority of stallions.[22]

Freezing Semen

Because a laboratory full of equipment and supplies is required for cryopreservation of stallion semen, this procedure is not readily adapted to most ambulatory practices. In addition to the freezing apparatus itself, refrigeration, incubators, microscopes, and assorted other supplies are needed. Handling semen and supplies in a temperature-controlled manner is critical for success, and as such, practitioners should consider referring this service to facilities experienced in the procedure: some of these facilities offer mobile laboratories as part of their service.

SUMMARY

The value of providing equine reproductive services in ambulatory setting is well established. Ambulatory practice has been, and will most likely continue to be, the primary provider of equine reproductive veterinary services. The limitations for performing various reproductive procedures in an ambulatory setting are those imposed by the amount of equipment and supplies that must be brought to the patient, as well as those imposed when procedures require additional assistance. This is analogous to human medical care: the ambulance cannot substitute for a hospital but it can certainly provide significant assistance. Similarly, although excellent reproductive service can be provided in ambulatory practice, a fair number of advanced techniques and procedures requiring laboratory conditions, equipment, and personnel are difficult to provide from the back of a vehicle.

REFERENCES

1. Asbury AC. Examination of the mare. In: Colahan PT, Merritt AM, Moore JN, et al, editors. Equine medicine and surgery, vol II. St Louis: Mosby; 1999. p 1088–93.
2. Shindeler RK. Rectal palpation. In: McKinnon AO, Voss JL, editors. Equine reproduction. Philadelphia: Lea & Febiger; 1993. p. 204–11.
3. McKinnon AO, Squires EL. Ultrasonic evaluation of the reproductive trac. In: Colahan PT, Merritt AM, Moore JN, et al, editors. Equine medicine and surgery, vol II. St Louis: Mosby; 1999. p. 1100–14.
4. McKinnon AO. Diagnosis of pregnancy. In: McKinnon AO, Voss JL, editors. Equine reproduction. Philadelphia: Lea & Febiger; 1993. p. 501–8.
5. Mckinnon AO. Twin reduction techniques. In: Samper JC, Pycock JF, McKinnon AO, editors. Current therapy in equine reproduction. Philadelphia: WB Saunders; 2007. p. 357–73.
6. Pascoe DR, Pascoe RR, Hughes JP, et al Management of twin concept by manual embryonic reduction: comparison of two techniques and three hormone treatments. Am J Vet Res 1987;48:1594–9.
7. Sheerin PC, Howard CE, LeBlanc MM, et al, Effects of operator, treatment, and mare age on the live foal rate of mares after manual twin reduction. Anim Repr Sci 2010; Suppl:S312–3.
8. LeBlanc MM. Advances in the diagnosis and treatment of chronic infectious and post-mating-induced endometritis in the mare. Reprod Domest Anim 2010;45 (Suppl 2):21–7.
9. Riddle WT, LeBlanc MM, Stromberg AJ. Relationships between uterine culture, cytology and pregnancy rates in a Thoroughbred practice. Theriogenology 2007;68: 395–402.
10. Pycock JF. Breeding management of the problem mare. In: Samper JC, editor. Equine breeding management and artificial insemination. Philadelphia: WB Saunders; 2000. P. 195–228.

11. LeBlanc MM. Tutorial article. The current status of antibiotic use in equine reproduction. Equine Vet Educ 2009;21:156–67.
12. LeBlanc MM. Vaginal examination. In: McKinnon AO, Voss JL, editors. Equine reproduction. Philadelphia: Lea & Febiger; 1993. p. 221–4.
13. Bergfelt DR. Estrous synchronization. In: Samper JC, editor. Equine breeding management and artificial insemination. Philadelphia: WB Saunders; 2000. p. 165–77.
14. Loomis PR, Squires EL. Frozen semen management in equine breeding programs. Theriogenology 2005;64:480–91.
15. Lyle SK, Ferrer MS. Low-dose insemination—why, when and how. Theriogenology 2005;64:572–9.
16. Frazer GS, Beard WL, Abrahamsen E, et al. Systemic effects of a polyethylene polymer-based obstetrical lubricant in the peritoneal cavity of the horse. In: Proceedings of the 50th Am Assoc Equine Prac. Denver; 2004. p. 484–7.
17. Frazer GS. Dystocia and fetotomy. In: Samper JC, Pycock JF, McKinnon AO, editors. Current therapy in equine reproduction. Philadelphia: WB Saunders; 2007. p. 417–35.
18. Brinsko SP. How to perform uterine lavage: indications and practical techniques. In: Proceedings 47th Am Assoc Equine Prac. San Diego; 2001. p. 407–11.
19. Blanchard TL, Macpherson ML. Postparturient abnormalities. In: Samper JC, Pycock JF, McKinnon AO, editors. Current therapy in equine reproduction. Philadelphia: WB Saunders; 2007. p. 465–75.
20. Hurtgen JP. Semen collection in stallions. In: Samper JC, editor. Equine breeding management and artificial insemination. Philadelphia: WB Saunders; 2000. p. 81–90.
21. Samper JC. Artificial insemination. In: Samper JC, editor. Equine breeding management and artificial insemination. Philadelphia: WB Saunders; 2000. p. 109–31.
22. Brinsko SP, Rowan KR, Varner DD, et al. Effects of transport container and ambient temperature on motion characteristics of equine spermatozoa. Theriogenology 2000; 53:1641–55.

Equine Wellness Care in Ambulatory Practice

Claudia Sandoval, DVM[a],*, Claudia True, DVM[b]

KEYWORDS

• Equine wellness • Vaccine • Deworming • Dentistry

Equine wellness care is changing. Vaccination and deworming, the traditional components of preventative medicine, are provided by veterinarians less often due to the availability of discounted vaccines and dewormers. To maintain a role in preventative medicine, it is important to show clients the value of veterinarians providing these services. In addition to vaccinations and deworming, wellness examinations, routine dental care, fecal egg counts, blood work, and nutrition consulting can improve the health of the horses that ambulatory veterinarians care for. Because many clients pay for animals' health services out of pocket, they want to know how services will benefit their horses.[1] Developing a wellness program that encompasses all aspects of preventative medicine, and effectively communicating it to clients, can be a valuable asset to the ambulatory practitioner.

Findings suggest that the cost of veterinary care is of low importance compared to other criteria for owners selecting a veterinary practice.[1] From the client's perspective, veterinary medicine should be a profession where patient care comes first and monetary aspects come second.[2] Making sure that clients and patients are seen on an annual or biannual basis will build a strong relationship with the client and patient—leading to more accurate data gathering, increased client satisfaction, and more client involvement in patient care.[3] Clients can easily understand and accept wellness visits if they are focused on the benefits of the services at financially competitive rates. An inadequate discussion of costs has been shown to be a specific area of concern for pet owners; failure to adequately discuss the cost of veterinary care makes it difficult for them to make informed decisions.[1,2]

WELLNESS PROGRAM

Through a wellness program, clients can better appreciate the advantages of their veterinarian playing an active role in maintaining their horse's health, not just restoring it after illness or injury. Since wellness visits get the veterinarian on the farm at regular

The authors have nothing to disclose.

[a] Fairfield Equine Associates, LLC, 32 Barnabas Road, Newtown, CT 06470, USA
[b] Woodside Equine, LLC, PO Box 989, Ashland, VA 23005, USA
* Corresponding author.
E-mail address: csandoval@fairfieldequine.com

Vet Clin Equine 28 (2012) 189–205
doi:10.1016/j.cveq.2012.02.001
0749-0739/12/$ – see front matter © 2012 Elsevier Inc. All rights reserved.

Table 1 Yearly wellness services available as packaged programs			
Wellness Program	**Bronze***	**Silver***	**Gold***
Services			
Wellness Exam & Consultation	1	2	2
Soundness Jog			2
Routine Motorized Dental w/Sedation	1	1	1
EWT Vaccine	1		
EWT/Rhino/Flu Vaccine (5 Way)		2	2
Potomac Horse Fever	1	2	2
Rabies Vaccine	1	1	1
WNV Vaccine	1	1	1
Coggins		1	1
Fecal Float	3	3	3
CBC Profile			1

* Numbers indicate the amount of services performed for the year.

intervals, the client and doctor can make individualized plans for each horse. In an era when spurious and potentially harmful information is easily available online, routine wellness visits help the veterinarian retain his or her role as the primary source of knowledge. A wellness visit allows for a comprehensive approach to the horse; all aspects of care—from weight management to proper foot balance to advice on supplements—can be discussed with clients. The wellness visit often reveals additional services the horse needs that the client might not be aware of. For example, if the veterinarian has any concerns about the horse's hoof balance, appropriate steps such as "foot balance" radiographs and a conversation with the farrier can be offered.

Services typically found in wellness programs include an annual or semiannual physical examination, nutrition consultation, yearly dental exam, Coggins test, and fecal egg count. For some practices, a wellness program consists of a bundled prepaid package of services. What is offered will vary with practice type and region; typical programs may include tiered levels of care based on potential for exposure to other horses. For example, a care level tailored to the show horse might include twice-yearly vaccines for equine herpes virus (EHV) and influenza, whereas the care level for the mature horse that does not travel may not need these vaccines. Some practices choose to add services, such as a yearly lameness examination in their performance level package or specialized lab work in a geriatric package (eg, fasting insulin and glucose, complete blood count, and chemistry). **Table 1** is an example of the wellness program offered by one author's clinic.

A practice may want to further incentivize client adoption of a wellness program by offering reduced stable call fees for multiple horses of the same owner, at the same barn, or in the same area. Discounts can be given on products or services with a yearly coupon (eg, $30 discount for any service) or a percentage discount throughout the year for additional services or products. Any additional expense for these services can potentially be offset by the incremental revenue. The discounts offered by these plans are advantageous for 2 reasons. First, wellness program fees for the entire year can be collected up front, and many clinics find it beneficial to have their enrollment period during late winter to early spring when accounts receivable are down. Second, discounting a package generates revenue on services that were not consistently used in the past.

Lack of promotion or an owner's inability to make a single large payment yearly can result in underutilization of a wellness program. If the economy is particularly depressed within a practice area, offering to split the wellness payments into regular intervals (eg, quarterly) might ameliorate the latter risk, as can requiring a credit card or a third party payer to be on file with the clinic.

It must be emphasized that everyone involved in the ambulatory practice needs to be actively involved in advancing the wellness program. A discussion between veterinarians and staff regarding standards of care should be the start of any wellness program—a consistent voice from doctors, technicians, and staff will help explain and promote program benefits to clients, and good client communication is key to a successful program. Practice employees are often a client's most regular contact with a practice. They can lay the ground work for conversations between clients and veterinarians, raising the client's awareness and interest before the veterinarian arrives at the farm. While mailers and client education brochures are traditional methods of client communication, newer technologies such as e-mail, practice websites, Facebook, and Twitter are less expensive and faster.

When the authors are vaccinating at a new farm, their clinics' wellness programs are always introduced and the advantages discussed. Wellness programs are a way of reinserting the veterinarian as a major voice in the horses' health care and effectively capturing untapped revenue at key times of the year.

VACCINES

Planning a vaccination strategy is based on a multitude of factors as seen in **Fig. 1**. The development of an effective vaccination program also requires a partnership between the veterinarian and the horse owner, as vaccines are only one aspect of preventing disease. Previous issues of *Veterinary Clinics of North America in Equine Practice* have evaluated the evidence and efficacy for many of the vaccines currently available, stressing that, with a couple of exceptions, published research for many of these vaccines is limited.[4] Since owners can obtain vaccines directly (online and in farm supply stores), it is important for veterinarians to demonstrate the value they add by being directly involved in all aspects of infectious disease control, including vaccine selection and administration. Understanding the science behind the available vaccine choices for each situation and communicating this expertise to clients is essential.

Vaccine Selection

The vaccination guidelines available on the Internet by the American Associate of Equine Practitioners (AAEP) has proved an excellent resource for veterinarians, not only for vaccination principles but also for discussing vaccine technology, label claims, vaccination schedules, adverse reactions, and other methods for infectious disease control.[5] The AAEP has established rabies, Eastern/Western equine encephalomyelitis (EEE/WEE), tetanus, and West Nile virus (WNV) as core vaccinations for horses using the American Veterinary Medical Association (AVMA) definition of a core vaccine. Core vaccines are those that protect from diseases that are endemic to a region, those with potential public health significance, those required by law, those that are virulent/highly infectious, and/or those posing a risk of severe disease. Core vaccines have clearly demonstrated efficacy and safety, and thus exhibit a high enough level of patient benefit and low enough level of risk to justify their use in the majority of patients.[5]

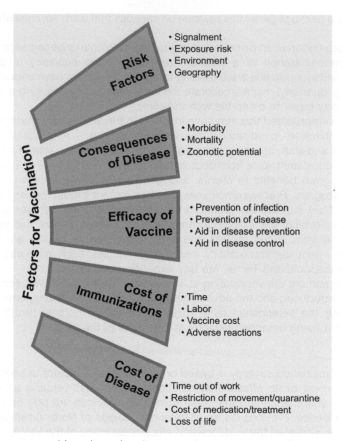

Fig. 1. Factors to consider when planning a vaccination program. (*Data from* the AAEP vaccination guidelines: principles of vaccination; http://www.aaep.org/vaccination_guidelines.htm. 2008.)

Ambulatory veterinarians can demonstrate their expertise by choosing effective vaccines and letting clients know the reasons for their choices. When making a vaccine selection, it is recommended to review the challenge models and comparison studies used to evaluate efficacy. WNV vaccines, for example, have different challenge models for vaccine licensing: mosquito feeding, needle inoculation, and intrathecal models.[6] If cost of vaccine is a concern, the least expensive vaccine may save horses' lives but may not be best at reducing morbidity. An in-depth understanding of vaccines and vaccine technology helps reinforce the perception of the veterinarian's expertise in equine care and helps facilitate dialogue on appropriate vaccine selection and intervals, both within the practice and with clientele. The AAEP guidelines also provide a list for risk-based vaccines, whose necessity varies due to factors such as signalment, exposure risk, environment, and geography (see **Fig. 1**). The risk-based vaccines include anthrax, botulism, EHV, equine viral arteritis, equine influenza, Potomac horse fever, rotaviral diarrhea, and strangles.[5]

The literature comparing vaccine products is sparse. Challenges can arise when comparing vaccines because immune responses to the products themselves can differ widely and the responses tested may not be representative of protection. For example, circulating antibody responses to intranasal equine influenza vaccination are minimal, suggesting that there are other factors, such as local protection at the nasal mucosa, that may be enhanced by this vaccine.[7] Some risk-based vaccines may only reduce clinical signs, which raises the question of whether it is worth vaccinating with a vaccine that is only partially effective, especially if there is a risk for an adverse event after vaccination. Regarding EHV and equine influenza virus, 2 of the risk-based diseases for which vaccination is most common, practitioners should be aware of the following:

1. EHV has received a great deal of attention due to the outbreaks of the myeloencephalitic form of EHV-1 (EHM). Currently, there are no vaccines that have a label claim to prevent EHM infection. According to the AAEP vaccination guidelines,[5] the high–antigen load vaccines may have the greatest potential to limit nasal shedding of EHV-1 and may assist in limiting the spread of outbreaks of EHM. Low–antigen load respiratory vaccines are variable in antibody production[8] but often lower in cost.
2. Recent findings on equine influenza from the 2010 OIE Expert Surveillance Panel have led to new conclusions and recommendations. They identified that all equine influenza virus isolates in 2008–2009 were of the American lineage and composed only of 2 clades: clade 1 (South Africa/03-like or Ohio/03-like viruses) was identified in North America and parts of Europe, and clade 2 (Richmond/1/07-like viruses) was identified in Europe and parts of Asia.[9] Since H7N7 viruses and H3N8 viruses of the Eurasian lineage were not detected in the surveillance, the panel concluded that these lineage viruses should not be included in vaccines. They recommend that vaccines should include both clade 1 and clade 2 viruses of the Florida sublineage[9]; however, at this moment, there are no vaccines in the North American market that contain both clades.

Adverse Events

All vaccines have to undergo safety testing prior to licensing, but when administering vaccines, local and systemic reactions can be seen. Ideally, the benefits of the vaccines outweigh the morbidity and mortality of the disease. Adverse reactions are not always predictable and there are inherent risks of vaccination. Vaccination has been demonstrated to elicit a prominent inflammatory response in horses, elevating white blood cell count, serum amyloid A, and fibrinogen.[10] The adjuvant alone, however, can also cause a response.[11] While an inherent risk, adverse reactions can be alarming to clients. They should be handled promptly, and with concern toward the client, as well as the horse.

Vaccines are meant to stimulate the immune system and with that come some potential side effects, which are usually non–life threatening. While evaluating an adverse event, what constitutes an adverse reaction should be considered—fever, malaise, and muscle soreness are expected side effects, as in human vaccinations. Educating clients on what to expect is key. When people are vaccinated, they often receive written information that outlines potential adverse reactions and what to do if any are noted. Providing this information to veterinary clientele can foster a conversation on what to expect and what is truly an "adverse" event and can help allay client fears should an adverse reaction occur.

In the authors' clinical experience, typical adverse reactions after intramuscular vaccines are localized muscular swelling and soreness and systemic signs of fever and/or lethargy. A retrospective study of adverse event reports for veterinary biologic products from 1999 to 2005 showed that systemic events were most commonly reported for equids.[12] The strangles vaccines (both intramuscular and intranasal), for example, have been documented to have adverse reactions such as fevers, nasal discharge, abscessation, lymphadenitis, and purpura hemorragica.[13] Additionally, a 2011 study demonstrated incomplete attenuation of the currently modified live virus strain, which was not found to be safe in young naïve ponies (<1 year old).[14] To minimize adverse events, it would be ideal to know the protective titers for equine diseases so vaccination could be performed only as needed. To date, however, strangles is the only disease with a recommended titer for when to consider vaccination (SeM <1:1600).[15] Thus, vaccinating based on titers for individual diseases cannot be generally recommended at this time. There is insufficient literature when evaluating equine immune reactions to multivalent versus monovalent vaccines, antigens and adjuvants, and adverse events. Similarly, studies examining differences in geriatric or metabolically compromised horses are rare. The only study in aged horses evaluating immune response to a vaccine showed a significantly reduced anamnestic response to influenza vaccination in comparison with younger adult horses.[16] This poses a challenge to evaluating vaccine efficacy for different age populations but does not assess the susceptibility of geriatrics to adverse reactions.

Safety and efficacy data are also not available regarding the concurrent use of multiple vaccines. Multivalent vaccines cannot be licensed without safety and efficacy data including potency testing of each antigen contained within the multivalent product. While each company's product has been deemed safe, the reactions of multivalent and monovalent vaccines when used concurrently are unknown.

With respect to adjuvants used in equine vaccines, some elicit more immune response than others,[10] but this may not correlate with its potential to create an adverse event. Furthermore, there is no research of the effect on the horse's immune system when administering different adjuvants simultaneously. Adjuvants have been linked to nonspecific adverse effects, which include fever, arthritis, uveitis, anorexia, soreness, and lethargy.[17] More often, though, they cause injection site reactions due to inflammation and, more rarely, granulomas or sterile abscesses.[17] It is of the authors' opinion and experience that if all vaccines (for any age horse) need to be administered in one visit, minimizing the adjuvants used (ie, using a multivalent product or a nonadjuvant product) may decrease the likelihood of adverse events.

In an attempt to limit adverse reactions, some of the information accumulated from various sources (Craig Barnett, DVM, Paola, Kansas, personal communication)[5,18] have been compiled in **Box 1** as recommendations for vaccine administration. If an adverse reaction does occur, veterinarians should report them to the vaccine's manufacturer and/or the US Department of Agriculture Center for Veterinary Biologics.

When considering the factors outlined here and the current lack of research, it is clear that vaccinations should be kept in the hands of veterinarians. Additionally, clients need to be made aware of the possibility for adverse events and contact their veterinarian when it occurs. Finding additional research or information about vaccine products can be challenging for equine ambulatory practitioners; however, the authors have had positive experiences reaching out for expert advice to other equine veterinarians with additional expertise in infectious disease, immunology, or vaccine development. Also, the aforementioned AAEP vaccination guidelines elaborate on the different vaccines available.

DENTISTRY

In the last decade, equine dentistry has come to the forefront for clients and veterinarians alike. Current equine veterinary literature teaches the value of a thorough

---

Box 1
Guidelines for administering equine vaccinations to reduce the likelihood of adverse events[5,18]

Proper care and handling

- Never mix vaccines in the same syringe.
- When using multidose vials, wipe the top of the vial with an alcohol pad before using and allow it to dry.

Accountability

- Consistently administer the same vaccine at the same location or record the location so the proper vaccination can be attributed to the event.
- Record the serial numbers of the vaccines administered.
- Educate clients with respect to proper expectation and potential problems.

Vaccine Selection

- Eliminate vaccines with marginal or questionable efficacy and/or safety.
- Administered non-adjuvanted vaccines if available.
- Administration of vaccines containing multiple antigens/adjuvants at the same time may increase the risk of adverse events, especially when combining those from different manufacturers.
- When adverse reactions have occurred, splitting the vaccines should be considered to identify the vaccine and reduce the adverse events.
- Avoid administering killed adjuvanted vaccines at the same location as modified live vaccines as certain adjuvants may inactivate certain modified live agents.

Administration

- Use a sterile needle and syringe at each injection.
- For a full-sized horse, use a 1.5-inch needle; use a 1-inch needle for miniatures to administer vaccines deep intramuscularly.
- Ensure the needle has not entered a blood vessel before injecting.
- Avoid administering multiple vaccines in the same location.
- To help reduce local injection site reactions, rub the injection site after vaccine administration.
- Do not inject over the croup or gluteal/hip region due to poor gravitational drainage.
- If splitting vaccines, wait 2 to 3 weeks between vaccines to get an effective immune response for the next vaccine.
- Horses should not be vaccinated in the 2 weeks prior to shows, performance events, sales, or domestic shipment.

---

routine oral examination. Studies indicate the rate of dental pathology is higher than what is clinically diagnosed.[19-25] What constitutes a thorough oral examination is detailed elsewhere,[26] but an examination of both soft tissue (lips, tongue, gingiva, mucosa, palate, lymph nodes, and salivary glands) and hard tissue (all bony structures of the head including the bars of the mouth and teeth) will increase the amount of pathology diagnosed by the practitioner. In addition to identifying sharp enamel points and Class 1 malocclusions (waves, hooks, overgrowths, as well as displaced and rotated teeth), an examination can find issues such as soft tissue trauma, periodontal disease, exposed pulp horns, fractured teeth, neoplasia, and other oral pathology.

Routine oral exams and dental care should be major components of a preventative medicine program. Not only do clients now expect this, but evidence confirms oral pathology is often present and has not been addressed. Conducting an oral exam with a speculum and mirror along with correcting routine abnormalities should be the norm in any equine practice. After gaining confidence in what to look for in the mouth and related structures, the veterinarian needs to bring this knowledge to the client. Whenever possible, the practitioner should take the time to show their findings of oral pathology to owners. Pictures or an endoscope linked to a monitor is an excellent way to educate the client as to what pathology needs to be addressed in the horse's mouth.

Several state legislatures and boards of veterinary medicine have dealt with contentious debates regarding who should be allowed to practice equine dentistry. Pathology identified in oral examination requires a diagnosis, treatment, and a plan to proceed. Since diagnosis and treatment fall squarely in the realm of veterinary medicine, veterinarians have an obligation to educate themselves in the basics of a good oral examination and dentistry at various continuing education forums, as well as from colleagues who have chosen to focus their practices on dentistry.

Equipment

While the needs of individual practitioners may vary, equipment needed to perform a good oral exam can include a full mouth speculum, a dental halter or head stand, a bright light source, and a mirror. To better evaluate pathology, a dental explorer, probe, and picks are also helpful.

Different types of speculums are available; a McPherson speculum is one commonly used model. It is usually constructed of stainless steel and opens with a ratchet system. Generally, the more teeth the ratchet has, the easier it is to comfortably open to a wider size and to use in a variety of horses' mouths. Wider bite plates or a bar plate is recommended when working on horses with incisor malocclusions. If a practitioner works on many ponies or miniature horses, a pony speculum is advised. Other, more expensive speculums do not use the ratchet system and offer the ability to fit almost any size equid, allowing the mouth to be easily opened with almost infinite adjustments.

Many practitioners assert that visual examination of the horse's oral cavity is easier when the head is elevated with a head stand or other head support. Using an owner's shoulder as a head support increases risk to the client and liability to the practitioner; horse heads, even when sedated, can cause serious injury, especially when a speculum is added. Head stands have a base that rests on the ground, allowing the practitioner to vary the height of the head; other head supports hang from a rope. Before purchasing either, consider that either system requires some accommodation; head stands require additional room in a vehicle, whereas the hanging halter needs a beam above the working area.

Mirrors and good lighting are imperative to complete a thorough oral examination. Periodontal disease and decay, abrasions to the tongue and cheeks, as well as small fractures are more easily seen, especially in the back of the mouth, with the assistance of these items. A mirror set at 35° to 45° allows for better visualization of the cheek teeth. Additionally, a bright light source, a head lamp or a light that attaches to the bite plate, allows for enhanced visualization of sharp enamel points. A rigid endoscope can be used to more thoroughly examine the entire dental arcade and its associated soft tissue structures.

Other pieces of equipment that can assist the practitioner in performing a thorough oral exam are an explorer, probe, and picks. An explorer allows the practitioner to determine if there are open pulp horns. A probe, which has measurements on it, is used to evaluate the depth and assess the severity of periodontal disease. A variety of picks and long-handled alligator forceps are available to remove feed and determine if a diastema (space between teeth) is causing periodontal disease. These can also be useful when cleaning out periodontal pockets and food from the center of a fractured tooth. Pressurized water, from either an inexpensive garden sprayer or more specialized equipment offered by equine dental companies, can make a big difference in getting these areas thoroughly cleaned for proper examination.

The "workhorse" of any dental practice is the equipment used to reduce enamel points and malocclusions. The choice of system should be considered carefully, since this is the biggest single expense when setting up for dentistry in a practice. Most wet labs allow the practitioner a chance to get a feel for a variety of equipment. Also, take time to speak with other veterinarians already using the equipment.

Hand floats, particularly those designed to address the last upper and lower cheek teeth, as well as short "S" floats to help with sharp edges on canines are recommended additions even if motorized equipment is used. If a practitioner chooses to use only manual floats, additional floats that are designed for incisors, premolars, and molars will need to be purchased. Many of these blades are made to be resharpened or re-gritted.

In the authors' opinion, the use of motorized equipment and diamond gritted burrs has vastly improved the ability to quickly and accurately reduce points and correct malocclusions. The majority of practitioners choose power instruments for their dental work due to the ease, speed, and wide selection of instruments. For example, power tools often have different units, shafts, and grinding wheels that allow access to different parts of the horse's mouth. If the veterinarian works at farms with no access to electricity, some of these units are battery operated.

With any power unit, there is the ability to quickly over reduce a malocclusion and possibly cause pulpal exposure or necrosis. Remaining on one tooth too long will also cause thermal damage to the pulp.[27] By keeping the mouth irrigated, not remaining on any tooth too long, visualizing the procedure, or purchasing a tool that has water-cooling capabilities, these risks can be kept to a minimum. When using motorized instruments, protecting the veterinarian's health is also important. This includes the use of examination gloves, eye protection, a dust-filtering mask, and ear plugs.

Radiography is also an essential part of dentistry as most of the equine tooth is not exposed in the oral cavity. Radiographs are used not only for dental pathology but also for evaluating skeletal structures such as the paranasal sinuses, which have an intimate relationship with the caudal cheek teeth. Intraoral and extraoral radiography is available, and it is recommended that common techniques are learned and practiced. There are several good references available with respect to equipment and the techniques associated with radiography.[28,29]

Extractions

Extracting permanent teeth in horses can be performed by the ambulatory practitioner. Keep in mind that offering intraoral extractions means an added commitment not only in additional equipment but also in further education regarding technique. Proper anesthesia, analgesia, radiography, and extraction technique can be found in multiple sources as well as through continuing education. A thorough knowledge of dental and skull anatomy also needs to be established before performing an extraction since crucial soft tissue structures, such as blood vessels and nerves can be damaged during extraction. If extractions are incorporated into practice, it is extremely important to educate the clientele on possible complications (and how those will be handled) as well as a thorough estimate. There should be a "plan B" in place in case the tooth fractures beneath the gingiva or other scenarios develop. For example, if general anesthesia is necessary (either for a fractious animal or one where a standing intraoral extraction or repulsion is not possible) and the horse needs to be referred, where will this take place? What are the additional costs? All of these questions need to be discussed with the client before the extraction.

Record Keeping

The findings of the oral examination, along with patient signalment, history, and brief physical, need to be recorded. This is most easily done by use of a standard dental record (**Fig. 2**). Dental terminology and abbreviations are established by the Academy of Veterinary Dentistry and the American Veterinary Dental College and can be found in equine dentistry texts.[26,30]

The Modified Triadan Tooth Numbering System, also shown in **Fig. 2**, should be used in oral and written communication pertaining to the equine teeth as a way of standardizing communication amongst peers. Photographs of the oral cavity demonstrating pathology can also be included into records as ways of monitoring changes between exams or documenting pathology before and after treatment.

The ambulatory practitioner should also be sure to point out any dental problems to clients and let them know how they will be addressed. They should also be advised that some dental procedures may need to be performed over a period of time (eg, addressing larger malocclusions on several visits to prevent pulpal exposure from the removal of too much tooth in a single procedure). Other abnormal findings that should be noted include periodontal pockets, asymptomatic slab fractures of a tooth, and feed packing between the teeth. Such findings should be recorded and prompt the practitioner to recommend further evaluation. If more involved care is needed, these cases can be referred to a veterinarian whose focus is dentistry.

It is not hard to imagine how including an oral examination with an annual visit for vaccines will consistently increase revenue. Dentistry can easily comprise 10% to 15% of a practice's revenue, with up to 30% having been reported.[31] Any ambulatory practitioner can add profit and benefit their patients by incorporating a routine oral examination into their yearly wellness protocols.

DEWORMING

Over the past decades, with the availability of deworming products and the pervasive client concern that "worms are bad," deworming has become a practice that is no longer the sole purview of veterinary practitioners. This is not without consequence; in the last 20 years, the literature on anthelmintic resistance has grown exponentially. Documented resistance to all classes of dewormers necessitates changing deworming practices to slow the resistance trend. Research has identified widespread resistance of cyathostomes to all 3 classes of dewormers[32–34]—benzimidazoles (BZ), pyrantel salts (PYR), and macrocyclic lactones (ML)—and of ascarids (*Parascaris equorum*) to ML.[35] The evidence for parasite resistance has been addressed previously[36]; developing a treatment plan is an important part of a wellness program.

Challenging the Dogma

Recently a parasitologist wrote, "The major parasite enemy of horses is no longer a particular species but rather anthelmintic resistance in general."[37] To compensate for decreasing drug efficacies, there has been a paradigm shift from treating gastrointestinal parasites on a rotational basis (every 8 weeks for example) to parasite surveillance and treatment as needed. A more-targeted approach of deworming based on fecal egg counts (FECs) has been proposed and is in use by some equine

EQUINE DENTAL CARE
ANIMAL CARE HOSPITAL, *8565 Hwy 64, Somerville, TN 38068, (901) 466-9224*

Equine Dental Examination/ Treatment Record

Horse:_____ Owner:_____ Barn:_____ Trainer:_____ Date:_____
Breed:_____ Age:_____ Sex:_____ Color/ Markings:_____ RDVM:_____
Use: □ Pleasure □ Breeding □ Retired □ Performance:_____ □ Other:_____
Complaint: □ Routine Dental Care □ Dental Recheck □ _____
History: Last Dental Work (Date/ Dentist):_____ Pasture Graze (hrs/day): □ 18+ □ 12+ □____
Current Medications: □ TMP/SMZ □ Bute _____ Other: _____
□ Wt. Loss □ Dropping Feed □ Abnormal Chewing □ Quidding □_____
Performance Problems: □ Head Tossing □ Head Tilt □ Resisting □_____
Physical Examination: □ Digital Pictures   □ Radiography: UI LI C 100s 200s 300s 400s
Condition: BCS:___/9 □ Underweight □ Normal □ Overweight □ Obese   T=____ P=____ R=____ GI: □ +4
Head: □ Normal □ Abnormal:_____   Feces: □ Not Examined □ Normal □ Large Stems
Poll Sensitivity: □ Normal □ Mild □ Moderate □ Severe **Odor**: □ Normal □ Oral □ Nasal _____
TMJ Sensitivity: □ Normal □ Mild □ Moderate □ Severe **Dissymetry**: L / R Larger_____
Other Findings/ Rads:_____

Sedation: Given IV, (CCs per drug/ Time) & Repeat Sedation.
Sedivet (10mg/ml)   Dormorsedan (10mg/ml) Torbugesic (10mg/ml) Diazapam (5mg/ml)   _____
_____ cc/_____   _____ cc/_____   _____ cc/_____   _____ cc/_____   _____ cc/_____
_____ cc/_____   _____ cc/_____   _____ cc/_____   _____ cc/_____   _____ cc/_____
_____ cc/_____   _____ cc/_____   _____ cc/_____   _____ cc/_____   _____ cc/_____
Reversal Agents: Yohimbine (5mg/ml):___cc/____ Atipamezole (5mg/ml): _____cc/____   □ **Banamine**____cc IV.
Local Anesthetic: Lidocaine 2%: _____ cc @_____, _____cc @_____, _____cc @_____
Oral Examination & Treatments: (All Measurements are in mm.)
Cheeks: □ Normal □ Buccal Laceration / Ulcer _____ □ Callous_____ □_____
Tongue: □ Normal □ Lingual Laceration / Ulcer _____ □ Callous_____ □_____
Palate: □ Normal □ Abnormal:_____   **Lips**: □ Normal □ Abnormal:_____
Gums: □ Normal □ Periodontal Pockets/ Diastemata:_____
Other Findings:_____
% Molar Occlusion: Right: Before____ After : <50 >90   Left: B_____ A: <50 >90
Molar Table Angles: Right: B____ A: 10-15 Degrees_____   Left: B_____ A: 10-15 Degrees_____
RostroCaudal Mobility (mm): B_____ A_____   EMC: (After) R:_____ L:_____
Points: □ Mild □ Moderate □ Severe

Teeth	Exam Findings	Treatment
Incisors		
Canines	□Tartar 1 2 3 4 □ Vestigial 1 2 3 4 □ TI 1 2 3 4 □ Prev. CR/OD	□ Scaled
Wolf		
100 CT		
200 CT		
300 CT		
400 CT		

M3	M2	M1	PM4	PM3	PM2	WT	C	I3	I2	I1	I1	I2	I3	C	WT	PM2	PM3	PM4	M1	M2	M3
										GINGIVA											
111	110	109	108	107	106	105	104	103	102	101	201	202	203	204	205	206	207	208	209	210	211
411	410	409	408	407	406	405	404	403	402	401	301	302	303	304	305	306	307	308	309	310	311
										GINGIVA											

Prescriptions: □ TMP/SMZ 960mg: Give __ pills twice daily for ____ days. □ CHX Soln 0.05% Oral Rinse BID for __ days.
□ _____   □ _____
Recommended Procedures: □ X-rays □ Extractions □ Other_____
Special Instructions: _____
Recheck/ Next Dental Appointment: □ 1 week □ 1 month □ 3 months □ 6 months □ 1 year □ Other _____
Please Call if You have any Questions or Concerns!!!   *Stephen S. Galloway, DVM, FAVD*_____
                              □ DC (emailed:_____) □ CaseLog □ ContSub Log □ Invoice □ Recall

Fig. 2. Sample dental record. (*Courtesy of* Dr Stephen Galloway, Somerville, TN.)

practitioners to decrease the likelihood of resistance.[32,38,39] It is important to remember that horses evolved with intestinal parasites and small numbers of most parasites do not cause significant health problems; instead, they can help stimulate immunity that protects the horse from a more severe worm burden.[37] Both owners and veterinarians need to change their mindset from one where all internal parasites are considered harmful to one where parasites are part of the normal flora of the equine gastrointestinal tract.

The species that are primarily targeted in adult equine deworming strategies include cyathostomins, large strongyles (*S vulgaris* and *Triodontophorus* spp), and tapeworms (*Anoplocephola perfoliata*). Other species such as *Dictyocaulus arnfieldi*, *Habronema* spp, *Draschia* spp, *Onchocerca* spp, and *Oxyuris equi* are thought to be addressed concurrently.[37] Ascarids should be targeted parasites in foals, as they can cause considerable pathology in young horses.

For adult equids, the prevalence of *S vulgaris* has decreased dramatically as a result of common deworming practices. The strongyle egg output of grazing horses consists of almost solely cyathostomes, which makes it the principal parasitic pathogen of adult horses.[40] It should be noted, however, that cyathostomins have a low pathogenicity; therefore, maintaining a modest population of these parasites in horses should be acceptable. The challenge for the ambulatory practitioner is finding the balance of what constitutes acceptable levels of parasitism. Research has documented that in a herd, the majority of cyathostomin populations (about 80%) are in a minority of the host population (20%–30%).[41]

A targeted deworming approach aims at controlling egg shedding in a herd by focusing treatments toward the moderate and high shedders, thereby creating refugia—that is, populations of parasites not exposed to dewormers (eg, parasites on pasture, parasites in untreated low shedders, and encysted cyathostome larvae).[32,37,39,42] Parasites in refugia can dilute the numbers of resistant worms, thereby creating nonresistant progeny and slowing down the propagation of anthelmintic resistant genes. FECs are then used to target treatment toward horses shedding above a predetermined cut-off value. Unfortunately, these cut-offs are recommendations from parasitologists, not evidence based. Recently, it was found that horses with strongyle FECs below 100 to 500 eggs/g (EPG) had significantly smaller worm burdens than horses above this range.[43] While this study was done in a young subset of horses (<2 years), it is the first evidence for using treatment cutoffs in the 0 to 500 EPG range.

FECs can be helpful in determining whether horses are shedding strongyle and ascarid eggs but less useful for determining the size of the worm burden, and they do not reflect the presence of migrating or encysted larvae. FECs show no linear relationship between egg counts and worm counts within the horse,[43] and variability has been identified in individual egg counts.[39] Over time, there is a strong level of repeatability of FEC levels; horses shedding at less than 200 EPG have a strong tendency to stay low at consecutive FECs.[44] FECs also are limited in differentiation of strongyle egg genera and species,[43] and there is poor sensitivity for *A perfoliata* eggs. Despite their challenges, FECs remain the primary method for identifying individuals for treatment.

FECs are most useful to determine the efficacy of anthelmintic treatment and monitoring the herd for resistance. The fecal egg count reduction test (FECRT) is currently the only method available for testing resistance. An FECRT is performed by taking a fecal before and 2 weeks after treatment to calculate the percentage of shedding reduction. If this reduction percentage is lower than a threshold (90% for BZ and PYR; 95% for ML),[41] resistance is likely present. Although a FECRT can identify anthelmintic resistance, a shortening of the egg reappearance period (ERP) can also represent an early warning sign of resistance.

While most anthelmintic resistance research has focused on strongyles and ascarids, *A perfoliata* has also become an important equine parasite as it has been linked with causing certain types of colic.[45] The diagnostic techniques for detection of tapeworm eggs include a modified McMaster and detection of antibodies using a serum enzyme-linked immunosorbent assay (ELISA) technique. The fecal test has low sensitivity, and while the ELISA is thought to be better, it can produce false positive results due to persisting antibodies from natural infection.[46,47] There are no practical methods for detecting resistance in tapeworms, as the persistence of antibodies when using serum ELISA discounts it for this purpose and egg count methods lack sufficient sensitivity to be used for drug efficacy evaluations.[37] Until further research is available, it has been recommended that horses be dewormed with praziquantel or double-dose PYR formulations once yearly.[35]

Developing a Plan

To challenge dogmatic rotational deworming practices, to implement more sustainable approaches, and to reassert the veterinarian's role in managing the horse's health, an effective deworming program needs to consider many different factors. When developing a targeted plan, the location, optimal transmission time of the parasite, and its life cycle should all be considered. Treatment timing and frequency can be impacted by these factors. For example, the time of year or seasonality impacts the transmission and life cycle of cyathostomes[48]; the Northeast has a decreased likelihood of shedding and transmission over the winter, while in the Southeast, it is at its peak. Tapeworm transmission may also display seasonality since the intermediate host is an oribatid mite. While little is known about the mite, it is assumed that it is not transmitting during cold temperatures.

Characteristics of the horse population on the farm, including age, density, and immune system status, should also be taken into account. For example, while small strongyles are the principal parasitic pathogen of adult horses, *P equorum* is considered to be the most important in foals and yearlings. Therefore, deworming practices should be focused on the age of the horses and the life cycle of the parasite to prevent large accumulations of worm burdens. In geriatric equids, a potential correlation was recently found between horses with pituitary pars intermedia dysfunction and increased FECs.[49]

Knowledge of the egg reappearance period of different dewormers and their differing spectra of activity, even within the same parasites' life cycle, can also aid in choosing the most effective anthelmintic. For example, encysted L3 strongyle larvae are not impacted by most dewormers, except by moxidectin and occasionally 5-day double-dose fenbendazole.[50]

While the goal of deworming is to control egg shedding, control of internal parasites should not be addressed by chemical dewormers alone. Manure and pasture management can often decrease the likelihood of transmission. Pasture maintenance including hygiene, harrowing, clipping, plowing, and interspecies grazing can reduce pasture parasite loads.[51,52] Clients often treat their horses without consideration of these factors, and veterinarians have both the obligation and the opportunities to educate clients, improve horse health, and provide a service that is needed.

Practical Application

A recent AAEP presentation describes how to implement a parasite control program in an equine practice based on FECs.[38] In summary, a program based on FECs was introduced to clients through a newsletter, while staff (including veterinarians, veterinary technicians, and veterinary assistants) were simultaneously trained on client communication. The program was well received by their clientele; however, as with any newly developed program, challenges arose. These challenges included training technicians and assistants to perform fecals, reminders for client compliance, and making management changes on those high shedders that require it. In this practice, despite the economic climate, there was a 15% increase in the participation of their modified wellness program over previous years. This example shows how client satisfaction can be achieved through client education and demonstrates that clients are willing to pay for services as long as it is clear how the services will benefit their horses.

Due to the limitations of FECs and anthelmintic resistance, the authors have adopted a compromise to the targeted approach. In this approach, all horses receive 2 anthelmintic treatments per year regardless of FEC, as *S vulgaris* can be managed with twice-yearly strategic treatments of an ML.[41] FECs are then performed 2 or 3 times per year, and the moderate and high shedders are identified and treated additionally as needed. While horses are infected by a variety of species, most gastrointestinal parasites, with the exception of tapeworms, are managed with targeted deworming using the 3 classes available (BZ, PYR, ML). The goal should not be to eliminate the parasites but to keep the parasite populations below the threshold of causing clinical signs.

Unfortunately, the "best" deworming practices remain a bit of an unknown. The amount of refugia needed to delay the development of resistance remains unknown, as well as the consequences of deworming selectively over time. But what is clear is that current deworming practices have led to this resistance crisis and veterinarians and clients need to be reeducated.

SUMMARY

Clients want dependable veterinary care and to understand how the services will benefit and meet their horse's needs. Wellness visits provide ambulatory practitioners with great opportunities to strengthen the doctor-client-patient bond; effective communication with clients during wellness visits, where new literature or facts can be presented, can offer opportunities for demonstrating the value of having the veterinarian maintain a primary role in disease control. The criteria for selecting vaccines, interpreting FECs, and diagnosing dental pathology require the continued need for veterinary involvement. When providing wellness services, veterinarians should discuss those services, the reasons for them, as well as the possibility of adverse reactions. In so doing, the veterinarian is able to clearly distinguish himself or herself from a technician who is merely giving a "shot." Although some of these services can be performed by clients and lay professionals, the knowledge and training that veterinarians bring to these tasks add benefits to the horse beyond the services provided. For example, by targeting treatment and conveying the goals and limitations of FECs and deworming to clients, the speed at which anthelmintic resistance occurs will be diminished, and veterinarians will regain control over equine parasite management. Additional client education, such as demonstrating dental pathology to clients and how veterinary treatment benefits their horse, will not only improve the health of the horse further but also solidify the veterinarian's role in preventative medicine.

While all components of a wellness program were not detailed here, services such as nutritional consultation, blood work, and lameness evaluation should be offered based on the practice's equine population. With the increasing population of geriatric horses, dentistry, nutrition, blood work, and lameness should be assessed annually or biannually. Each practice has its own set of criteria that could be included under the umbrella of "preventative medicine." It is during these times, when the client is most relaxed and not concerned about a serious health problem, that it is easiest to demonstrate the significance of veterinarians in equine wellness care.

ACKNOWLEDGMENTS

The authors would like to thank the following doctors for their advice and expertise in the preparation of this work: Craig Barnett, Ryland Edwards, Martin Nielsen, Ronald Schultz, and Wendy Vaala. Also, a special thanks to Ian Berke, David True, and Karen Luscombe for their help.

REFERENCES

1. Coe JB, Adams CL, Bonnett BN. Prevalence and nature of cost discussions during clinical appointments in companion animal practice. J Am Vet Med Assoc 2009;234: 1418–24.
2. Coe JB, Adams CL, Bonnett BN. A focus group study of veterinarians' and pet owners' perceptions of veterinarian-client communication in companion animal practice. J Am Vet Med Assoc 2008;233:1072–80.
3. Shaw JR, Adams CL, Bonnett BN, et al. Veterinarian-client-patient communication during wellness appointments versus appointments related to a health problem in companion animal practice. J Am Vet Med Assoc 2008;233:1576–86.
4. Barquero N, Gilkerson JR, Newton JR. Evidence-based immunization in horses. Vet Clin North Am Equine Pract 2007;23:481–508.
5. American Association of Equine Practitioners. Vaccination guidelines. Available at: http://www.aaep.org/vaccination_guidelines.htm. Accessed October 23, 2011.
6. Seino KK, Long MT, Gibbs EPJ, et al. Comparative efficacies of three commercially available vaccines against West Nile virus (WNV) in a short-duration challenge trial involving an equine WNV encephalitis model. Clin Vac Immunol 2007;14:1465–71.
7. Daly JM, Newton JR, Mumford JA. Current perspectives on control of equine influenza. Vet Res 2004;35:411–23.
8. Holmes MA, Townsend HG, Kohler AK, et al. Immune responses to commercial equine vaccines against equine herpesvirus-1, equine influenza virus, eastern equine encephalomyelitis, and tetanus. In: Proceedings of the 52th Annual Convention of the American Association of Equine Practitioners. Lexington (KY): The American Association of Equine Practitioners (AAEP); 2006. p. 224–6.
9. Cullinane A, Elton D, Mumford J. Equine influenza: surveillance and control. Influenza Other Respi Viruses 2010;4:339–44.
10. Andersen SA, Petersen HH, Ersbøll AK, et al. Vaccination elicits a prominent acute phase response in horses. Vet J 2012;191:199–202.
11. Mills PC, Auer DE, Kramer H, et al. Effects of inflammation-associated acute-phase response on hepatic and renal indices in the horse. Aust Vet J 1998;76:187–94.
12. Frana TS, Elsken LA, Karli SA. Summary of adverse event reports for veterinary biologic products received by the USDA from 1999 through 2005. J Am Vet Med Assoc 2006;229:1100–2.
13. Waller AS, Jolley KA. Getting a grip on strangles: recent progress towards improved diagnostics and vaccines. Vet J 2007;173:492–501.
14. Borst LB, Patterson SK, Lanka S, et al. Evaluation of a commercially available modified-live Streptococcus equi subsp equi vaccine in ponies. Am J Vet Res 2011;72:1130–8.
15. Sweeney CR, Timoney JF, Newton JR, et al. Streptococcus equi infections in horses: guidelines for treatment, control and prevention of strangles. J Vet Intern Med 2005;19:123–34.
16. Muirhead TL, McClure JT, Wichtel JJ, et al. The effect of age on the immune response of horses to vaccination. J Comp Pathol Suppl 2010;142:S85–90.

17. Spickler AR, Roth JA. Adjuvants in veterinary vaccines: modes of action and adverse effects. J Vet Intern Med 2003;17:273–81.
18. Barnett CD. Adverse events reported followng the use of a commercially available equine vaccine line. Compan Anim Tech Rep 2000;18.
19. Dixon PM, Tremaine WH, Pickles K, et al. Equine dental disease, part 1: a long-term study of 400 cases: disorders of incisor, canine and first premolar teeth. Equine Vet J 1999;31:369–77.
20. Dixon PM, Tremaine WH, Pickles K, et al. Equine dental disease, part 2: a long-term study of 400 cases: disorders of development and eruption and variations in position of the cheek teeth. Equine Vet J 1999;31:519–28.
21. Dixon PM, Tremaine WH, Pickles K, et al. Equine dental disease, part 3: a long-term study of 400 cases: disorders of wear, traumatic damage and idiopathic fractures, tumours and miscellaneous disorders of the cheek teeth. Equine Vet J 2000;32:9–18.
22. Dixon PM, Tremaine WH, Pickles K, et al. Equine dental disease, part 4: a long-term study of 400 cases: apical infections of cheek teeth. Equine Vet J 2000;32:182–94.
23. Dixon PM. The gross histological and ultrastructural anatomy of equine teeth and their relationship to disease. In: Proceedings of the 48th Annual Convention of the American Association of Equine Practitioners. Lexington (KY): The American Association of Equine Practitioners (AAEP); 2002. p. 421–37.
24. du Toit N, Burden FA, Dixon PM. Clinical dental examinations of 357 donkeys in the UK. Part 2: epidemiological studies on the potential relationships between different dental disorders, and between dental disease and systemic disorders. Equine Vet J 2009;41:395–400.
25. van den Enden MSD, Dixon PM. Prevalence of occlusal pulpar exposure in 110 equine cheek teeth with apical infections and idiopathic fractures. Vet J 2008;178:364–71.
26. Easley J, Tremaine W. Dental and oral examination. In: Easley J, Dixon P, Schumacher J, editors. Equine Dentistry. 3rd edition. Edinburgh (UK): Saunders Elsevier; 2010. p. 186–98.
27. Baker G, Allen M. The use of power equipment in equine dentistry. In: Proceedings of the 48th Annual Convention of the American Association of Equine Practitioners. Lexington (KY): The American Association of Equine Practitioners (AAEP); 2002. p. 438–41.
28. Baratt R. Equine dental radiography. In: Proceedings of the American Association of Equine Practitioners Focus on Dentistry. Lexington (KY): The American Association of Equine Practitioners (AAEP); 2011.
29. Barakzai SZ. Dental Imaging. In: Easley J, Dixon P, Schumacher J, editors. Equine Dentistry. 3rd edition. Edinburgh (UK): Saunders Elsevier; 2010. p. 199–221.
30. Tremaine W. Rach D. The business of equine dentistry. In: Easley J, Dixon P, Schumacher J, editors. Equine Dentistry. 3rd edition. Edinburgh (UK): Saunders Elsevier; 2010. p. 43–7.
31. Tremaine W, Rach D. The business of equine dentistry. In: Easley J, Dixon P, Schumacher J, editors. Equine Dentistry. 3rd edition. Edinburgh (UK): Saunders Elsevier; 2010. p. 43–7.
32. Kaplan RM. Anthelmintic resistance in nematodes of horses. Vet Res 2002;33:491–507.
33. Kaplan RM. Drug resistance in nematodes of veterinary importance: a status report. Trends Parasitol 2004;20:477–81.
34. Molento MB, Nielsen MK, Kaplan RM. Resistance to avermectin/milbemycin anthelmintics in equine cyathostomins: current situation. Vet Parasitol October 18, 2011. DOI:10.1016/j.vetpar.2011.10.013.

35. Reinemeyer CR. Anthelmintic resistance in non-strongylid parasites of horses. Vet Parasitol. October 18, 2011. DOI:10.1016/j.vetpar.2011.10.009.
36. Uhlinger CA. Evidence-based parasitology in horses. Vet Clin North Am Equine Pract 2007;23:509–17.
37. Nielsen MK. Sustainable equine parasite control: perspectives and research needs. Vet Parasitol October 18, 2011. DOI:10.1016/j.vetpar.2011.10.012.
38. True CK, Dewitt SF, Dennison LF, et al. How to implement an internal parasite-control program based on fecal egg counts. In: Proceedings of the 56th Annual Convention of the American Association of Equine Practitioners. Lexington (KY): The American Association of Equine Practitioners (AAEP); 2010. p. 258–60.
39. Uhlinger CA. Uses of fecal egg count data in equine practice. Comp Cont Educ Pract Vet 1993;15:742–8.
40. Lyons ET, Tolliver SC, Drudge JH. Historical perspective of cyathostomes: prevalence, treatment and control programs. Vet Parasitol 1999;85:97–111.
41. Kaplan RM, Nielsen MK. An evidence-based approach to equine parasite control: it ain't the 60's anymore. Equine Vet Educ 2010;22:306–16.
42. Stratford CH, McGorum BC, Pickles KJ, et al. An update on cyathostomins: anthelmintic resistance and diagnostic tools. Equine Vet J Suppl 2008;43:133–9.
43. Nielsen MK, Baptiste KE, Tolliver SC, et al. Analysis of multiyear studies in horses in Kentucky to ascertain whether counts of eggs and larvae per gram of feces are reliable indicators of numbers of strongyles and ascarids present. Vet Parasitol 2010;174:77–84.
44. Nielsen MK, Haaning N, Olsen SN. Strongyle egg shedding consistency in horses on farms using selective therapy in Denmark. Vet Parasitol 2006;135:333–5.
45. Proudman CJ, French NP, Trees AJ. Tapeworm infection is a significant risk factor for spasmodic colic and ileal impaction colic in the horse. Equine Vet J 1998;30:194–9.
46. Abbott JB, Barrett EJ. The problem of diagnosing tapeworm infections in horses. Equine Vet J 2008;40:5–6.
47. Abbott JB, Mellor DJ, Barrett EJ, et al. Serological changes observed in horses infected with Anoplocephala perfoliata after treatment with praziquantel and natural reinfection. Vet Rec 2008;162:50–3.
48. Nielsen MK, Kaplan RM, Thamsborg SM, et al. Climatic influences on development and survival of free-living stages of equine strongyles: implications for worm control strategies and managing anthelmintic resistance. Vet J 2007;174:23–32.
49. McFarlane D, Hale GM, Johnson EM, et al. Fecal egg counts after anthelmintic administration to aged horses and horses with pituitary pars intermedia dysfunction. J Am Vet Med Assoc 2010;236:330–4.
50. Reinemeyer CR, Farley A, Clymer B. Comparisons of cyathostome control and selection for benzimidazole resistance using larvicidal regimens of moxidectin gel or fenbendazole paste. Int J Appl Res 2003;1:7–13.
51. Herd RP. Epidemiology and control of parasites in northern temperate regions. Vet Clin North Am Equine Pract 1986;2:337–55.
52. Matthee S, Krecek RC, Milne SA, et al. Impact of management interventions on helminth levels, and body and blood measurements in working donkeys in South Africa. Vet Parasitol 2002;107:103–13.

Prepurchase Examination in Ambulatory Equine Practice

Harry W. Werner, VMD

KEYWORDS

- Prepurchase examination • Liability risk management
- Operational processes • Service mapping
- Standards of care • Client communications

Prepurchase examination can be a valuable service to the equine industry, strengthen client loyalty, foster practice growth, and increase profitability. This article suggests strategies to structure, manage, and perform prepurchase examinations successfully in a pleasure and performance horse ambulatory practice.

Within the equine veterinary profession, a significant number of skilled practitioners choose not to perform prepurchase examinations. Their decision may be influenced by a common perception that difficulties exist linked to offering a prepurchase examination in a general equine practice. Typically, the perceived difficulties are associated with devising ways to manage client expectations, concerns linked to increased liability risk exposure, and confusion about how to achieve timely, effective communications with all parties involved in the service.

Requirements and protocols for performing prepurchase examinations at auction sales and for breeding stallions and mares differ significantly from those associated with pleasure and performance horse disciplines. This chapter addresses only pleasure and performance horse disciplines. Specific elements of the physical examination component of prepurchase examination vary greatly among equine disciplines, intended uses, patient breeds, individual practitioners, etc, and are not discussed here. Detailed technical descriptions of recognized standards of care for prepurchase physical examination are easily found in other sources.

When offering prepurchase examination as a service in equine practice, one must address the following tasks:

- Clearly define the goals for your practice's standards of patient care and client service that are linked to prepurchase examination (**Fig. 1**).

This article was written with practice manager Susan H. Werner, who designed the operational processes and materials associated with prepurchase examination at Werner Equine. The author also wishes to thank valued mentors, Drs Bill Moyer, Midge Leitch, Tom Vaughan, Andy Anderson, Dan Marks, Kent Carter, and Willie McCormick, who influenced this approach to prepurchase examination. Please contact Dr Werner regarding any questions about these materials or processes.
The author has nothing to disclose.
Werner Equine, LLC, 20 Godard Road, North Granby, CT 06060, USA
E-mail address: hwwvmd@wernerequine.com

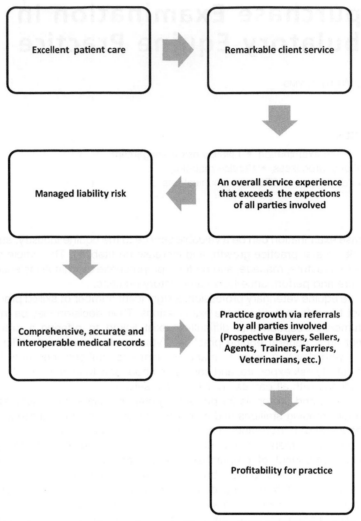

Fig. 1. Prepurchase examination service goals. (Copyright 2001–2012 Werner Equine, LLC. All rights reserved.)

- Ensure that the examining veterinarian has thorough knowledge of the equine discipline in which the patient will be involved (ie, intended use).
- Understand your market and client base; that is, know what your clients expect regarding this service.
- Map out each point of practice interaction with the primary parties involved in the prepurchase examination process (**Figs. 2–6**).
- Structure the operational processes you will use to deliver the service. Consider the client's perspective, the roles and perspectives of each staff member, and the tools you have at your disposal. Gather and document information pertinent to the examination from all parties involved.
- Perform a high-quality physical examination and ancillary studies.

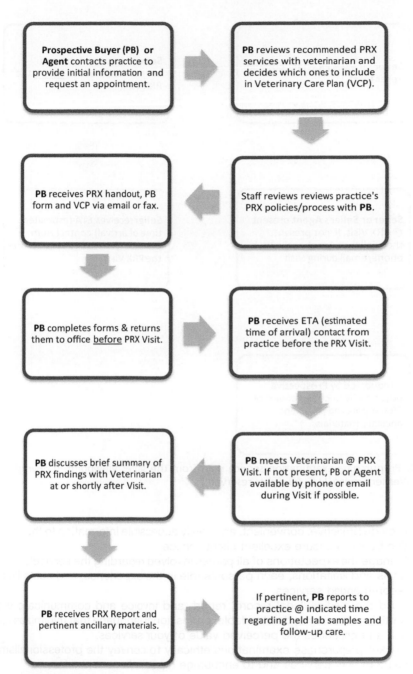

Fig. 2. Prepurchase examination service map from the prospective buyer (PB) viewpoint. (Copyright 2001–2012 Werner Equine, LLC. All rights reserved.)

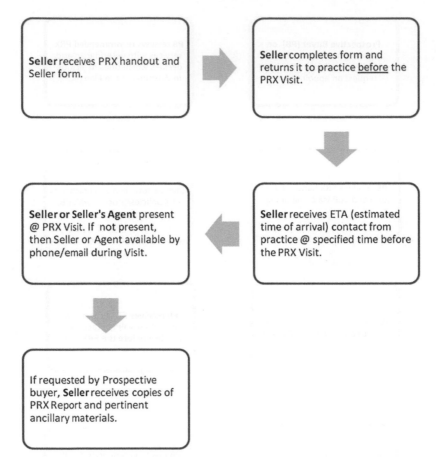

Fig. 3. Prepurchase examination service map from the seller viewpoint. (Copyright 2001–2012 Werner Equine, LLC. All rights reserved.)

- Provide proactive, convenient, and easily accessible information to the prospective buyer to ensure excellent client service.
- Manage the expectations of all parties involved regarding the service's value, its goals and limitations, each person's role in the experience, and costs linked to recommended services.
- Build the medical/legal record, report, and invoice and communicate with all participants using understandable, professional language that minimizes liability risk and enhances the perceived value of your services.
- Market prepurchase examinations ethically to convey the professionalism and value of your services and to encourage repeat client contacts.

In equine practice, one management strategy "does not fit all." As such, this article should be thought of an information template that can be adapted for use in individual practices.

HISTORY

Archeological evidence dates domestication of equines as early as 4000 BC in what we know today as Ukraine.[1] As equines were domesticated to meet specific and

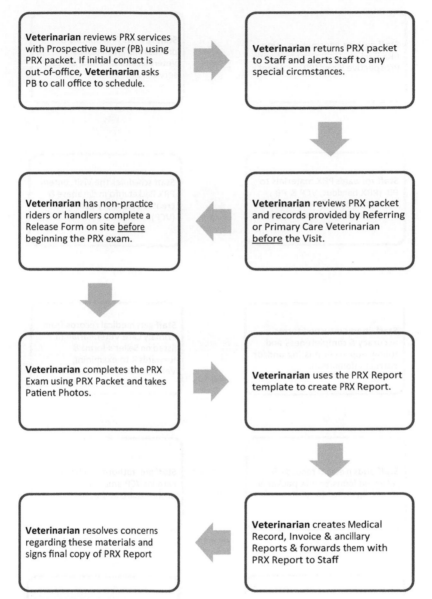

Fig. 4. Prepurchase examination service map from the veterinarian viewpoint. (Copyright 2001–2012 Werner Equine, LLC. All rights reserved.)

diverse needs (eg, draught, riding, battle, power vs speed, etc), transfer of ownership occurred and the concept of "intended use" emerged as the general directive for the prospective buyer. In 1868, English veterinary surgeon William Youatt suggested: "The buyer can discern, or ought to know, whether the form of the horse is that which will render him likely to suit his purpose . . . ."[2]

The veterinary profession did not truly come into its own until the late 18th century. Advisors (or examiners) for many horse acquisitions included farriers, farmers, and

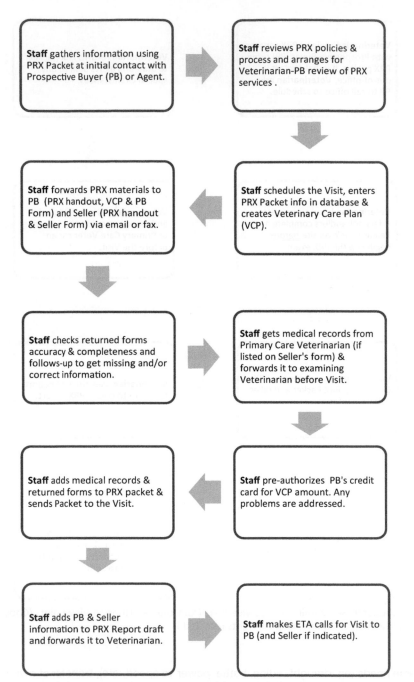

Fig. 5. Prepurchase examination service map from the staff viewpoint, part 1(Copyright 2001–2012 Werner Equine, LLC. All rights reserved.)

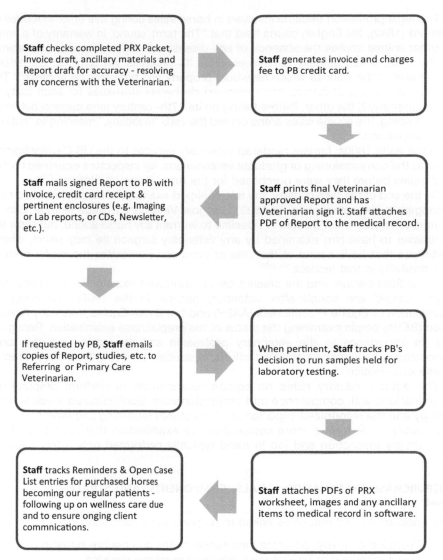

Staff checks completed PRX Packet, Invoice draft, ancillary materials and Report draft for accuracy - resolving any concerns with the Veterinarian.

Staff generates invoice and charges fee to PB credit card.

Staff mails signed Report to PB with invoice, credit card receipt & pertinent enclosures (e.g. Imaging or Lab reports, or CDs, Newsletter, etc.).

Staff prints final Veterinarian approved Report and has Veterinarian sign it. Staff attaches PDF of Report to the medical record.

If requested by PB, Staff emails copies of Report, studies, etc. to Referring or Primary Care Veterinarian.

When pertinent, Staff tracks PB's decision to run samples held for laboratory testing.

Staff tracks Reminders & Open Case List entries for purchased horses becoming our regular patients - following up on wellness care due and to ensure onging client commnications.

Staff attaches PDFs of PRX worksheet, images and any ancillary items to medical record in software.

Fig. 6. Prepurchase examination service map from the staff viewpoint, part 2. (Copyright 2001–2012 Werner Equine, LLC. All rights reserved.)

others. For example, Ireland's Travelers have long been known for their involvement in horse sales and as expert judges of horse flesh. They often serve at fairs and sales as "tanglers" (ie, individuals who mediate between a prospective buyer and seller until a deal is reached, usually for a fee ["luck money"]).[3]

As formal 19th-century veterinary education and practice focused directly on the horse, the value of a veterinarian's perspective regarding a horse for sale was increasingly recognized. It was believed that "there are few sources of greater annoyance, both to the buyer and the seller of the horse, than disputes with regard to the soundness of the animal . . . ."[4] Hence, the equine practitioner's opinion was sought to resolve, if not preclude, such disputes.

The legal profession became involved in horse sales during this time. In *Kiddell vs Burnard* (1842), the English courts held that "The term 'sound' in warranty of a horse or other animal implies the absence of any disease or seed of disease in the animal at the time, which actually diminishes or in its progress will diminish his natural usefulness in the work to which he would properly and ordinarily be applied."[5] The buying and selling of horses often involved deliberate strategies for each party to outwit (defraud?) the other. Before taking on its 17th- century (and current) definition of race riding, the equine sales arena coined the verb "to jockey," meaning to "out do" the competition.[6]

In the early 1800s, farriers rendered veterinary services to the US Cavalry horses. Prior to the commissioning of graduate veterinarians, lay inspectors examined horses and mules before they were purchased for the Army Remount Stations.[7,8]

By the end of the 19th century, the role of expert examiner of horses for sale clearly belonged to the veterinarian. In 1893, Glasgow Veterinary College lecturer George Armatage wrote: "most dealers . . . decline to warrant any horse sound, but allow the purchaser to have him examined by any veterinary surgeon he may select, whose certificate that he is sound at the time of purchase exonerates the dealer from all responsibility in that respect."[9,p43]

In the 20th century and the present day, prepurchase examination has become a highly valued and sought-after veterinary service. In the 1960s, the American Association of Equine Practitioners (AAEP) and the British Equine Veterinary Association (BEVA) began examining the status of the prepurchase examination. Recognizing its importance to the veterinary profession and the equine industry, both associations have made significant efforts to educate their members about prepurchase examination.

The equine industry relies on equine veterinarians to perform prepurchase examinations with competence and professionalism. Sophisticated medical technology and the recognized importance of structured recording and reporting make it possible to perform a more comprehensive examination that is a far cry from the cursory inspection and jog in hand typically performed only a few decades ago.

PREPURCHASE EXAMINATION: GOALS, COMPONENTS, AND STRATEGIES
Goals

The goals or desired outcomes linked to prepurchase examination include:

- Provision of timely, accurate information to the prospective buyer in a professional manner that facilitates an informed purchase decision
- Generation of positive perceived value of the prepurchase examination services for all parties involved
- Reduction of liability risk exposure
- Creation of comprehensive, accurate, and interoperational medical records
- Encouragement of repeat client contact that stimulates practice growth and profitability.

Components

Like all professional veterinary services, prepurchase examinations have 2 interdependent components: *patient care* and *client service.*

Standards of patient care include history, general observations, physical examination, and associated ancillary diagnostics. Physical examination elements and diagnostics vary with each case since they reflect the veterinarian's recommendations of care for a specific horse and the prospective buyer's choices of what services to include or exclude. Factors such as costs and timely reporting of examination and ancillary diagnostic findings can also affect what services the prospective buyer chooses to include in prepurchase examination.

Standards of client service involve every interaction the practice has with all parties involved in the prepurchase examination process: prospective buyer, seller, designated agents for those parties, other veterinarians, and nonemployees, such as drivers, riders, handlers, farriers, etc. How and when the practice interacts with each party involved have ramifications for the overall experience.

Strategies

Once the practice defines standards of patient care and client service for prepurchase examination, it must then define the strategies used to market, price, document, communicate about, and effectively deliver those services to all parties involved. Remaining sensitive to changes in your client and patient base and in the general equine industry is critical to offering a service that is perceived as valuable and fair in your marketplace. The manner in which a practice handles the expectations of all parties involved in prepurchase examination is critical to a successful outcome.

STRATEGIES: CLIENT SERVICE
Managing Expectations: The Prospective Buyer

What do the prospective buyer and/or agent expect of the prepurchase examination experience? Typically, they want information about the horse that can help them make an informed purchasing decision. They expect a competent, thorough examination. They want timely communications that they can easily understand before, during, and after the examination process. Most want to know if the horse they are considering is suitable for their intended use(s). These expectations determine which services the veterinarian recommends be included in the overall examination, how the services are executed, and how findings are reported.

Intended use may not always be the prospective buyer's only concern. In recent years, many prospective buyers lack in-depth equine experience and may not grasp the limitations of a prepurchase examination. Many of them are not familiar with the realities of horse ownership and the sometimes fragile nature of equine health. In 1893, Glasgow Veterinary College lecturer George Armatage wrote: "And first, I must caution all purchasers against a very common fault – that of wanting and expecting to find perfection in any horse: there is no such thing either in man or horse; all that can be done is to select one as nearly as possible approaching the standard required."[9,p42]

Here are some examples of expressed concerns and expectations reported by prospective buyers; such comments require a response by the equine practitioner:

- **"Safety is my paramount concern."** Any activity on or around horses carries inherent risk. Regardless of how placid the horse may be during examination, no assurance of future safety should ever be made or implied. In fact, the veterinarian's medical record and report should include the prospective buyer's stated concern and the examining veterinarian's response. If the horse is sedated during the course of the examination, the prepurchase examination report should state why the sedation was used (eg, to facilitate radiography, etc) in order to avoid any future misinterpretation that the horse was dangerous to handle if unsedated.

- **"This is an investment horse; I plan to resell it for a profit after my child leaves for college."** The prepurchase examination should be properly structured, executed, and reported without any consideration of current or future value.
- **"I am not interested in her current reproductive status."** Many prospective buyers of performance and pleasure mares give no thought to the horse's reproductive status. To avoid their unwitting acquisition of a pregnant mare, one should raise the possibility of pregnancy with the seller, record the seller's response, and suggest that the prospective buyer include an examination for pregnancy in the standard of care. Always document the prospective buyer's response to this discussion in the medical record and the prepurchase examination report.
- **"I need assurance that this horse will compete successfully over four foot fences."** The prepurchase examination is not intended to evaluate athletic ability.

A practice's failure to understand and address the prospective buyer's expectations and concerns can result in a disgruntled client. To achieve a better outcome (ie, a satisfied client who recommends your practice to others), a practice must provide timely, proactive communications. The practice must deliver a consistent message that helps all parties understand the purpose, limitations, advantages, costs, and scope of prepurchase examination.

Conflicts of Interest

For many years, it has been an axiom that a veterinarian should refuse to perform the prepurchase examination if the seller is an existing client. This recommendation attempts to avoid conflict of interest: perceived, if not real conflict. While this axiom appears reasonable, the realities of the equine marketplace are not so tidy. In the author's opinion, this recommendation can ethically be ignored in 2 instances:

1. A prospective buyer may have great faith in and respect for the veterinarian, considering her/him to be the individual most qualified to deliver the service regardless of any relationship with the seller.
2. The veterinarian may have thorough and current knowledge of the horse's medical status, thereby being in a stronger position to fully inform the prospective buyer.

In each instance, full disclosure of any relevant relationship between the examining veterinarian and the seller must be made to the prospective buyer prior to agreeing to examine the horse. This conversation should be documented in the medical record. Additionally, the seller must grant the examining veterinarian the right to disclose the horse's full medical record to the prospective buyer. Providing only an à la carte medical record that excludes certain items is unethical and unacceptable.

However, under any circumstances, if a veterinarian has any financial interest in the horse to be examined, he/she should decline to perform the prepurchase examination.

Managing Expectations: The Seller

The veterinarian–client relationship in prepurchase examination is between the examining veterinarian and the prospective buyer. However, it is important for the examining veterinarian to gain the goodwill and cooperation of the seller and/or agent. This process begins with thorough, accurate, and timely communication between the veterinarian and seller to:

- Agree on the specific date, time, and location of the examination
- Obtain a seller-signed statement of the horse's history

- Secure the seller's written permission for the examination and for the following services
  - Sedation
  - Clipping
  - Pulling of shoes
  - Blood collection
  - Pupil dilation
  - Administration of diuretic for drug testing
- Agree on who will handle the horse on the ground and who will ride or drive the horse.

The practice should insist that any handler, rider or driver of the horse be a practice employee, the seller, or the seller's employee. Any handler, rider, or driver of the horse who is not a practice employee should sign a liability release prior to handling the horse. For optimal liability risk management, one should require that any handler, rider, or driver of the horse be 18 years of age or older.

If the seller refuses to cooperate with the veterinarian's reasonable requests and/or gives the veterinarian significant reason to doubt the seller's integrity, the examining veterinarian should consider declining to perform the examination.

STRATEGIES: STANDARD OF PATIENT CARE

The prepurchase examination should be customized to fit the needs and expectations of the prospective buyer. This approach assumes that those needs and expectations are reasonable and that the examining veterinarian has the knowledge, experience, and clinical tools to accomplish the task.

Intended Use

The prospective buyer's expressed intended use of the horse directly influences which examination elements the examining veterinarian recommends, his/her interpretation of examination findings, and which services the client will be willing to pay. For example, upper airway endoscopy may not necessarily be recommended for a horse intended for weekend pleasure trail riding if the horse does not display abnormal respiratory noise during the examination. However, upper airway endoscopy may be appropriate for a horse intended to compete as a hunter under United States Equestrian Federation rules, as these rules allow for dismissal from the show ring of any horse making an abnormal respiratory noise.

The intended use of a horse often determines the significance of an abnormality detected during the clinical examination. For example, in team roping, total blindness in the left eye of the header is usually insignificant. However, in the heeler, such a finding would be career-ending. For safety reasons—real or perceived—partial blindness often causes parents seeking a mount for a child rider to reject a sales horse, even if the horse is otherwise acceptable to them.

To recommend an individualized standard of patient care, the examining practitioner must possess a thorough knowledge of the expressed intended use for any given horse presented for prepurchase examination. The veterinarian must also have access to diagnostic technology (radiology, endoscopy, etc) necessary to successfully perform the prescribed examination. Absent such knowledge and/or diagnostic capability, one should refer the prospective buyer to an examiner who is familiar with the proposed use and suitably equipped to perform the examination.

Physical Examination

Dr Abraham Verghese, a noted physician and author, asserts that: "a proper examination . . . earns the patient's trust . . . and serves as a ritual that transforms two strangers into a doctor and patient."[10] This comment on the transformative value of physical examination holds true in veterinary medicine regarding relationship building between clients and veterinarians. Physical examination is the key skill linked to almost every professional service we offer as doctors.

In prepurchase examination, the physical examination is typically detailed by body system. Findings and information generated on-site should be recorded on customized prepurchase examination worksheets to document every action by the veterinarian and other parties at the visit. In the author's practice, the prepurchase examination packet is printed on various colors of paper keyed to the item's use: white for in-house use, blue for paperwork completed at the visit, etc. The packet is also available for use as a pdf document to use on a laptop or tablet.

While this article does not itemize specific elements of physical examination for prepurchase examination, some general comments and strategies are appropriate:

- **Previsit forms:** The physical examination should not begin until all administrative documents are completed and in the possession of the examining veterinarian or his/her office.
- **Examination format:** Introduce the desired examination format prior to beginning the examination. Give a brief introduction of what is intended to be accomplished and certain simple ground rules to all attendees. By doing so prior to beginning the examination, the examining veterinarian can usually prevent circumstances developing which might otherwise compromise confidentiality or safety.
- **Safety:** The safety of the horse and all attendants is of paramount importance. The prepurchase examination venue has a tendency to attract onlookers, such as family members, unaffiliated boarders, other animals, etc. They can distract the horse, the handler, and the examiner. It is the veterinarian's responsibility to establish and maintain order.
- **Refusal to examine:** When environmental conditions preclude a meaningful and safe examination, one should refuse to examine the horse.
- **Geldings and stallions:** While most geldings or stallions will prolapse the penis to urinate at some time during the examination, some may not. Always advise the prospective buyer and seller that the penis must be visually inspected to ascertain that it is normal; they should be advised that sedation will be required to do so. Lesions such as melanoma, papilloma, and squamous cell carcinoma, especially in their early stages, can easily escape detection if the penis is palpated through the sheath.
- **Be discreet:** The examining veterinarian is working for the prospective buyer. All communications regarding examination findings, interpretations, concerns, and opinions are the proprietary property of the prospective buyer and the practice. Such information should not be shared without the prospective buyer's knowledge and written consent. All practice employees must understand that any aspect of the examination that they witness or hear is to be kept strictly confidential. Secure a written release from the prospective buyer to provide such information to additional parties.

  When the prospective buyer chooses not to purchase the horse, the seller often requests access to the examination report. While this request is understandable, it should not be granted by the veterinarian without the written permission of the prospective buyer.

Ancillary Services

- **Sedation:** Some ancillary services require sedation to achieve best results or to ensure the safety of the horse and/or human(s). In all cases, sedation should only be administered with the written permission of the seller. Additionally, always obtain blood samples to be submitted for drug testing before you sedate the horse.
- **Shoe removal:** While shoe removal is often required for proper radiographic imaging and examination of the foot, the seller should agree in writing to pulling of shoes. If indicated, the hoofs can be taped after the examination for protection until the shoes can be reset. If foot films are taken and shoes are not pulled, the record and report should state why the shoes were not pulled and note if the quality of the radiographic studied was compromised as a result.
- **Hair clipping:** Clipping may be indicated for ultrasonographic imaging or for close inspection of suspected surgical scars. Written consent to clip should be obtained from the seller.
- **Pupil dilation:** Secure permission from the seller to perform pupil dilation to facilitate ophthalmic examination.
- **Administration of diuretic:** Some veterinarians may administer a diuretic when needed to facilitate urine collection for drug testing. Written consent to do so should be obtained from the seller.
- **Upper airway endoscopy:** Even if a horse makes no abnormal respiratory noise during the motion segment of physical examination, upper airway endoscopy should be recommended whenever the respiratory demand in training or competition is significant (combined training, stadium jumping, carriage driving, etc). The author also recommends upper airway endoscopy when intended use includes showing as a hunter under United States Equestrian Federation regulations.
- **Immunoassays:** In some areas of the country, prospective buyers commonly request that blood be submitted for a *Borrelia* profile as part of the prepurchase examination. In such areas, the veterinarian should advise the prospective buyer that, given the very high percentage of clinically normal horses carrying measurable antibodies against *Borrelia*, they should consider the result as a reference rather than requiring a negative test as an absolute criterion for purchase.
- **Unrelated services at the time of examination:** Prospective buyers frequently ask the veterinarian to perform services at the prepurchase examination visit that are unrelated to the prepurchase examination. In the author's practice, these services are limited to preparation of an interstate health certificate, completion of an insurance examination form, immunizations required for the horse to gain entry to its destination facility, and any laboratory work necessary for interstate or foreign transport. Requests for "routine" immunizations, deworming, and dental care are referred to the prospective buyer's primary care veterinarian for 1 reasons: (1) any adverse reaction or consequence of such treatment can easily complicate or jeopardize completion of the sale and (2) such services provide an opportunity for the primary care veterinarian to meet the horse and begin its wellness care regimen.

PREPURCHASE EXAMINATION STRATEGIES: OPERATIONAL PROCESS

Once a practice defines its standards of patient care and client service for any service, it must then define the operational process that will most effectively deliver that service to all parties involved. Considering tools, people, and workflow—with input from veterinarians and staff—a system to deliver the service (ie, value) to the client can be designed. Operational processes are dynamic. They evolve as new standards of care, tools, skills, and strategies become available. As business writer Michael Port aptly notes, a "documented system can help you stay competitive, improve production, control costs and respond to the customer's changing needs."[11] Every point of interaction between the practice and all parties involved should be mapped. Each person's viewpoint should be considered. The goal should be to design a fluid process that can be adjusted as needed.

In the author's practice, forms and other communication tools and technologies in the prepurchase examination process were created using ideas suggested by processes used in the airline industry and human medicine. Pilot and human hospital surgical error prevention checklists[12] influenced the checklist coversheet on the prepurchase examination packet. The checklist and packet also reflect what was learned by mapping the service through each participant's lens. The checklist details each person's responsibilities to ensure that each requirement is met (**Appendix 1**). The packet includes examination on-site worksheets, the rider/handler release form, completed prospective buyer and seller agreements, and ancillary materials provided to the examining veterinarian (see **Appendix 1**).

Initially, when mapping out the prepurchase examination service, the author focused only on services performed at the patient visit. Recognizing the importance of previsit and postvisit communications and tasks, the operational process and packet were updated to reflect each participant's role *before, at, and after* the visit (**Fig. 7**). When possible, tasks were delegated to staff members to improve efficiency and to free the veterinarian to focus on patient care and direct client communications. The packet and most materials are templates in Microsoft Word (Redmond, Washington, USA) or Adobe Acrobat (San Jose, California, USA); they are easy to use and evolve to meet changing needs.

PREVISIT TASKS
Marketing

A practice's website, brochures, newsletters, handouts (**Appendix 2**), and other marketing communications should reflect a consistent message using language and images that clients can easily understand. These tools should be simple to use; provide basic information about the practice (not fees) and encourage clients to contact the practice directly. As noted by 2011 AAEP Convention keynote speaker Dennis Snow, "Direct, one-to-one contact between people (ie, between the client and a veterinarian or staff member) remains the best opportunity for a practice to deliver value and service."[13]

Initial Direct Contact with the Practice

Leveraging the skills of your trained support staff and maintaining a consistent message in every client interaction are critical to the success of any service in your practice, especially prepurchase examinations. Staff includes technicians, assistants, receptionists, managers, or whoever comes into contact with clients.

The first direct interaction with your practice linked to prepurchase examination is usually between a prospective buyer (or designated agent) and a staff member. The quality of that first interaction sets the tone for the client's overall experience. At this time, the staff should briefly review the practice's policy and process regarding prepurchase examination with the client. Using predesigned packets, they can gather preliminary information about the prospective buyer, the horse, and the seller, in

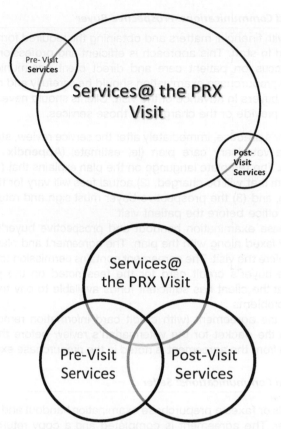

Fig. 7. Prepurchase examination service focus: old and new business models. (Copyright 2001–2012 Werner Equine, LLC. All rights reserved.)

addition to the desired appointment date, time, and location. Staff can arrange for the client to discuss the menu of prepurchase examination services with the examining veterinarian. Ideally, if the veterinarian is away from the office, staff can e-mail or text preliminary information to the veterinarian, who can then contact the prospective buyer directly. Responding to the prospective buyer in a timely manner throughout the process is important to a successful outcome of a prepurchase examination.

Veterinarian–Prospective Buyer Review of Services

After reviewing the horse's signalment and expressed intended use with the prospective buyer, the veterinarian should record any additional information, such as the prospective buyer's degree of familiarity with the horse, the intended use, and any specific concerns. Disclosed conflicts of interest and any obvious impediments to proceeding with the examination should be discussed. The veterinarian recommends his or her detailed standard of care for the specific horse; associated fees are reviewed. The prospective buyer ultimately indicates which services are to be included in the overall examination, and the veterinarian should note which services may have been declined. All information, including services that were declined by the prospective buyer, should be recorded on the packet. Ideally, support staff then confirms the appointment and reviews financial issues.

Previsit Tasks and Communications: Prospective Buyer

Ideally, dealing with financial matters and obtaining the required forms are tasks that can be delegated to staff. This approach is efficient and professional and frees the veterinarian to focus on patient care and direct client communication. Financial policies linked to prepurchase examination should be carefully and clearly discussed with prospective buyers in advance of the visit. Clients should never be surprised by the services you provide or the charges for those services.

- In the author's practice, immediately after the service review, staff uses software to create a veterinary care plan (ie, estimate) (**Appendix 3**) using packet information. The template language on the plan explains that (1) fees noted are the minimum that will be charged; (2) actual fees will vary for the reasons listed on the plan, and (3) the prospective buyer must sign and return a copy of the plan to the office before the patient visit.
- A prepurchase examination handout and prospective buyer's agreement are e-mailed or faxed along with the plan. The agreement and plan are signed and returned before the visit. The agreement contains permission to preauthorize the prospective buyer's credit card for the fees noted on the plan. This policy ensures that the client has sufficient funds available to pay the bill and avoids collection problems.
- Staff adds the agreement (with credit card information removed for security reasons) to the packet for the veterinarian's review before the visit. Pertinent information from the agreement is noted in the prepurchase examination report.

Previsit Tasks and Communications: Seller

- Staff e-mails or faxes a prepurchase examination handout and seller agreement to the seller. The agreement is completed and a copy returned to the office before the patient visit.
- If the seller lists a veterinarian in the history and gives permission to contact that practice, staff asks the practice to forward a medical history before the visit. Such communications are made via e-mail using template forms.
- Staff includes the agreement in the packet for the veterinarian's review before the visit. pertinent information from the agreement is noted in the prepurchase examination report.

In rare circumstances, a previously well-known prospective buyer, seller, or their agents are not able to return the required forms by fax or e-mail. In these situations, the forms may be accepted at the visit before the examination begins.

Visit Day Tasks and Communications

- Staff provides the prospective buyer and seller with an estimated time of arrival communication via phone, e-mail, or text.
- The veterinarian uses the packet to record examination details, findings, and all interactions with involved parties at the visit.
- After introductions of all relevant personnel, all forms providing permission to proceed and liability releases are completed and retained by the veterinarian.
- Relevant data (eg, laboratory test results, registration papers, etc) provided by the seller are added to the packet.

- As the examination proceeds, findings are detailed on the packet worksheet (**Appendix 4**). If height is measured, a disclaimer is included in the report stating that the measurement is unofficial for competition purposes.
- Abnormal findings are brought to the attention of the prospective buyer; advice is rendered as to their potential significance.
- If expert opinions or advanced diagnostics are indicated, referral of cases to specialists is recommended.
- After completing the physical examination, digital photographs are taken of the horse. These photographs document physical appearance and certain examination findings. The photos provide added value to the prepurchase examination report and are especially appreciated by prospective buyers when a decision is made not to purchase the horse.
- The veterinarian discusses the examination findings to date with the prospective buyer in person or by phone. All comments, questions or concerns made by either party are recorded in the packet. Regardless of cause, any element of the veterinarian's recommended standard of care for the horse's examination that either the prospective buyer declines to have performed, is not permitted by the seller, or is not possible to perform for any reason, must be clearly identified in the medical record, in the packet, as well as in prepurchase examination report.
- Ancillary studies scheduled by prearrangement at the initial services review or recommended on-site are agreed upon and completed. The author's practice advises prospective buyers that interpretation of diagnostic images on-site is "unofficial," pending a second interpretation performed in a quiet environment with no distraction.
- It is not advisable to "pass or fail" the horse. Instead, the practitioner should provide the prospective buyer with a clear explanation of all significant findings, as well as an opinion as to how each may, or may not, possibly impact the intended use. The written report to the prospective buyer should state that the practitioner's opinion is not a directive to purchase—or not purchase—the horse. For this reason, in the prepurchase examination report, the overall service performed is described simply as a "physical examination."
- At the end of the visit, the prospective buyer should be told when outstanding laboratory results will be available, Further, they should be informed that a detailed written report of all procedures and findings, patient photographs, a CD of any radiographic or ultrasonographic image studies performed at the visit, and a copy of the paid invoice will be mailed to them.
- If the prospective buyer requested that a blood sample be drawn and held for future submission for drug screen testing, the report should specify a date when they must notify the practice regarding their decision to have the laboratory testing performed.
- Errors made when entering information in medical records: The author's practice follows the liability risk reduction recommendations made by Gregg Scoggins, DVM, JD, in his presentation at the 2005 AAEP Convention: "correct errors by drawing a single line through the erroneous entry, designating the entry as an 'error', dating the correction and initialing the entry."[14]

Postexamination Tasks and Communications

- Using a document template, the veterinarian completes the prepurchase examination report.

- The veterinarian submits the completed packet and all ancillary materials (uploaded report draft, invoice and patient photographs, imaging study CDs, etc) to the office manager.
- The office manager reviews all materials for accuracy, consistency of content, completeness, and clarity from the client's perspective. The invoice is compared to the veterinary care plan (estimate) for accuracy. Any discrepancies are reviewed with the veterinarian. The veterinarian approves and signs the final copy of the report; see example (**Appendix 5**).
- If the prospective buyer has requested it, a copy of the report and images can be forwarded to the primary care veterinarian.

Reducing Liability Risk Associated with Prepurchase Examination

In "A Review of Equine Malpractice Claims, Dennis Meagher, DVM, MS, PhD, Diplomate American College of Veterinary Surgeons, states that" claims associated with purchase examinations have been one of the most common types of claims presented to the [American Veterinary Medical Association Professional Liability Insurance Trust]." Dr Meagher suggests that "liability related to purchase examination can be reduced by complete medical records and a detailed . . . report."[15]

Dr Meagher's presentation at the 2005 AAEP convention includes valuable steps one can take to reduce liability risk in equine practice. His advice influenced many of the tools, forms, and processes mentioned in this article. Proactive preparation and communications reduce liability risk and help manage client expectations.

- Support staff must have a thorough understanding of the purpose, process, and value of the prepurchase examination. They have to understand the "why" of each task and its implications for patient care for client service and the benefits it brings to the practice.
- Ongoing training and scripted responses to frequently asked questions can give your staff confidence. A consistent message reassures clients and can prevent confusion. Many of the best ideas for scripts come directly from staff. Terms used in all communications should be accurate and appropriate. For example, referring to the client as the "prospective buyer" reinforces the concept in the client's mind that prepurchase examination involves a potential purchase; it is not a recommendation to buy or not to buy.
- Clients appreciate speaking directly with the veterinarian before the prepurchase examination visit. This opportunity allows clients to voice their concerns; it enables the veterinarian to educate and recommend an appropriate standard of patient care.
- Creating standardized processes for gathering information, examining the horse, communicating with all parties before, during, and after the visit, and delivering a comprehensive report[16,17] can make the overall prepurchase examinations service a manageable, efficient—and pleasant—experience for everyone involved.

Finally, there are additional steps one can take to deliver value-laden prepurchase examinations:

- Invest in continuing education to perform the best prepurchase examination possible.
- Attend equestrian competitions to enhance your understanding of specific intended use.
- Listen carefully to the prospective buyer's concerns and expectations (wants, needs, and wishes); work with them to recommend an appropriate standard of patient care.

- Convey a consistent, ethical, and understandable message regarding prepurchase examination in every instance and type of interaction with everyone involved in the service. Language counts; it must be professional, easily understood, and consistent throughout all communications to deliver value, educate, and minimize liability risk. Medical records should use accepted terminology that is interoperable among practices.
- Ensure that all forms and financial matters are handled respectfully, professionally, and with confidentiality.
- Insist on proactive, timely communications.
- Provide the seller and prospective buyer with an estimated-time-of-arrival call prior to the visit.
- Perform a detailed examination that is documented accurately and completely.
- Offer to draw and hold drug screen samples for processing in the near future if needed.
- Include patient photographs in the report.
- If the prospective buyer cannot be present at the visit, arrange to speak to them by phone during the examination (if needed) and at its conclusion.
- Deliver an understandable, complete report that is professional in appearance and language.
- Provide copies of the report, imaging studies, etc to the prospective buyer and designated parties.
- Remind the prospective buyer to provide insurance examination forms to the veterinarian for completion in a timely manner.

SUMMARY

Prepurchase examination provides a significant opportunity for veterinarians to offer an important professional service to the equine industry. When the service is performed competently and ethically, prospective buyers and sellers will recommend the examining veterinarian to fellow horse owners and professionals.

To become comfortable with and skilled at performing prepurchase examinations, a veterinarian must understand the operational challenges associated with this service—and master them. Veterinarians performing prepurchase examinations should address the needs and manage the expectations of the prospective buyer, treat the seller and all parties with professional courtesy, be familiar with the intended use of the horse, competently perform a thorough physical examination, and pay close attention to the medical record and report. Communicate clearly with all parties before, during, and after the examination.

Feedback from staff and colleagues is critical to improving and refining the services offered. The veterinarian should work with staff to evaluate the processes used to deliver the prepurchase examination experience to clients and consult with mentors who are skilled in performing these services. Sharing your ideas for improving prepurchase examination with equine colleagues is a service to the veterinary profession and to the horse.

Performing a prepurchase examination in the way described may sound like a "tall order," but once patient care and service goals have been established, staff has been trained, and the process has been defined—the challenges become opportunities. The rewards include satisfied clients, reduced liability risk, increased profitability, and the satisfaction of having performed an interesting, valuable task to the best of one's abilities.

WERNER EQUINE, LLC   PRX CLIENT _____ PATIENT _____ APPT _____

SERVICE PROTOCOL: Pre-Purchase Examination

OFFICE MANAGER

@ Initial contact to set appointment

___ **Complete pages 1-2 Packet. Review spelling** of all information with caller for accuracy.
___ **Arrange for Vet-Prospective Buyer Services Review; give Vet packet** for review.
___ **Database entries:**

- *New Client*: Complete all fields; send newsletter "Yes". Check with Practice Manager if questionable.
- *New Patient:* Follow New Patient protocol for data entry.
- *Agents/Trainers/Sellers/Barns/Farriers/Referring-Primary Care Vets*: Enter in database. Follow protocol to indicate if someone referred client to us. Send Newsletter = "Yes". See Practice Manager if questions. Send thank you for referrals.

___ **Enter visit on Appointment Clipboard:** allow 2-3 hours; ask Vet if time frame questionable. Add ETA call to Open Case List.

After Vet reviews Veterinary Care Plan (VCP) with PB or Agent:

___ **Create VCP;** use Packet pg 3 and template estimate language in software. **Print VCP as unalterable PDF** (Adobe® PDF Creator)

___ **Send Pre-Appointment Materials (PDFs) via email/fax; use communication templates:**

  To PB/Agent: PB Agreement, VCP & PRX Handout.   **To Seller/Agent:** Seller Agreement & PRX Handout

___ **Check returned forms! Completed forms <u>must</u> be returned before Visit**

- Compare information on forms/packet/database. If not accurate/complete: follow-up and get complete/accurate info.
- Make corrections as needed in database. No changes allowed on PB/Seller signed forms. Follow protocol for correcting errors.
- If Seller lists Vet or previous medical/surgical/lameness, etc. history and gives permission on Agreement:
  - Contact practice for patient history using communication templates
  - Scan info as PDF; attach to medical record; forward to vet for his review before PRX visit; add hard copies to Packet

___ **Copy completed PB form with credit card information obscured. Retain original in client file; put copy in PRX packet.**
___ **Pre-Authorize PB credit card** for VCP amount. <u>All PRX paid by credit card</u>.
___ **PRX Report draft: Pre-fill** Addressee & PB/Seller information on Report draft ; for Report draft to Vet before appointment.
___ **Send Packet to Appointment with Vet**

After the Visit

___ **Review Packet:** compare info on worksheet, ancillary materials, Report draft, forms, database entries for accuracy/completeness.
___ **Ancillary materials:** secure originals (insurance forms, test reports, imaging study CDs, etc.) in Packet for archiving. Send copies to PB with Report if Vet indicates it is appropriate.

___ **Update Client/Patient information in database**

  E.g. Client/Patient Notes, Reminders, Open Case List, Reports, database info, patient classification and veterinary care needed post-visit (e.g. whether horse purchased, wellness care needed, etc.) These efforts affect patient care, client base, etc.

___ **Invoice:** Create STAT; charge credit card. Include paid invoice & credit card receipt with Report mailing.

Report Letter:

___ **Review** draft; use Track Changes/Comments in Word®. Watch accuracy, completeness, readability. See Vet and/or Practice Manager with concerns.

___ **Worksheet errors:** Vet must address in his handwriting on worksheet; e.g. single line out; reason noted; initialed.

___ **Vet must approve all changes to Report** before version finalized; i.e. Click on Accept All Change; Save final document.

___ **Print** Vet-approved final Report on letterhead paper; **have Vet sign** original Report.

___ **Scan final, signed Report as unalterable PDF;** attach to Patient in database.

___ **Mail** Report & Enclosure to Prospective Buyer. If New Client (not referred) for practice; enclose New Client Packet & newsletter.

___ **Email** unalterable PDF copies to Agents, Referring or Primary Care Vets if requested by Prospective Buyer (document request).

___ **Reminders, Reports, Recalls, new Client/Patient info, other case actions:** Enter in database & on Open Case List per protocols

___ **Scan entire Packet as unalterable PDF; attach to Patient file in database. File hardcopy in client's paper file.**

Appendix 1.

WERNER EQUINE, LLC   PRX CLIENT _____   PATIENT _____   APPT _____

SERVICE PROTOCOL: Pre-Purchase Examination

VETERINARIAN

Before Visit

__ Review VCP with PB/Agent (Use pg 3 of Packet)

__ Return Packet to the Office Manager

__ Review received history, PB/Seller form, ancillary information; follow through as needed with Office Manager/PB/Seller

@ Visit

__ Rider/Handler Release form: get fully completed <u>before</u> beginning examination

__ **Complete Exam Worksheets.** Check off areas examined; note findings. Enter NA if not examined or performed.
      Errors: single line-out, make correction, initial, note reason for change

__ **Take Patient Photographs; save on laptop to forward to Main Server**/PRX Materials Folder for Office Manager review.

__ **Create Imaging Study(ies) and CDs if pertinent:** 1 copy for PB (indicate on worksheet if given @ Visit); 1 copy for file.

__ **Make brief verbal report to PB/Agent** regarding PRX findings; **Record communication on sheet** in Packet.

@ or immediately after Visit

__ **Complete PRX packet; attach all ancillary paperwork.**

__ **Create medical record and invoice (Visit) in software.**

__ **Complete template PRX Report draft; save** in PRX Materials Folder on main server for Office Manager review.

__ **Return Packet/ancillary materials to Office Manager for review/ prompt creation of invoice/Report.**

__ **Sign final PRX Report.**

__ **Delete patient photos from laptop. Forward images that you wish archived for future educational use to Practice Manager.**

Appendix 1. (*Continued*).

WERNER EQUINE, LLC   PRX CLIENT _____   PATIENT _____   APPT _____

This confidential worksheet is intended to help a veterinarian complete a Pre-Purchase Examination in an orderly manner. It is not a report to any party. It lists services that are not necessarily indicated or possible for every examination. In fact, some items may be contraindicated or not permitted by the Seller or Seller's Agent. Absence of a comment or mark at any line item is not an error of omission by the veterinarian.

Preliminary Information from Initial Contact for Pre-Purchase Examination Appointment

DATE/TIME: _____ @ ____ AM PM   **FROM** (Contact) _____   **TO** (Staff Member) _____

PROSPECTIVE BUYER _____   **Present @ appointment?** Yes   No

Address _____ City _____ State _____ Zip _____

Home Tel. _____ Work Tel. _____ Cell _____

Email _____ Fax _____

PROSPECTIVE BUYER'S AGENT _____   **Present @ appointment?** Yes   No

Address _____ City _____ State _____ Zip _____

Phone _____ Email _____ Fax _____

SELLER _____   **Present @ appointment?** Yes   No

Address _____ City _____ State _____ Zip _____

Tel. _____ Email _____ Fax _____

SELLER'S AGENT _____   **Present @ appointment?** Yes   No

Address _____ City _____ State _____ Zip _____

Phone _____ Email _____ Fax _____

APPOINTMENT LOCATION

Barn _____   Address _____

City _____ State _____ Zip _____ Phone _____

HOW DID YOU LEARN ABOUT WERNER EQUINE? _____

Tel. _____ Email _____

PATIENT _____ **Breed** _____ **YOB** _____ **Sex** ____ **Color** _____

COMMENTS:

Appendix 1. (*Continued*).

WERNER EQUINE, LLC   PRX CLIENT _____   PATIENT _____   APPT _____

VETERINARIAN-PROSPECTIVE BUYER VETERINARY CARE PLAN REVIEW

Veterinarian _____   **Prospective Buyer or Agent** _____

Conversation Date/Time _____ AM/PM via ____ Phone   ____ Email   ____ Other _____

_____ **Declined to review Veterinary Care Plan**   **Reason** _____

ADDITIONAL INFORMATION REPORTED BY PROSPECTIVE BUYER OR AGENT DURING THIS CONVERSATION:

Intended Use _____   **Current level training/competition** _____

Vices/Behavior Concerns _____

Medical/Surgical/Lameness episodes _____

Corrective shoeing _____   **Rx to assist performance** _____

Other comments:

SERVICES (in order they appear on VCP/invoice)	FEES	#Advised	Declined	Comments
On Farm or Outpatient Appointment	$			
Physical Examination	Aborted: Average: Extended:			
Ancillary Studies (Base time noted)				
Electrocardiogram	$0			
Clinical Laboratory (blood draw)				
Drug Screen Sample/Process/Hold 30 days	$0			
Drug Screen/Submit >Hold; Express Ship	$0			
Drug Screen; Express Ship	$0			
CBC/Platelets/Fibrinogen	$0			
Equine Screen/CBC/Fibrinogen	$0			
EIA (AGID Coggins)	$0			
Lyme disease test; Express ship/handle	$0			
Thermography	$0			
Pull Shoes (per shoe)	$0			
Foot Prep (per foot)	$0			
Diuretic Admin (for urinalysis)	$0			
Sedation (IV)	$0			
Radiography procedure fee/Initial View	$0			
Subsequent views - Rads (note #)				
Fore digits | Carpi | Tarsi | Stifles	$0			
Endoscopy (non-video)	$0			
Ultrasonography	$0			
Dilation of Pupils (for ophthalmic exam)	$0			
IV Injection Propantheline Bromide	$0			
Rectal Examination	$0			
Clinical Lab – (non blood draws)				
Fecal, Biannual $0 or Shedder type (2 tests) $0	$0			
HYPP & Express Ship	$0			
STAT processing of Lab Testing	$0			
Extra Copy Imaging Study on CD (per CD)	$0			
Insurance Binder Complete/Process	$0			
Insurance Claim Form; Complete/Process	$0			
USA Interstate Health Certificate	$0			
Other:	$0			

Appendix 1. (*Continued*).

WERNER EQUINE, LLC

RELEASE OF LIABILITY BY HANDLER, DRIVER AND/OR RIDER OF HORSE

I, _____ , am 18 years of age or older

                (PLEASE PRINT YOUR NAME)

and have been asked by _____

to handle, drive and/or ride _____

for the purpose of veterinary examination and/or treatment.

I am competent to perform these tasks that have been asked of me by the individual noted above in regards to veterinary examination and/or treatment.

I understand the inherent risks involved in engaging in equine activities – including handling, driving and/or riding a horse for veterinary examination and/or treatment.

I hereby release *WERNER EQUINE, LLC* and any and all employees and principals of *WERNER EQUINE, LLC* from any consequences to myself, any other humans, animals and/or property that may arise from my handling, driving and/or riding of the horse(s) described above for veterinary examination and/or treatment.

| _____ | _____ | _____ | _____ |
| DATE | TIME | SIGNATURE | PRINTED NAME |

WITNESSED BY: _____   _____

                                        SIGNATURE   PRINTED NAME

20 Godard Rd. · N. Granby, CT 06060 · Tel (860) 653-5088 · Fax (860) 653-5080 · www.wernerequine.com

Appendix 1. (*Continued*).

WERNER EQUINE, LLC

Please complete each section of this form and return it to our office by fax or email <u>before the Examination appointment</u>.

PROSPECTIVE BUYER: AGREEMENTS REGARDING PRE-PURCHASE EXAMINATION

I, _____, am the Prospective Buyer of the horse named on this form.

Address _____ Tel _____ Email _____

Authorization for an Agent to Act on Prospective Buyer's Behalf:

I hereby grant authority to _____ to act as my Agent regarding all aspects of the Pre-Purchase Examination of the horse named on this form. This authority includes, but is not limited to, decisions regarding veterinary services and fees, as well as discussion of Examination findings, services and reports with any veterinarian(s) and/or designated staff, agents or representatives of *Werner Equine, LLC.*

Prospective Buyer's signature _____

HORSE _____ Age ____ Breed _____ Sex: G F S Color _____

Please circle intended use(s) for the horse named on this form:

English: Pleasure   Hunter   Jumper Dressage   Cross country Driving   Combined training/Eventing

Western: Pleasure   Trail   Rodeo   Reining   Cutting   Team Penning Barrel Racing   Roping

Other: Trail Riding Draft Pulling (in harness)   Miniatures   Breeding Other _____

Please list any specific concerns you have about the horse that is to be examined:

Please note if you want an <u>extra</u> copy of the Pre-Purchase Examination ____ Report ____ Radiographic Study
Emailed to _____ at _____

I hereby authorize Harry W. Werner, VMD to perform a Pre-Purchase Examination of the horse named on this form. I understand and agree that:

- Dr. Werner reviewed the Veterinary Care Plan (*VCP*) for Pre-Purchase Examination services with me or my Agent. I (or my Agent) received a copy of the *VCP*. Any questions I had were answered to my satisfaction.

- I am financially responsible for payment of all fees for Pre-Purchase Examination services to *Werner Equine, LLC. Werner Equine, LLC* will pre-authorize the credit card noted below for the estimated fees listed on my *VCP* once their office receives a *VCP* signed by me (or my Agent). After the Pre-Purchase Examination is completed, Werner Equine, LLC will charge the actual fees for services provided to the credit card listed on this document.

- If I (or my Agent) arrange for someone to ride, drive and/or handle the horse named above for the Pre-Purchase Examination, that person must be 18 years of age or older and must sign a *Release of Liability* at the Examination appointment before the Pre-Purchase Examination can begin.

PROSPECTIVE BUYER CREDIT CARD INFORMATION

Circle card Type: Visa   MasterCard Discover   Name on Card _____

Card Billing Address (include house # and zip)_____
Card
_____   Expiry Date _____

Cardholder's Signature _____

I am 18 years of age or older and have the authority to execute this document. To the best of my knowledge, the information I provided on this document is true.
Date/Time   Signature: Prospective Buyer or Agent   Printed Name: Prospective Buyer or Agent

20 Godard Road ▪ Box 5 ▪ North Granby, CT 06060 ▪ Tel 860-653-5088 ▪ Fax 860-653-5080 ▪ linda@wernerequine.com

© 2000-2012 Copyright Werner Equine, LLC All Rights Reserved.

Appendix 1. (*Continued*).

WERNER EQUINE, LLC

Please complete each line on this form & return tour office by fax or email <u>before the Examination appointment</u>.

SELLER: AGREEMENTS and INFORMATION REGARDING PRE-PURCHASE EXAMINATION

I,_____, am the SELLER and present owner of the horse named below.

Seller Address _____

Email_____ Tel _____ Fax _____

Seller's authorization for an AGENT to act on the Seller's behalf

I hereby grant authority to_____ to act as my Agent regarding all

aspects of the Pre-Purchase Examination of the horse named on this form.

Seller's signature _____

Agent Address _____

Agent Email _____ Agent Tel _____ Agent Fax _____

PATIENT INFORMATION

Name_____ Age_____ Breed _____ Sex M F G Color_____

Registration/Microchip # _____ Tattoo _____ Height _____

Present Use _____

Duration present ownership _____ Duration present custody/care _____

Has horse competed?   Yes   No   Unknown

If Yes, note level & date of last competition _____

Last vaccinations (note month/year) _____ Unknown history of vaccinations

_____ Eastern-Western Encephalitis/Tetanus _____ Potomac Horse Fever _____ West Nile Virus

_____ Rhinopneumonitis/Influenza _____ Strangles _____ Rabies

Last de-worming (Date & product) _____ ____ Unknown de-worming history

Has insurance coverage ever been denied? (Circle one):   No   Not to my knowledge   Yes

If coverage denied, reason for denial _____

Behavioral problems or concerns: None Yes: _____

_____

Medical episodes: None Unknown Yes: _____

_____

Surgical episodes: None Unknown Yes: _____

_____

Lameness episodes: None Unknown Yes: _____

_____

HYPP certification (circle one)   Unknown   Negative/Negative   Negative/Positive   Positive/Positive

20 Godard Road ▪ Box 5 ▪ North Granby, CT 06060 ▪ Tel 860-653-5088 ▪ Fax 860-653-5080 ▪ linda@wernerequine.com

Appendix 1. (*Continued*).

WERNER EQUINE, LLC

Seller Agreements and Information Regarding Pre-Purchase Examination - Continued

Reproductive history/Mare _____ __Not applicable

Possible current pregnancy? Yes   No   History of infertility? No   Not Known   Yes _____

Reproductive history/Stallion _____ __Not applicable

History of infertility?   No   Not Known   Yes: _____

Corrective Shoeing: No   Not Known   Yes: _____

Current Diet: _____

Supplements: None   Not Known   Yes: _____

Medications used to assist performance: None   Yes: _____

Is horse possibly under effects of any medication at this time?   No   Yes

If yes, specify: _____

_____

Veterinarian of record _____

Email_____   Tel _____

Farrier of record _____

Email_____   Tel _____

I hereby authorize Harry W. Werner, VMD to perform a Pre-Purchase Examination of the horse named on this document. I understand and agree that:

- The Pre-Purchase Examination will include physical examination; it may also include diagnostic and ancillary services recommended by Dr. Werner and approved by the Prospective Buyer or designated Agent of the Prospective Buyer.

- I consent to use of sedation, clipping and/or pulling of shoes as deemed necessary by Dr. Werner in the course of the Pre-Purchase Examination.

- I consent to the release of all medical records pertaining to the horse named on this document to the Prospective Buyer and Werner Equine, LLC; such records include those records available from any veterinarian(s) and farrier(s) of record.

- If I (or my Agent) arrange for someone to ride, drive and/or handle the horse named on this document for the Pre-Purchase Examination, I understand that person must be 18 years of age or older and must sign a *Release of Liability* at the appointment before the Pre-Purchase Examination can begin.

- I hereby release Werner Equine LLC and any veterinarians, employees and principals of Werner Equine, LLC from any consequences of the Pre-Purchase Examination to any humans, animals or property.

**I am 18 years of age or older and have the authority to execute this document.
To the best of my knowledge, the information I provided on this document is true.**

_____	_____	_____
Date/Time	Signature: Seller or Seller's Agent	Printed Name: Seller or Seller' Agent

---

20 Godard Road • Box 5 • North Granby, CT 06060 • Tel 860-653-5088 • Fax 860-653-5080 • linda@wernerequine.com

Appendix 1. (*Continued*).

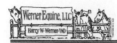 *Since 1979 – Providing veterinary care that improves the health and welfare of the Horse*

PRE-PURCHASE EXAMINATION

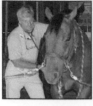

What is the purpose of a Pre-Purchase Examination?
Our goal when performing a Pre-Purchase Examination is to protect the interests of the Prospective Buyer by determining, as much as circumstances permit, the current health status of the horse offered for sale.

What factors affect the services included in a Pre-Purchase Examination?
Pre-Purchase Examination may be limited to physical examination of the horse or expanded to include additional supportive diagnostic studies and ancillary services. Dr. Werner will recommend particular components of Pre-Purchase Examination for a specific horse after considering such factors as:

- Intended use
- Age
- Breed
- Medical history
- Competition history
- Present level of training

In addition to physical examination, supportive diagnostic studies and ancillary services can provide additional, valuable information about the horse's current health status. Ancillary services include radiography, endoscopy and ultrasonography, drug screening and other pertinent laboratory tests. The Prospective Buyer can choose to include or exclude specific services.

Other factors can modify the Pre-Purchase Examination on-site at the visit. These factors include:
- inadequate working conditions;
- refusal of the Seller/Seller's Agent to permit performance of a service;
- exceptionally unruly behavior of the horse and/or
- absence of a qualified adult to handle, drive or ride the horse.

As with any diagnostic procedure, the fees associated with a Pre-Purchase Examination are dependent on:
- the level of complexity of each procedure
- the duration of the examination process
- the nature of the supporting diagnostic technology we employ
- environmental conditions on site
- complications or patient response to medications and/or procedures

How much time is involved in a Pre-Purchase Examination?
In medicine, we cannot know precisely how much time and what diagnostic procedures will be required until the actual examination process begins. We schedule a minimum of two hours for Pre-Purchase Examination. A Prospective Buyer or designated Agent is usually present at or reachable by phone during the visit and can make informed decisions about the examination.

What information is required from a Prospective Buyer and Seller before the visit?
We email an Agreement/Information document and a Veterinary Care Plan (a description of anticipated services and their approximate costs) to the Prospective Buyer. We also email an Agreement to the Seller to gather details of the horse's medical history, permission to perform the examination, etc. Completed forms must be returned to our office by email or fax before the Pre-Purchase Examination visit.

What if you have additional questions about Pre-Purchase Examination?
We welcome your questions about Pre-Purchase Examinations. Please call our office or contact Dr. Werner directly at (860) 653-5088 during his 8-9am weekday Phone Time to discuss specific questions or concerns. Our website www.wernerequine.com displays additional information about Pre-Purchase Examinations.

 Member, American Association of Equine Practitioners

20 Godard Road · North Granby, CT 06060 · Tel (860) 653-5088 · Fax (860) 653-5080 · www.wernerequine.com

Appendix 2.

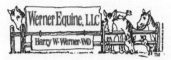

20 Godard Road · Box 5
North Granby, CT 06060
Tel 860-653-5088
Fax 860-653-5080
www.wernerequine.com

Since 1979 – Providing veterinary care that improves the health and welfare of the Horse

Test Client		
Test		
Street		
North Granby CT 06060		

Date	01/20/2012
Reference	Harry Werner, VMD
Patient	TEST HORSE

Details

This Veterinary Care Plan (VCP) describes minimum fees for services proposed for this patient at this time: Pre-Purchase Examination, Digital Radiography (8 views) and associated services listed on this document. Services are to be provided on-farm in Avon.

Fees associated with Pre-Purchase Examination reflect the level of complexity & duration of each procedure and the nature of supporting diagnostic technologies or care. This VCP is based on the veterinarian's verbal review of recommended services with the Prospective Buyer or designated Agent. Fees noted on the VCP are for those services selected by the Prospective Buyer/Agent for inclusion in the overall Pre-Purchase Examination. ACTUAL FEES CHARGED WILL VARY from those noted on this VCP due to variables at the visit such as environmental conditions, patient response to procedures, any complications that occur and/or decisions about services made on-site by the Prospective Buyer or designated Agent.

Veterinary Care Plan presented to Mr. Smith via email on 1/20/12 by Linda, Office Manager.

Estimation of Professional Services

Service Provided	No	Amount
Medical Appt. Avon On-Farm		0.00
Pre-Purchase Physical Examination		0.00
Pre-Sedation Evaluation/Intravenous Sedation		0.00
Foot Preparation For Radiography		0.00
Digital Radiographic Study, Initial View		0.00
Digital Radiographic Study, Subsequent Views		0.00
Equine Infectious Anemia Testing (Coggins)		0.00
IV Blood Draw; Process/Hold For Drug Screen		0.00
	Total:	0.00

PLEASE SIGN BELOW TO ACKNOWLEDGE YOUR RECEIPT OF AND AGREEMENT TO THIS VETERINARY CARE PLAN:

OWNER/AGENT _____ DATE _____

PLEASE RETURN A COPY OF THIS ENTIRE DOCUMENT TO WERNER EQUINE BEFORE THE APPOINTMENT (Fax 860 653-5080).

Please call us before the appointment if you have questions about this Veterinary Care Plan.

This VCP expires 30 days from the date shown on this document.

THANK YOU FOR GIVING US THE OPPORTUNITY TO CARE FOR THIS PATIENT

Appendix 3.

WERNER EQUINE, LLC   CLIENT _____   PATIENT _____

PRE-PURCHASE EXAMINATION WORKSHEET

This confidential worksheet is intended to help a veterinarian complete a pre-purchase examination in an orderly manner. It is not a report to any party. It contains line items that are not necessarily indicated or even possible for every examination. In fact, some items may be contraindicated or not permitted by the Seller or Seller's Agent. Absence of a comment or mark at any line item in no way represents an error of omission by the veterinarian. Notations may include free text as well as the following codes: √ = Performed   U = Unable to Perform   NA= Not Applicable

PHYSICAL EXAMINATION   DATE: _____   TIME: Start: _____   Stop: _____

CONDITIONS

Weather _____   Indoor _____   Outdoor _____

Hoof/Shoeing status _____   Patient Behavior _____

Horse handled by _____   Horse ridden/driven by _____

Also present _____

ADDITIONAL INFORMATION PROVIDED VERBALLY AT THE APPOINTMENT (including declined services)

Reported By: _____

PATIENT IDENTIFICATION

Name _____   Breed _____   YOB _____   Sex _____   Color _____

Microchip _____   Tattoo _____   Brand _____

Registration # _____   Unofficial Height (shod/unshod) _____

Markings:

NB When deemed relevant,, record scars (e.g. sinusotomy, lymph node incision, laryngotomy, laryngoplasty, digital neurectomy, patellar desmotomy, cunean tenotomy, laparotomy, vulvoplasty, cryosurgery, wounds) and conformation faults at the appropriate worksheet sites.

Appendix 4.

WERNER EQUINE, LLC   CLIENT _____   PATIENT _____

PHYSICAL EXAMINATION

___ **Behavior** _____

___ **Ophthalmic**   Environment: dark   dim   bright   Instrument: penlight   ophthalmoscope

Mydriatic? _____ Corneal anesthesia? _____ Corneal stain? _____

L _____   R _____

Temperature ____ °F   **Pulse** ____ per minute   **Respirations** ____ per minute   **BS** ____ /9

___ **Cardiovascular at rest**

Arrhythmia? _____   Murmur? _____

Jugular   L _____   R _____   Mucosal Color _____   CRT ____ Secs

___ **Respiratory at rest**   Bagged _____ ?

Upper Airway _____

Left Chest _____   Right Chest _____

___ **Integument** _____

___ **Oral Cavity** _____

___ **Skull** (Inspection/Palpation/Percussion) _____

___ **Ears - external**   L _____   R _____

___ **Throatlatch** _____

___ **Neck**

Flexion   L _____   R _____   V _____

Extension _____

___ **Nuchal Crest** _____   ___ **Withers** _____

___ **Thoracolumbosacral**

Axial _____

Left epaxial _____   Right epaxial _____

___ **Croup** _____   ___   **Tail** _____

___ **Perineum** _____   ___   **Abd. Ventrum** _____

___ **External Genitals** _____   Dropped? _____

___ **Left Forelimb**

Inspection _____

Palpation _____

Ranges of motion _____

Hoof Testers _____   Heel Sensation _____

Hoof Condition _____   Shoeing _____

PRX APPOINTMENT WORKSHEETS 2/6

Appendix 4. (Continued).

WERNER EQUINE, LLC   CLIENT _____   PATIENT _____

___ **Right Forelimb**

Inspection _____

Palpation _____

Ranges of motion _____

Hoof Testers _____   Heel Sensation _____

Hoof Condition _____   Shoeing _____

___ **Left hindlimb**

Inspection _____

Palpation _____

Ranges of motion _____

Hoof Testers _____   Heel Sensation _____

Hoof Condition _____   Shoeing _____

___ **Right hindlimb**

Inspection _____

Palpation _____

Ranges of motion _____

Hoof Testers _____   Heel Sensation _____

Hoof Condition _____   Shoeing _____

___ **In Hand**   Walk _____   Jog _____

___ **On Longe**   Walk _____   Trot _____   Canter _____

___ **Saddling/Mounting** _____

___ **Ridden**   Walk _____   Trot _____   Canter _____   Over Jumps _____

___ **In Harness** _____

___ **Way of going** _____

___ **Flexion Tests**   LF _____   RF _____

                          LH _____   RH _____

___ **Respiratory in exercise**   Tachypnea? _____   Noise? _____   Insp _____   Exp _____

Appendix 4. (*Continued*).

WERNER EQUINE, LLC   CLIENT _____   PATIENT _____

___ **Neurologic**

Cranial nerves	_____	Tight Circles	_____
Backing	_____	Tail Lift	_____
Sway	_____	Anal Sphincter	_____
Foot Placement	_____	Cutaneous	_____
Blinded	_____	Hopping	_____
Other	_____		

___ **Cardiovascular Post-Exercise**

Arrhythmia? _____   Murmur? _____

Jugular   L _____   R _____

___ **Respiratory Post-Exercise**

Upper Airway _____

Left Chest _____   Right Chest _____

___ **Palpation per Rectum** _____ **Propantheline bromide IV** ___ ml

ANCILLARY STUDIES

___ **SEDATION** Acepromazine ___ ml Detomidine ___ ml Xylazine ___ ml Butorphanol ___ ml Diazepam ___ ml

___ **RADIOLOGY** (See Radiology worksheet page)   ___ **PULL SHOES** (Note # shoes @ right)   _____

___ **ENDOSCOPY**

Upper Airway _____   Other _____

___ **ULTRASONOGRAPHY**   MSK _____   Other _____

___ **THERMOGRAPHY** _____

___ **VIDEO** _____   ___ **PHOTO(S)**

___ **EKG** _____

___ **INSURANCE EXAM FORM**   (Attach form to packet.)

___ **HEALTH CERTIFICATE FORM**   (Attach form to packet.)

___ **LABORATORY TESTING**

Entry of SO indicates sample collected/held for possible testing. Note STAT if applicable.

___ Lyme disease test (ELISA/WB)	___ EIA AGID	___ Equine Screen CBC Fibrinogen (L040)	___ HYPP
___ Drug Screen	___ Fecal	___ Equine Inflammatory profile (L070)	___ CBC
___ Other diagnostic testing:	_____		

___ **OTHER ANCILLARY SERVICES** _____

Appendix 4. (*Continued*).

WERNER EQUINE, LLC   CLIENT _____   PATIENT _____

RADIOGRAPHY

____ # of Foot Preps   __ Extra CD of Study Created per pg 6 or PB form for: _____

	Hoof	Pastern	Fetlock	Cannon	Carpus	Elbow	Shoulder	Tarsus	Stifle	TL vert	C vert	Skull	Tibia	Radius	#
PV															
LM															
DP															
DLPMO															
DMPLO															
DLVMO															
DMVLO															
DV															
LM/f															
DPDD															
PA															
ML															
PLAMO															
PLAMO/f															
LL															
RDLVO															
LDRVO															
PPDP															
#															

RADIOGRAPHY FINDINGS:

Appendix 4. (*Continued*).

WERNER EQUINE, LLC   CLIENT _____   PATIENT _____

VERBAL REPORT OF PRE-PURCHASE EXAMINATION RESULTS TO PROSPECTIVE BUYER OR AGENT

DATE _____ TIME _____AM/PM   VETERINARIAN_____

MEANS OF COMMUNICATION _____TO _____

COMMENTS:

_____

_____

_____

_____

_____

_____

_____

_____

RESPONSE: _____

_____

_____

_____

AUTHORIZATION TO RELEASE PRE-PURCHASE EXAMINATION INFORMATION

I hereby authorize release of the Pre-Purchase Examination:

_____ Report   _____ Radiographic Study   _____ Other _____

To: _____

_____ Via Email (complimentary)   Email address: _____

_____ Via Hard Copy @ appx.$/copy   Mailing address: _____

_____   _____
   Printed Name: Prospective Buyer/Agent   Signature: Prospective Buyer/Agent

Appendix 4. (*Continued*).

WERNER EQUINE, LLC
Since 1979 – Providing veterinary care that improves the health and welfare of the Horse

March 3, 2011

Mr. David Duncan
38 West 43rd Street
Lansing, Michigan 48906

Re: COMMANDER 2007 bay Hanoverian gelding
Markings: right hind ½ sock with medial black spot

Dear Mr. Duncan:

At your request, I performed a physical examination of COMMANDER on February 27, 2011 at 2:30 pm in your presence at Hillside Farm. Sarah Collins presented the horse and rode the horse for the examination. My veterinary assistant, Martha Clark, handled the horse on the ground. Your trainer, Mark Evans, was also present at the examination

Intended Use
You stated that you intended to use this horse for English Pleasure/hunter.

Expressed Concerns: None

Disclosed History
Ms. Collins, the Seller, disclosed the following information regarding COMMANDER:

- Present Use: as green broke hunter
- Duration of present ownership: since birth
- Duration of present custody/care: since birth
- Current competition level/Date of last competition: None
- Last vaccinations:
    - 10-10-10: EHV1&4, Influenza, rabies
- Last de-worming: 1-6-11 ivermectin/praziquantel oral paste
- Denials for Insurance Coverage: None
- Behavioral problems/concerns: None
- Medical episodes: None
- Surgical episodes: 6-6-2008: routine castration
- Lameness episodes: 9-1-2008: left fore subsolar abscess; full recovery
- HYPP certification: Unknown

Member, American Association of Equine Practitioners   1/5

20 Godard Road • P.O. Box 5 • North Granby, CT 06060 • Tel (860) 653-5088 • Fax (860) 653-5080 • hwwvmd@wernerequine.com

Appendix 5.

WERNER EQUINE, LLC
Since 1979 – Providing veterinary care that improves the health and welfare of the Horse

- Reproductive history: NA
- Possibility of current pregnancy: NA
- History of infertility: NA
- Corrective shoeing: None
- Current diet: grass hay; 12 % protein pellet concentrate
- Supplements: None
- Medications to assist performance: None
- Is horse possibly under the effects of medication at time of examination: No
- Veterinarian of record: Allen Williams DVM
- Farrier of record: Francis Taylor CJF

Examination

I examined **COMMANDER** at rest and in motion in hand, on longe and under saddle on flat and over jumps. Due to icy conditions, I was unable to include a jog on hard surface outside as part of this examination.

Physical examination included evaluation of the following elements:

- Behavior
- Ophthalmic
- Vital Signs
- Body condition
- Cardiovascular at rest and after exercise
- Respiratory at rest and during/after exercise
- Skin and hair coat
- Oral cavity
- Head and neck
- Neurologic
- Trunk
- Pelvic girdle and tail
- Perineum and external genitals
- Each limb: inspection, palpation, ranges of motion, hoof condition, hoof tester response heel sensation, shoeing

 Member, American Association of Equine Practitioners   2/5

20 Godard Road • P.O. Box 5 • North Granby, CT 06060 • Tel (860) 653-5088 • Fax (860) 653-5080 • hwwvmd@wernerequine.com

Appendix 5. *(Continued).*

WERNER EQUINE, LLC

Since 1979 – Providing veterinary care that improves the health and welfare of the Horse

- Motion examination: in hand, on longe, saddling and mounting, under saddle way of going, flexion tests (all limbs)

Ancillary services included:

- Digital radiography of each fore digit, tarsus, stifle and fetlock

- Coggins testing

- Drug screen blood draw and processing/express shipping of samples for drug screen testing

- Sedation was used to ensure the quality of the ancillary testing results

- Insurance form completion

- A Health Certificate was completed and processed for travel within the United States. A copy of the form was forwarded to the appropriate regulatory agent.

Declined Services: I recommended that upper airway endoscopy be included in the standard of care of Pre-Purchase Examination for COMMANDER. However, you declined to include this service in this Pre-Purchase Examination.

Observations/Findings

COMMANDER did not exhibit lameness, ataxia, abnormal respiratory sounds or fatigue.

From examination of those organ systems made available to me for evaluation, I note the following:

- On radiography, there are two osteochondral (bone/cartilage) fragments within the right hind fetlock.

I interpret this observation of COMMANDER as follows:

- The osteochondral fragments represent a significant risk of future lameness.

  If such fragments are removed surgically before the onset of secondary intra-articular pathology, the patient's prognosis is excellent.

Clinical Laboratory Test Results/Interpretation

- The Coggins test result was negative.

- The Drug screen test results were negative.

Member, American Association of Equine Practitioners   3/5

20 Godard Road • P.O. Box 5 • North Granby, CT 06060 • Tel (860) 653-5088 • Fax (860) 653-5080 • hwwvmd@wernerequine.com

Appendix 5. (*Continued*).

WERNER EQUINE, LLC

Since 1979 – Providing veterinary care that improves the health and welfare of the Horse

---

Copies provided of Pre-Purchase Examination information

- A copy of the digital radiographic study was created and archived on the enclosed CD to facilitate future veterinary and/or farrier care.

- At your request, we e-mailed a copy of the Report and digital radiographic study to Dr. Allen Lee.

This Pre-Purchase Examination Report is a record of the examination findings and my interpretation of those findings; it is not a recommendation to purchase or not to purchase COMMANDER .

If you have any questions or concerns, please be sure to contact me.

We appreciate having had the opportunity to examine COMMANDER on your behalf.

Sincerely,

Harry W. Werner VMD

Harry W. Werner VMD

Encl.   Coggins Test Report; Drug screen Report; Insurance examination form; Health Certificate; Pre-Purchase Examination patient photos; Imaging Study CD

C.   File; Dr. Allen Lee

 Member, American Association of Equine Practitioners   4/5

20 Godard Road ● P.O. Box 5 ● North Granby, CT 06060 ● Tel (860) 653-5088   ● Fax (860) 653-5080   ● hwwvmd@wernerequine.com

Appendix 5. (*Continued*).

WERNER EQUINE, LLC
Since 1979 – Providing veterinary care that improves the health and welfare of the Horse

PRE-PURCHASE EXAMINATION PATIENT PHOTOGRAPHS

Date: 2/27/11   Prospective Buyer: David Duncan   Horse: COMMANDER

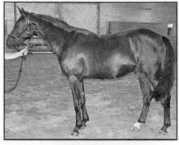
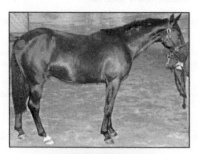
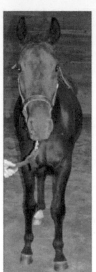
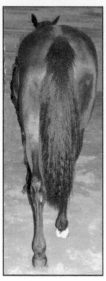

20 Godard Road • P.O. Box 5 • North Granby, CT 06060 • Tel (860) 653-5088 • Fax (860) 653-5080 • hwwvmd@wernerequine.com

Appendix 5. (*Continued*).

REFERENCES

1. International Museum of the Horse. What we theorize: when and where did domestication occur? Available at: www.imh.org. Accessed March 9, 2012.
2. Youatt W. History, treatment and diseases of the horse. Philadelphia: JB Lippincott; 1868. p. 361.
3. Bhreatnach C, Bhreatnach A. Portraying Irish travelers: histories and representations. Newcastle upon Tyne (England): Cambridge Scholars Publishing; 2006. p. 15.
4. Stevart DR. The law of horses family library of veterinary medicine. Medford (MA): Cummings School of Veterinary Medicine, Tufts University.
5. Beeman GM, Soule SG, Swanson TD. History and philosophy of the medical examination of horses for purchase VCNA: Equine Practice 1992;8(2);258.
6. Online Etymology Dictionary. 2010 Douglas Harper. Available at: www.etymonline.com. Accessed March 9, 2012.
7. US Army Medical Department: Office of Medical History. Available at: www.history.amedd.army.mil. Accessed March 9, 2012.
8. Vaughan JT. Professional liability in equine practice, risk management and loss control. AAEP Proc 2008;54:112.
9. Armatage G. MRCVS: the horse: management in health and disease. London (England): Frederick Warne & Co; 1893.
10. O'Grady D. Physician revives a dying art. The New York Times, October 11, 2010.
11. Port M. Everybody's doing it. American Express Open Forum Small Business. Available at: www.openforum.com. Accessed February 3, 2010.
12. Haynes AB, Weiser TG, Berry WR, et al. A surgical safety checklist to reduce morbidity and mortality in a global population. N Engl J Med 2009;360:491–9.
13. Snow D. Service Excellence in Veterinary Practice: It Does Matter. 57th Annual Convention of the American Association of Equine Practitioners. San Antonio, TX, November 17–20, 2011.
14. Scoggins G. Legal considerations concerning patient medical records. AAEP Proc 2005;51:515–9.
15. Meagher D. A review of equine malpractice claims. AAEP Proc 2005;51:508–14.
16. Moyer W, Werner H. Risk reduction in the reporting of the purchase examination. AAEP Proc 1999;45:24–6.
17. Moyer W, Werner H. Purchase examination guidelines for risk reduction. In Forensics and Risk Management Proceedings of the 70th Western Veterinary Conference. Las Vegas (NV); 1998. p. 92–8.

Index

Note: Page numbers of article titles are in **boldface** type.

Vet Clin Equine 28 (2012) 249–261
http://dx.doi.org/10.1016/S0749-0739(12)00024-7
0749-0739/12/$ – see front matter © 2012 Elsevier Inc. All rights reserved.

vetequine.theclinics.com

Moving?

Make sure your subscription moves with you!

To notify us of your new address, find your **Clinics Account Number** (located on your mailing label above your name), and contact customer service at:

Email: journalscustomerservice-usa@elsevier.com

800-654-2452 (subscribers in the U.S. & Canada)
314-447-8871 (subscribers outside of the U.S. & Canada)

Fax number: 314-447-8029

Elsevier Health Sciences Division
Subscription Customer Service
3251 Riverport Lane
Maryland Heights, MO 63043

*To ensure uninterrupted delivery of your subscription, please notify us at least 4 weeks in advance of move.

Printed and bound by CPI Group (UK) Ltd, Croydon, CR0 4YY

03/10/2024

01040350-0003